For my son Raffael Singh Aujla.
Remember, your energy is limitless,
and your potential is infinite.
Always believe in yourself.

Dr Rupy Aujla

Healthy High Protein

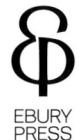

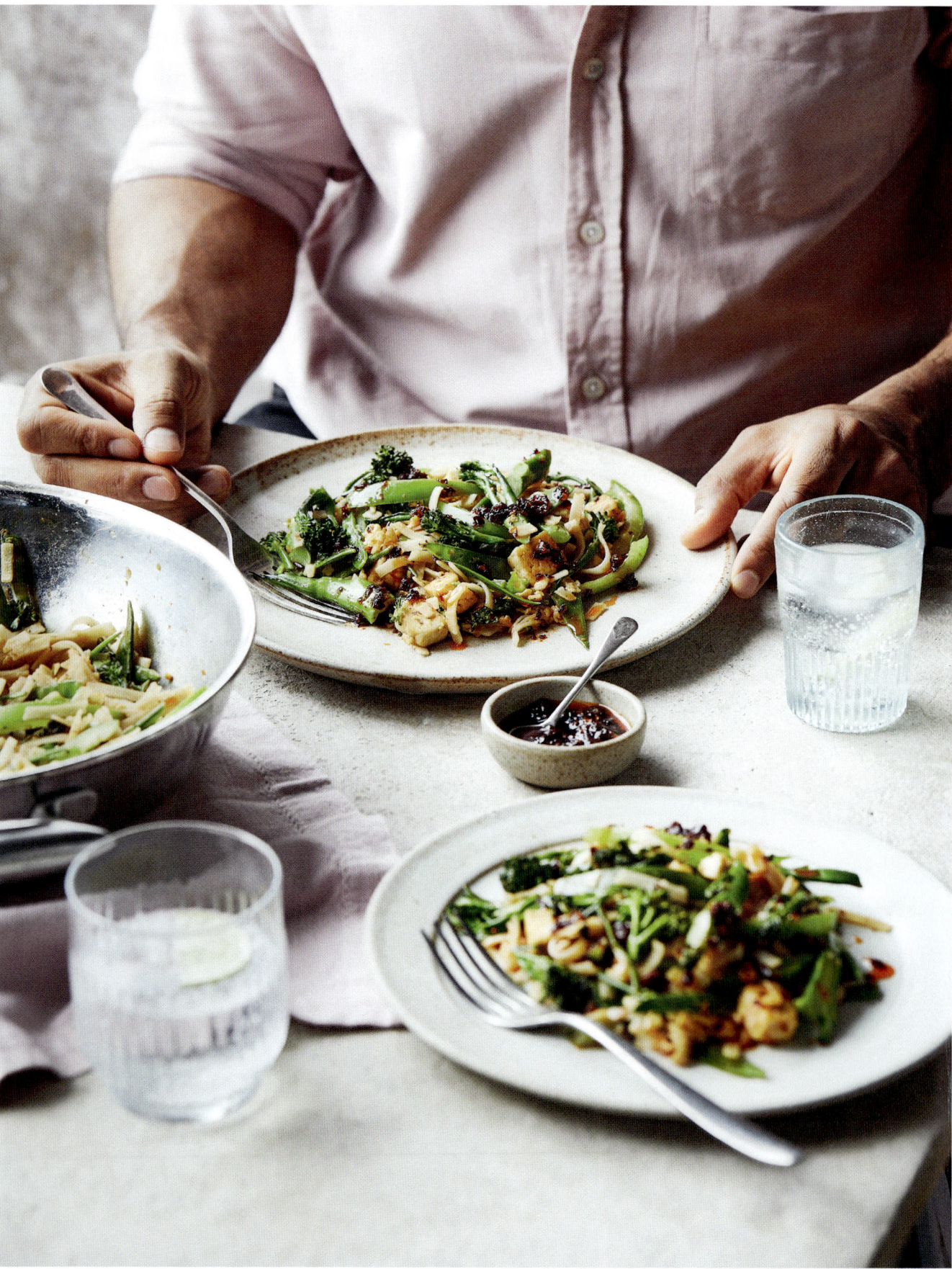

CONTENTS

Introduction	4
Healthy High Protein	12
Better Gut Health	32
Lowering Inflammation	54
Breakfast & Brunch	70
One-pan Dinners	104
High-protein Diversity Bowls	142
Fresh & Light Plates	168
Meatless Midweek	188
Midweek Meat & Fish	222
Snacks, Toppers & Drinks	260
Resources	272
Nutritional analysis of recipes	274
Nutrition tables	276
Index	280
References	284
Acknowledgements	286

THIS BOOK WILL REFRAME THE WAY YOU THINK ABOUT PROTEIN

INTRO-DUCTION

When you think of 'high-protein' recipes, I imagine you picture boiled, overcooked chicken with a side of limp broccoli and sludgy brown rice. A bland, muscle-centric, calorie-counting, obsessive approach to food that strips any emotion and joy from mealtimes.

Such was my experience at medical school, when I committed to finally getting the 'six-pack abs' that so many glossy magazines assured me were just six weeks away. It was a miserable process; slopping out the same tasteless, prepped meals, meticulously weighed and optimised for macros and calories. It's forever stained my opinion of anything to do with fitness food.

Typical high-protein recipes and cookbooks also tend to be high protein at the expense of everything else. Full of meat and dairy at nearly every mealtime with little or no consideration for gut health, fibre requirements, the need for ingredient variety or the inflammation potential of animal-protein-rich diets.

I want to reassure you that this is not one of those cookbooks. In fact, this book will reframe the way you think about protein because most of us don't understand the critical role that it plays beyond supporting the health and function of our muscles.

Having good amounts of quality protein in our diet:

- Is essential for hormonal health.
- Can support weight loss and weight maintenance.
- Can reduce cravings and balance blood sugar levels.
- Can even improve your energy levels, support menopausal health and enhance longevity.

I'm going to teach you where you can get good-quality protein beyond red meat, chicken and fish, as well as how you can easily calculate your individual needs. You will learn how much you need to consume each day, how to spot the foods that can boost your protein intake and how to easily get your protein while being mindful of your overall health and longevity.

You'll begin to recognise the variety of protein sources on your plate and approximate whether you have enough for your needs. You'll also understand how to create a balanced plate and meet your own personal protein needs by adding a little extra nuts, seeds or some unusual high-protein ingredients that you may not have come across before.

Whether you choose to be fully plant based or not, I'll explain how you can maintain high protein intake in a healthy way that's also considerate of your gut health, lowering inflammation, and increasing longevity, your energy levels and overall wellbeing.

If you get these elements of your diet on track, you'll be supporting your heart and brain health and even preventing some of the most serious diseases that I see as a doctor, such as cancer and type 2 diabetes.

Why protein is so important

Protein is the most important molecule for life and this book is going to become your go-to guide, unlocking everything you need to know about this vital nutrient. The introductory chapters explain:

- How to calculate your unique protein requirements.
- Why protein is more than just about muscle building.
- The role of protein in hormonal, bone and skin health and metabolism.
- Why consuming enough protein can reduce cravings, help you feel fuller for longer and help you naturally lose weight.
- How protein can support your energy levels, strength and longevity.
- How protein can be found in a multitude of healthy sources, beyond chicken and beef.
- Why real foods are much better sources of protein than heavily marketed protein shakes, supplements and bars.

You'll also learn about the importance of gut-supportive and anti-inflammatory foods in more detail and why ensuring optimal protein intake, supporting gut health and controlling inflammation are essential for your wellbeing and for feeling great every day.

Eating this way doesn't require a new list of foods or ingredients to invest in. In fact, you probably have the best gut-friendly staples in your kitchen cupboards already.

By the end of this book you'll know the foods, tips and tricks you can use to put your health on the right foot every time you sit down to eat, plus a host of delicious recipes to get you started.

Food as medicine

The recipes in this cookbook are all high protein, but they're also healthy. In other words, they are also full of gut health-supporting colourful vegetables, and a range of fibres and anti-inflammatory ingredients. Typical of my style of cooking, this book is about taste as well as the functional benefits of eating well. It also acknowledges global cuisines, traditional flavour pairings and the benefits of good food for our health.

People's understanding of food over the last ten years has evolved and the message is out there: our plates are powerful tools of change. We're all becoming increasingly enthusiastic about a move to a more conscious plate that is as much about the planet as it is about personal nutrition. Rather than six-pack abs and rapid weight loss for beach-body summer holidays, which can actually be detrimental to our bodies, we're becoming more interested in longevity, better mental health and vitality.

The conversation around 'food as medicine' is becoming commonplace. It's no longer a quirky idea popularised by fringe doctors, but instead a mainstream concept that global governments, including that of the United States, are championing. More people are recognising that the simple act of eating well every day is one of the most powerful forms of medicine.

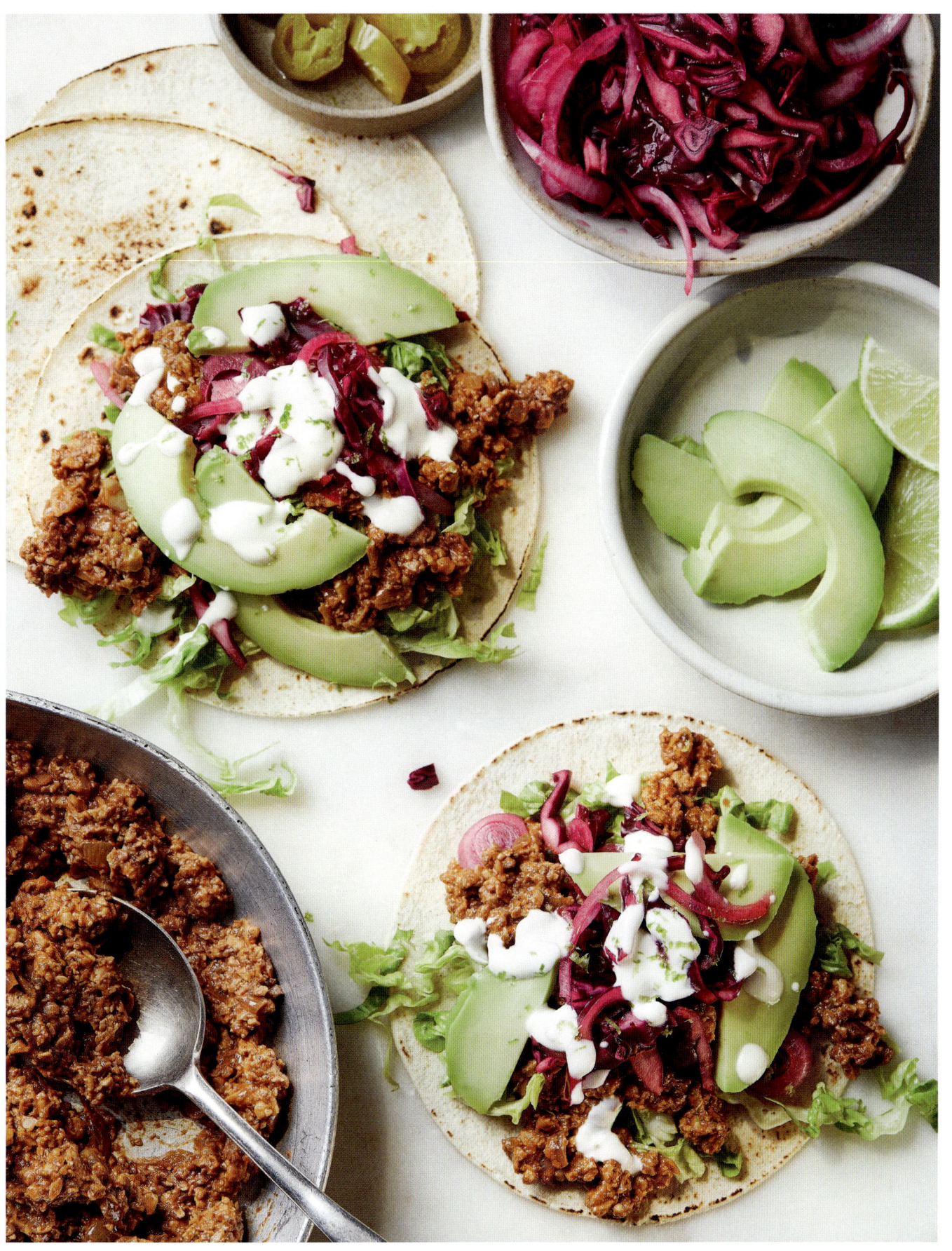

Plant-based protein

I'm also noticing a trend towards enjoying more varied plants and fibre, a theme that I welcome from an environmental perspective, as well as a health stance. Multiple studies published in top-tier scientific journals have demonstrated the benefits of eating more wholefood, plant-based, fibre-rich diets. But alongside this enthusiasm for 'more plants' and 'only plants', some concerning trends have emerged.

First is the rise of faux meats that are introducing more ultra-processed ingredients into our supermarkets, which may be worse for health than the meat products they're replacing. And secondly, there is the replacement of traditionally protein-rich animal products with lower-quality proteins that mimic the texture instead of the nutrition of animal protein. Jackfruit instead of pork. Mushrooms instead of steak. Aubergine instead of chicken. These may resemble each other, but the protein and nutrients are far from alike.

I'm a fan of nodding to the texture and flavours of food if you choose to eat only plants. It's important to not feel as if you're having to sacrifice the enjoyment of food to save the planet or maintain your ethics. But you DO need to be more conscious of protein if you choose to replace animal proteins in your diet and especially if you are 100% plant based.

I say this as a doctor with over 15 years of clinical experience, treating thousands of patients, and with deep respect and compassion for those who choose not to eat animal products for ethical reasons. The reality is that if we shift our eating patterns we need to be more considerate of protein, one of the most important features of our diet.

Simply stating that 'all plants contain protein' and insinuating that it's therefore not necessary to worry about protein intake is not helpful. While it is true that all plants contain protein, it is disingenuous to people and their individual health and wellbeing requirements to suggest that they do not need to concern themselves with ensuring adequate protein intake.

It's very easy to undereat protein on a plant-centric diet and there are even more critical circumstances, which I detail in this book, where people should be more aware of their requirements. Our needs for protein change with age, and there is also fresh debate around what the minimum thresholds for protein intake should be.

On the flipside, there is ample evidence that it is possible to eat a varied and protein-rich diet from mostly plants (or even solely plants) to thrive and ultimately improve health. But it takes careful planning and consideration of where you get your protein from and your unique requirements. Simply having some beans or a plant-based source of protein on your plate is not enough. You need to know the correct amounts that are relevant to you and your individual needs.

I think the move towards 'wholefood' and 'plant forward' is brilliant to see, but we need to anticipate what's down the road. A swing too far in the opposite direction away from meat and animal protein-centric diets can potentially have caveats, just one of which is protein inadequacy.

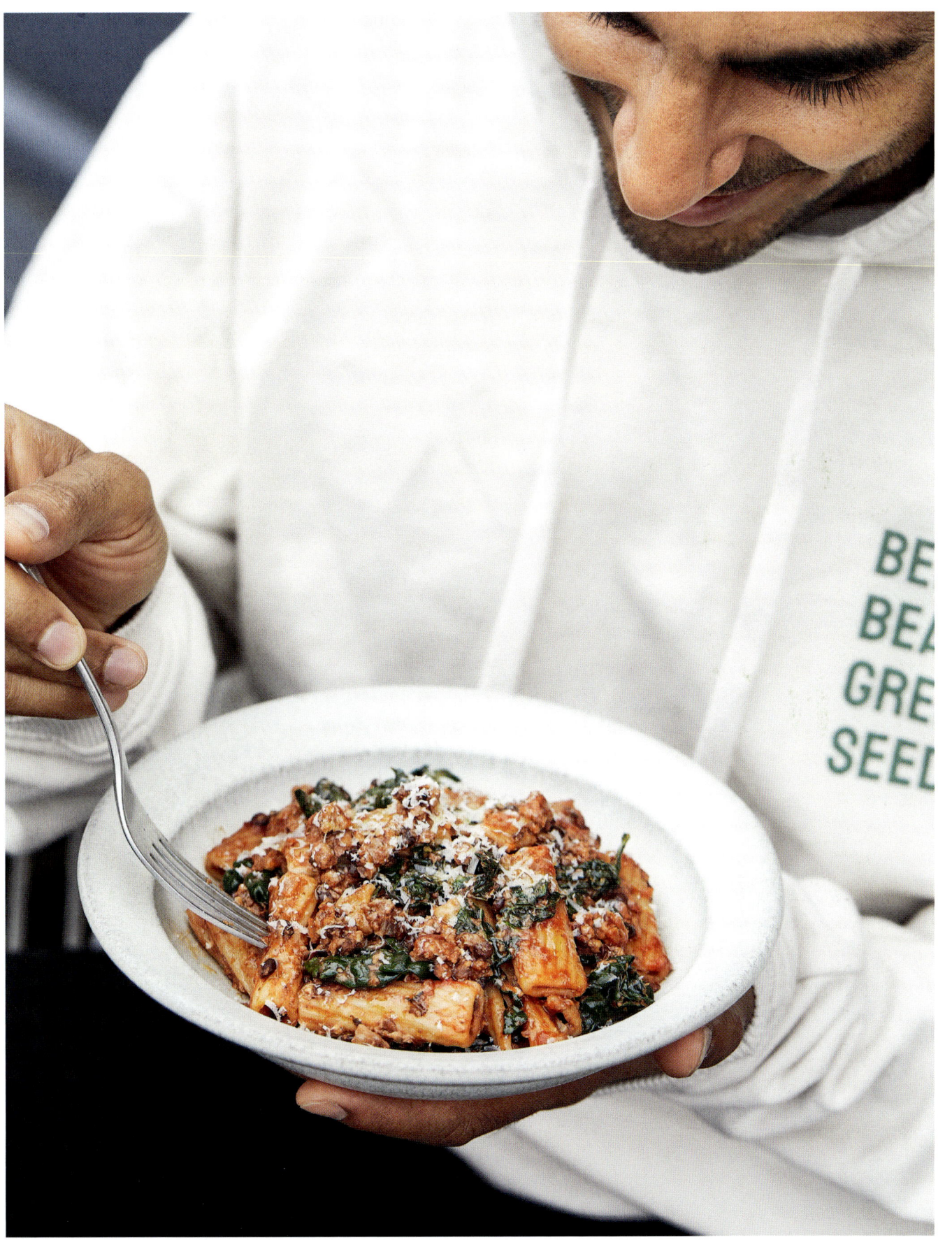

Understanding nutrition

The humble goal of my work is to simplify healthy eating for you, just as I've done for thousands of my patients.

I want to help you put into practice food as medicine every day. And hopefully, with every delicious meal you prepare in your kitchen pharmacy, you can become more resilient instead of reliant on doctors like me.

The world of nutrition is evolving. For example, we now understand a lot more about blood sugar and how it affects our eating behaviour. Eating sugar-laden food or refined carbohydrates that create large rises in blood sugar, and corresponding crashes, can result in increased sensations of hunger that lead to overeating.

We are also continuing to develop a more robust understanding of the gut microbiota and how our unique population of microbes can affect mood, weight control and the likelihood of disease. Inflammation is another area of growing interest and I foresee more people learning about the tactics to bring this natural process into balance, which I discuss in later chapters.

The excitement around personalised nutrition continues to inspire more people to trial wearable devices such as blood glucose monitors and breath analysers and to regularly check their vitamin levels using at-home blood tests. The rapid fall in the cost of testing such as full-body MRI scans has encouraged many of us (myself included) to regularly check our body composition which can help dictate our exercise and eating habits.

But, even for somebody who loves diving into the science, reading the literature and engaging in discussions with academics on a weekly basis, this can all feel horribly overwhelming.

It's easy to get lost in the minor details; I want you to focus on the core pillars.

Three core pillars

Focus on three core pillars of what makes your diet nutritious and medicinal, and you'll succeed in your goal of feeling healthier and happier. Do this consistently and I guarantee you'll feel and enjoy a clearer mind, more energy and better digestive health. It really comes down to these three key requirements:

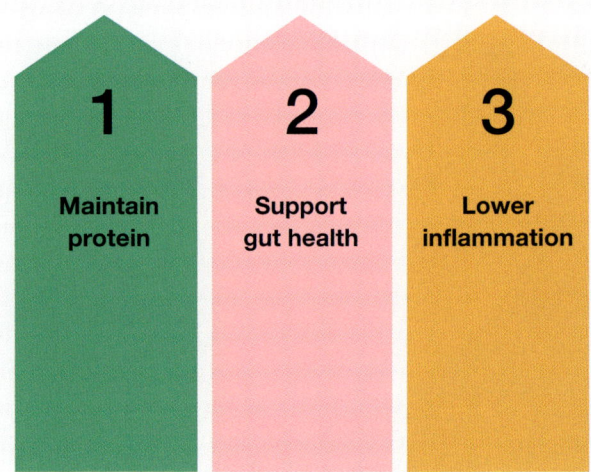

1 **Maintain protein**

2 **Support gut health**

3 **Lower inflammation**

In this book, I'm going to help you to answer three simple questions every time you cook a meal or sit down to eat:

1
Is there <u>enough protein</u> on my plate to meet my requirements?

2
Are there ingredients in this meal that are supporting my <u>gut health</u>?

3
Is the overall impact of this meal going to be <u>anti-inflammatory</u>?

If you can answer 'yes' to all these when assessing a recipe that you're making at home, a dinner that you're ordering when out, or even deciding what breakfast to choose when you're rushing out the door, then you're onto a winner for your health.

I want you to learn these questions to ask yourself at mealtimes, and I'm also going to teach you which simple, delicious ingredients to add to your plate to tip the balance in favour of health and vitality.

Included in this book are gut-boosting ingredients that support your microbes, the strategies that balance your diet from pro- to anti-inflammatory and how to quickly build up more protein on your plate without necessarily having to rely on animal-based ingredients.

If we prioritise our intake of protein and gut health-boosting foods, that also reduce inflammation, we can begin to thrive. Eating according to these principles has been shown to improve lifespan, health span, longevity, immune health and even mental wellbeing. And the best thing about it is that it can be absolutely delicious as well as super easy.

HEALTHY HIGH PROTEIN

YOUR BODY IS ALMOST ENTIRELY MADE UP OF PROTEINS.

Take yourself back to your childhood when you first encountered a Lego set. The magic of Lego was that, as long as you had enough pieces to build with, the possibilities were seemingly infinite. Even if you had only 20 different types, with enough of them, you could still build magnificent and intricate structures. Everything from St Paul's Cathedral to a Ferrari was in the realm of possibility with basic blocks of Lego arranged and organised in a specific way. Lego are the building blocks in the world of toys, just like proteins are the building blocks in the world of biological materials.

Proteins themselves are made up of even smaller blocks called amino acids. There are 20 amino acids in total, nine of which are labelled 'essential'. It's imperative to get these specific essential aminos from your diet because your body cannot produce them. Your body can generate the remaining 11 amino acids, so you don't necessarily need to consume them from food.

Some foods contain all nine essential amino acids in good amounts that we can absorb when we eat them, like animal-based proteins such as chicken, fish and beef, and special plant-based ingredients such as hemp seeds and tempeh (fermented soya beans). Other plant-based ingredients need to be combined to get all nine in sufficient quantities, such as rice paired with lentils, or nuts paired with beans. Ensuring you get enough total protein as well as the correct collection of nine essential amino acids in good amounts is crucial.

The sequence of how these amino acids are arranged, and how they're folded into 3D structures, will determine the function and purpose of a protein. Everything from microstructures like enzymes and hormones to macrostructures like your nails, skin, muscles, bones and organs is largely constructed from proteins built from the same 'Lego-like' building blocks of 20 amino acids.

What is protein used for?

If you ask most people what they think protein is used for in the body, many of us would incorrectly assume that it is largely used for muscles on our arms and legs. This naive assumption disregards the importance of protein as the most critical biomolecule.

Aside from water and fat, your body is almost entirely made up of proteins. They are the central molecules of life with the most diverse functions and roles in your body.

When you consume protein from food, only about 25% is actually used for muscle building and maintenance. The rest of the proteins from your diet are broken down and utilised for a variety of other uses such as repairing cells, building connective tissues and manufacturing immune cells.

In fact, a vital function of your liver is actually to produce proteins. Everything from lipoproteins (proteins that transport cholesterol in your blood) to globulins (proteins that carry immune cells around the body) is produced in the liver. The insatiable need for protein is constant.

For this reason, whether you're in your 20s or your 60s, your body actually churns through around 300g of protein each day. That's the equivalent protein content of 1.5kg of beef steak every single day. Your protein turnover is so high, you actually replenish every protein in your body four times over, every single year!

Now before you start planning your week full of red meat-filled dinners or trying to eat six chicken breasts a day, let me make very clear, I'm not suggesting that we need to physically consume 300g of protein each day. It is not necessary to consume that amount of protein from food because your body is like an intelligent recycling plant that is constantly moving and repurposing proteins in circulation.

Your liver is tasked with breaking down and reusing existing proteins in the body every single minute of the day. Whether you're asleep or in the gym, your liver is continually generating proteins that are transported around the body and utilised for various functions.

But while the recommended protein intake is nowhere near 300g per day, the threshold for daily protein is higher than most people realise. And from what I have seen in the academic literature over the last five years, it's also higher than what I used to believe myself.

Another important thing to remember is, unlike fats that can be stored in tissue, or sugar (glucose) that can be stored in your muscles and liver to be called upon when you need it, there is no storage facility in your body for protein. For example, you can't rely on a very high-protein meal from Monday to support your protein needs on Thursday. Any excess protein you consume is simply excreted from the body via the urine. Hence, you need to be consuming enough protein *daily* to meet your requirements and preferably at each mealtime.

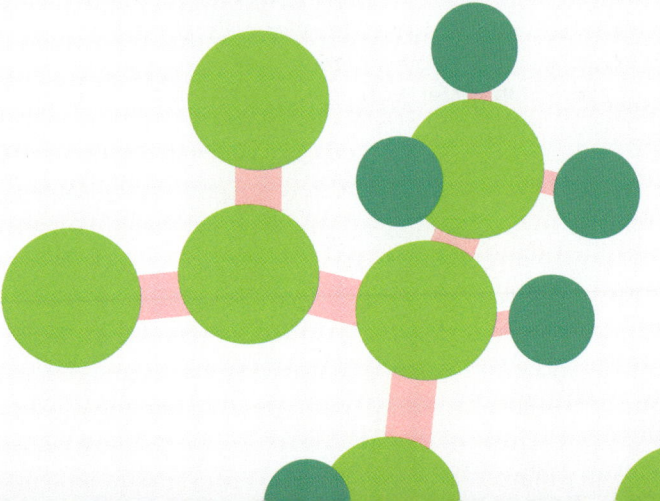

Why is protein so important now?

A 'plant-forward' diet is a concept that I wrote about in my first book. It's an evidence-based way of eating and protecting your health by focusing your plate on wholefood plant-based ingredients with judicious use of animal products.

Since I first wrote about this eight years ago, there has been an explosion of interest across the world. Championed by both sustainability and health experts, they all appear to agree: fewer animal products in the diet correlate with better health outcomes and may even benefit the planet.

However, shifting your diet from an omnivorous diet that includes animal proteins on a daily basis, to one that uses meat, fish and dairy sparingly, can come with a downside. And that downside is potentially underconsuming protein.

Now, I just want to state from the very beginning: all plants contain protein, and it is absolutely possible to ensure more than adequate protein intake from plants alone. Just ask plant-based tennis super champion Novak Djokovic, whose protein needs are incredibly high. He's managing to support his daily requirements, as are many other fully plant-based professional athletes.

However, the convenience and availability of obtaining those proteins from plants alone is more challenging than if one opted to include animal sources in their diet. Even for omnivores such as myself, if the proportion of plants on our plate increases, there is the real potential and common pitfall of not consuming enough daily protein.

My position on this has evolved. I used to think consuming minimal protein in one's diet was more than sufficient to ensure a healthy and happy body. But the research tells me otherwise and as a home cook and a medical doctor, I have adapted my diet accordingly.

I still believe that adopting a 'plant-forward' diet has benefits, and it's a way of eating I still recommend and enjoy myself. But without careful planning and a broad understanding of where you obtain your dietary protein from, it can be quite tricky to meet your protein requirements.

I suspect that not incorporating enough plant-based proteins from food has led to a lot of people feeling unwell and lacking in energy when they cut out animal products partially or completely. I've also personally seen this in many plant-based patients of mine.

Careful attention to how much and where you get your protein from is necessary to thrive on a plant-forward diet that still has many benefits to overall health and wellbeing.

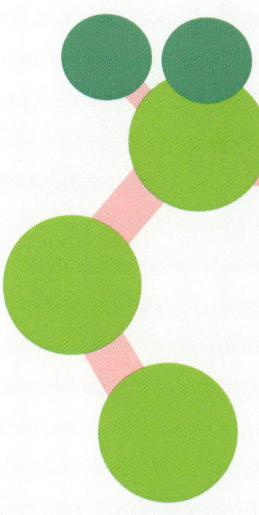

What are the benefits of eating enough protein?

Aside from ensuring that you have adequate protein to prevent muscle loss and age more healthfully, you may experience some immediate, tangible benefits when you start consuming more protein. These include:

Fewer sugar cravings

Cravings appear to diminish because protein is very satiating and you're less likely to crave sugary foods. This effect can be magnified if you incorporate more protein at breakfast, which keeps you fuller for longer and less likely to crave mid-morning snacks.

Weight loss

Protein requires more energy than carbohydrates and fat to be broken down. This extra effort during digestion can marginally increase your total energy burn each day which can aid weight loss. The extra satiation that protein makes you feel leads to less snacking and reduces your total daily energy consumption which can improve weight management without consciously having to count calories.

More energy

You may notice your energy levels are higher and you're able to sustain longer bouts of exercise. More protein in your diet, coupled with exercise, can improve muscle strength, recovery and help you achieve a leaner, stronger body.

Better focus

Incorporating more protein in meals can keep your blood sugar levels steady, which may have a positive effect on your ability to focus and avoid energy crashes as a result of fluctuating blood sugar levels.

Better sleep

Proteins form the building blocks of melatonin and other hormones that are involved in different stages of sleep. There is a tentative link for plant-based proteins potentially being beneficial for sleep, but the studies are generally of poor quality.

While these short-term wins sound great, it's also imperative that you understand the long-term longevity, health and wellbeing benefits of healthy high protein consumption, which include...

Bone and muscle health

Above 55 years of age, we absorb less protein and over the age of 40 we have a greater risk of sarcopenia (loss of muscle mass and strength) and less bone mass (referred to as bone mineral density). More protein in the diet, especially in older adults, is associated with greater bone mineral density and a lower loss of bone cells (referred to as bone cell turnover). This could be because protein enhances calcium uptake and stimulates a growth hormone (called IGF-1) which helps lay down bone cells, creating stronger bones that are less likely to fracture on impact.

While more muscle may sound like a vanity metric in the realm of how aesthetically pleasing you appear, having enough muscle is critical in older age as you become more prone to falls and loss of balance. Making sure you eat enough protein helps maintain and preserve lean muscle mass and can improve bone density when coupled with appropriate exercise.

Metabolic health

Your muscles also serve as an important store of sugar. The less muscle you have, the higher the risk of metabolic health issues like type 2 diabetes, because more sugar has to be stored as fat. This magical combination of protein and exercise will contribute to better metabolic health, which is precisely the medicine that people require.

Longevity

A meta-analysis of over 700,000 adults found that higher protein intake (particularly from plant-based sources) was associated with lower deaths from all causes, including cancer and cardiovascular disease. Making sure you consume enough protein supports your liver and other organs and ensures your bodily processes are working optimally. Having enough protein is important for ageing as healthily as possible.

Healthy menopause

After menopause, women become deficient in the key hormones oestrogen and testosterone which have protective roles for cardiovascular and brain health and much more.

Multiple studies have shown that women with a lower protein consumption (around 0.8g per kg of bodyweight) have higher fat mass and less lean muscle compared to those with a higher protein intake. Even during perimenopause, adequate protein may ward off weight gain. Higher protein consumption is associated with less frailty in older women and large studies, such as The Women's Health Initiative, have established this connection.

I hope you are convinced that you need to be aware of how much protein you eat daily and that having enough brings multiple benefits. Let's dive into some tactics to help you achieve this easily every day.

How much do I need?

Calculating how much protein you need to consume each day requires a little arithmetic. But I think there's merit in doing some simple math and getting an overall idea of how much your individual requirements are.

The amount of protein an individual requires is expressed as 'number of grams of protein per kilogram of bodyweight'. Officially the standard minimum requirement for protein is 0.8 grams per kilogram of bodyweight per day for a healthy adult.

Putting this into context, this equates to about 60g of protein per day for a 75kg individual. Split across a typical eating pattern of three meals a day, this results in a requirement of 20g of protein per meal.

Looking at population data for both the US and UK, most people (both omnivores and plant-based eaters) more than meet this requirement. However, on closer inspection, 0.8g per kilogram of bodyweight is the *minimum* requirement to prevent protein deficiency.

Considering everything I've explained about the importance of protein thus far, underconsuming this critical nutrient is something you want to avoid. And remember, your body cannot store protein, so you have to consume sufficient amounts each day.

Because this nutrient is so important, if you do underconsume protein, your body will start to break down its own muscles (referred to as 'lean mass') as a source of amino acids. This means your body will essentially pull protein out of your muscles and break it down into the fundamental amino acids that are required for all those vital functions. This is the metabolic equivalent of dipping into your pension savings account to pay the weekly bills.

In the same way this is not a good idea for your retirement plan, it is not a good idea for your longevity. If this continues to happen it can lead to loss of muscle from your legs and arms, which you need to rigorously preserve as you age.

To avoid this deficiency, the World Health Organization (WHO) and many other organisations have stipulated 0.8g per kilogram of bodyweight as the base level of protein intake. But most of us don't just want to avoid ill-health as a result of deficiency, and my guess is that if you're reading this book, you're interested in optimising your health and wellbeing, not simply evading illness.

There is a growing consensus that the target for 'optimal health' is much higher than 0.8g, and instead we should be aiming for a minimum of 1.2g per kilogram of bodyweight, for both sexes. This is 50% higher than the previous recommendation.

Using the same example of a 75kg individual, this now equates to 90g of protein per day, or 30g of protein at each meal in a standard three meal a day pattern of eating.

To make things slightly more complicated, an individual's protein requirements will vary depending on various factors, such as age, whether they are pre- or post-menopause, medical conditions, activity level and health goals (such as weight loss or muscle gain). With these in mind, an optimal protein intake may be anywhere between 1.2g and 1.6g per kilogram of bodyweight.

Here are some examples to give you an idea:

Amandeep is a 65-year-old woman, who works out occasionally during the week doing home-based aerobic exercise and walks regularly. She's post-menopausal, does not take HRT and has no other medical conditions. She's 65kg and at her desired weight. Her protein requirements would be:

1.2g x 65kg = 78g protein per day
(an average of 26g at each meal)

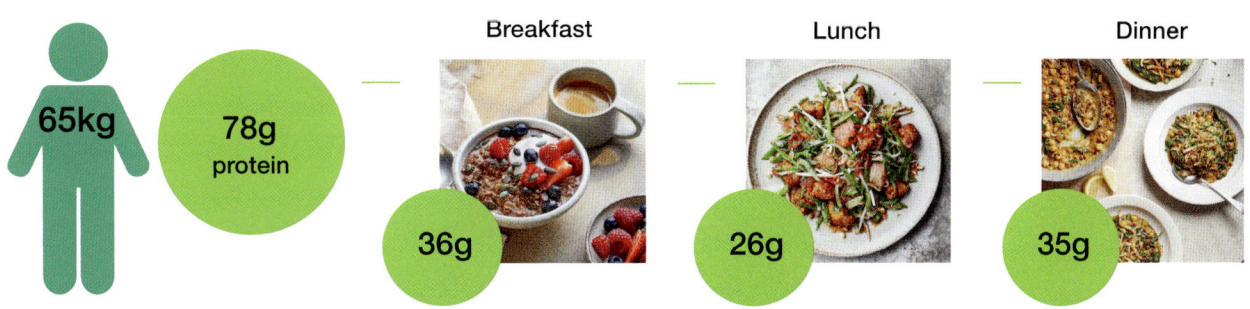

Mary is 33 years old. She trains regularly at the gym and is interested in gaining some lean muscle as she's training for a CrossFit competition. She weighs 50kg. Her protein requirements would be:

1.6g x 50kg = 80g protein per day
(an average of 27g at each meal)

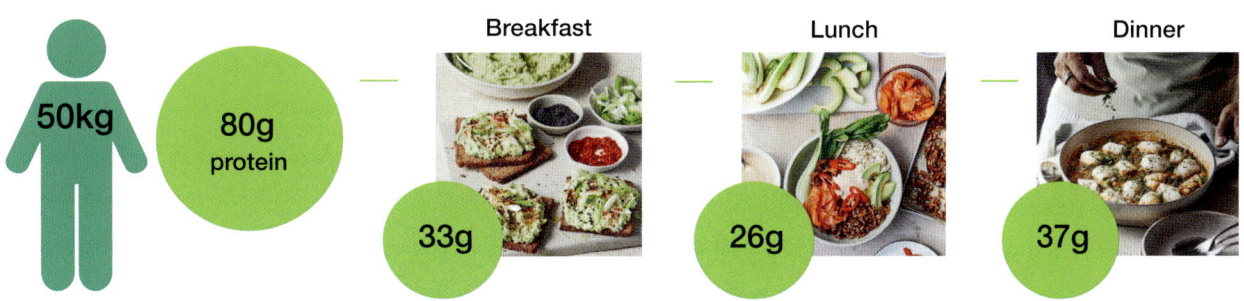

To save you the hassle of doing further math, I've linked to a handy protein calculator here that will incorporate your needs based on your health goals.

For anyone with medical conditions and especially for those with kidney disease, I highly recommend speaking with a medical professional before making any changes to your protein consumption, and any changes to your diet in general.

HEALTHY HIGH PROTEIN

YOUR BODY CANNOT STORE PROTEIN, SO YOU HAVE TO CONSUME SUFFICIENT AMOUNTS EACH DAY

The bottom line is, for most people who do not have any special circumstances and are not looking to build large amounts of muscle, I think a minimum of 1.2g per kg of bodyweight is a good, evidence-based starting point. The same formula applies regardless of your sex as it's based on weight.

Even if you were to opt for a higher amount and consume more protein than required, your body is very efficient at excreting excess protein via the kidneys. There do not appear to be any negative effects of excess protein intake (even as high as 2.5g per kilogram of bodyweight), as long as you're not overconsuming energy or excess amounts of saturated fats.

Additionally, if your protein intake comes from largely plant-based sources, as I recommend, there are extra benefits from the consumption of nutrients such as fibre, anti-inflammatory phytochemicals and micronutrients that are commonly found in plant proteins.

For these reasons, most recipes in this book have a minimum of 20g of protein per serving, coming mostly from plant proteins, coupled with ideas for how to 'boost your protein'. By simply adding more of an ingredient or adding a new ingredient to increase the protein per serving, you can flex your meals to suit your personal requirements. And just like my other cookbooks, the recipes are also perfectly fine for families and children, who, incidentally, also happen to have higher protein requirements.

However, I want to make an important caveat. You do not need to be prescriptive with your food. I personally do not weigh or measure my food and I do not recommend people do so, unless you're an athlete or body builder and your appearance or performance depend on it.

Pages 24–7 show what portions of protein-rich foods generally look like, so you can 'guesstimate' the protein content of your meals without having to conform to rigid practices that are so often recommended in the fitness and health industry.

I want you to have a relaxed and enjoyable relationship with food, rather than a 'fuel-like' mentality that discounts the beauty and joy of sitting down to eat a wonderful meal.

When should I eat protein?

A number of common myths, perhaps seeded and perpetuated by fitness communities, have made protein consumption overly complex. Online you can find a mix of elaborate protocols for when you should be consuming protein, supplement guides for specific amino acids and suggestions for the best-quality proteins from collagen, whey and vegan sources.

The evidence suggests that it does not need to be this elaborate. Simply meet your protein requirements from wholefoods, mostly plants, and consistently every 24 hours, and you'll experience all the benefits protein has to offer.

When you eat your protein doesn't seem to matter as long as you get *enough* each day. However, I will add two caveats. First, consuming good amounts of protein in the first meal of your day seems to have benefits. Secondly, there appear to be advantages to having good amounts of protein at each meal to support steady blood sugar levels.

As we have already discussed, protein at breakfast can maintain satiety and stave off cravings and, above all, will prevent you from overeating which is the most important and commonest problem that people face each day. Specific timing around workouts does not appear to be important, even for those looking for muscle gain benefits.

Since fasting has become an attractive method for people to control what and how much they eat, I'm often asked if it's possible to fast and still maintain protein intake. The honest answer is yes, but it depends.

If you can still consume the required amount of protein per day in your reduced eating hours, such as a 16:8 fasting protocol, that's fine. However, if you fast for a few days at a time, with no intake of food at all, you may find that you are under consuming protein, which can reduce lean muscle mass over time. This is something I would avoid or approach with caution, particularly if you're above the age of 40.

In short, keep it simple. Eat enough protein at every meal and pay particular attention to prioritising protein at breakfast. I have plenty of recipe ideas to make this achievable.

Plant v. animal: where should I get my protein from?

This is perhaps the most important question and contentious part of the whole protein debate! I suspect many nutritionists and doctors of a plant-based persuasion avoid this area because of an uncomfortable truth: it is harder to get good amounts of quality protein from plants alone.

That's not to say it's unachievable. It's just more of a challenge.

I tend to get most of my own protein intake from wholefood, plant-based sources because there appear to be extra longevity and general health benefits with more protein consumption coming specifically from plants. A large study published in the *British Medical Journal* (*BMJ*), examining several hundred thousand people, found that eating more protein was significantly associated with a lower risk of mortality and health problems. The benefit of higher protein consumption was further enhanced when more of the protein came from plant-based sources.

This may be because of the added fibre, phytonutrients and plant chemicals that wholefood plant-based proteins contain, and for this reason it's also what I would advise people to consider as well.

It's up to you what proportion of your protein comes from plants. But deciding between both categories of proteins, animal- versus plant-based, is confusing because there is no simple solution, and everything comes with a trade-off.

Animal proteins

Animal proteins, such as dairy, poultry, meat and fish, are great because, according to various measures of protein bioavailability – such as the Protein Digestibility Corrected Amino Acid Score (PDCAAS) and Digestible Indispensable Amino Acid Score (DIAAS) – they deliver easily accessible amino acids that your body can readily use, in high amounts for very little quantity of food. They also contain all nine essential amino acids. But, depending on the cut of meat, these products can also contain high amounts of saturated fats, cholesterol and other components. When consumed in high quantities, these extras can be problematic for health and linked to higher cardiovascular disease and diabetes risk.

Plant-based proteins

Good sources of plant-based proteins, such as soya, lentils, nuts and seeds, are fantastic because of the extra nutrients they contain. These include phytosterols that reduce cholesterol, fibres that support your gut health, and minerals such as zinc and magnesium. However, the quantity and bioavailability of these proteins tend to be lower than in animal proteins, which makes it more challenging to meet your daily protein needs.

Let's use an example comparing beans and chicken. The digestibility of proteins from beans and the quantity of specific amino acids they contain are both much lower than chicken. This requires you to eat far more beans, coupled with other plant-based

Show me the protein

proteins (like nuts and seeds), to ensure you're getting all the amino acids you require. Chicken on the other hand, has all the amino acids you need packaged in an easy-to-digest format that your body can use, and so therefore less planning is required. However, depending on the cut, the chicken might contain high amounts of cholesterol and saturated fat that could increase your risk of cardiovascular disease if eaten in excess. In addition, the chicken has no beneficial fibre or phytonutrients to protect you.

For omnivores, there is an ideal solution: a wholefood, plant-focused diet. One that includes small amounts of lean meat and fish, coupled with a variety of plant-based proteins. It enables you to easily consume enough protein at the higher requirements while also benefiting from all the gut-health and inflammation-lowering benefits of plants. Plus it has the strongest evidence base for longevity and general health benefits.

For vegetarians and vegans, it is still possible to eat enough protein, but you need to be more cognisant of how much and where you're getting them from. Depending on your weight and activity level, you may also want to consider supplementation with whey, soy and pea products, which I discuss on page 31.

If this information is new to you, it can all seem overwhelming. Calculating how much protein you need each day, carefully planning diverse proteins if you're vegetarian or vegan, making sure you don't eat too much or too little of each ingredient. I confess, it sounds like a lot.

Remember, don't let perfect be the enemy of good.

I do not expect anyone to regularly track their food, weigh it, take pictures of it and monitor their calorie intake. I've seen how destructive and unhealthy those behaviours can become when people are simply trying to follow a healthier lifestyle in the real world.

Over time, using these quick references on the next pages, you'll become a good 'guesstimator' of the protein content of your meals. This will enable you to casually keep an eye on how much protein you have at each meal, and whether you need more or less.

Just like keeping an eye on how many glasses of water you've drunk each day, cups of coffee or even mouthfuls of sugary treats, it's important to have a general idea of your protein intake. But, I don't think it's something you need to fastidiously measure every day. This section will help you develop a general hunch as to whether you need to bump it up a bit.

As a rule of thumb, there is lower protein content per serving of plant-based ingredients compared to animal sources. These images will give you a quick reference of how much protein you're getting from different ingredients, as well as typical serving sizes that we tend to consume them in.

HEALTHY HIGH PROTEIN

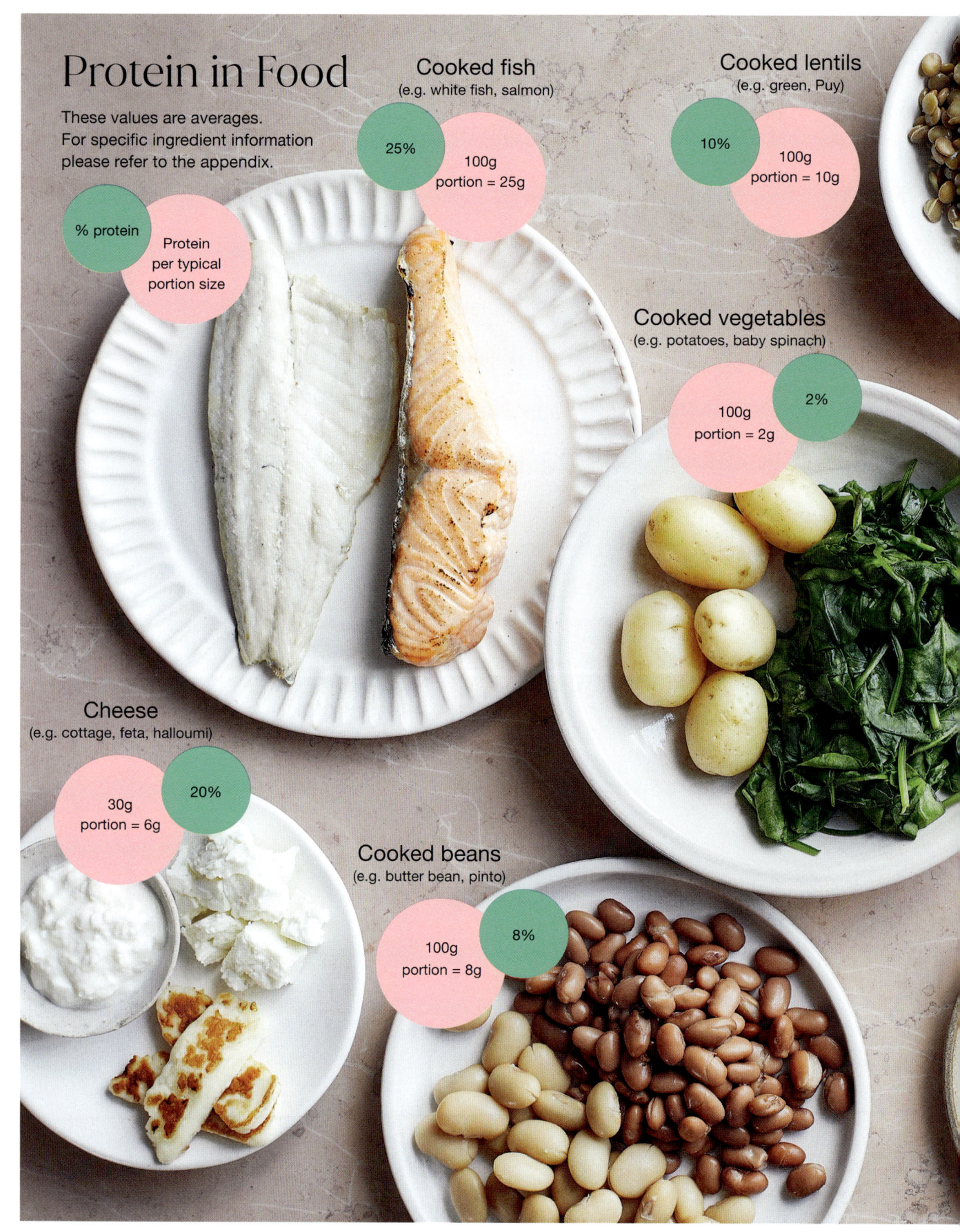

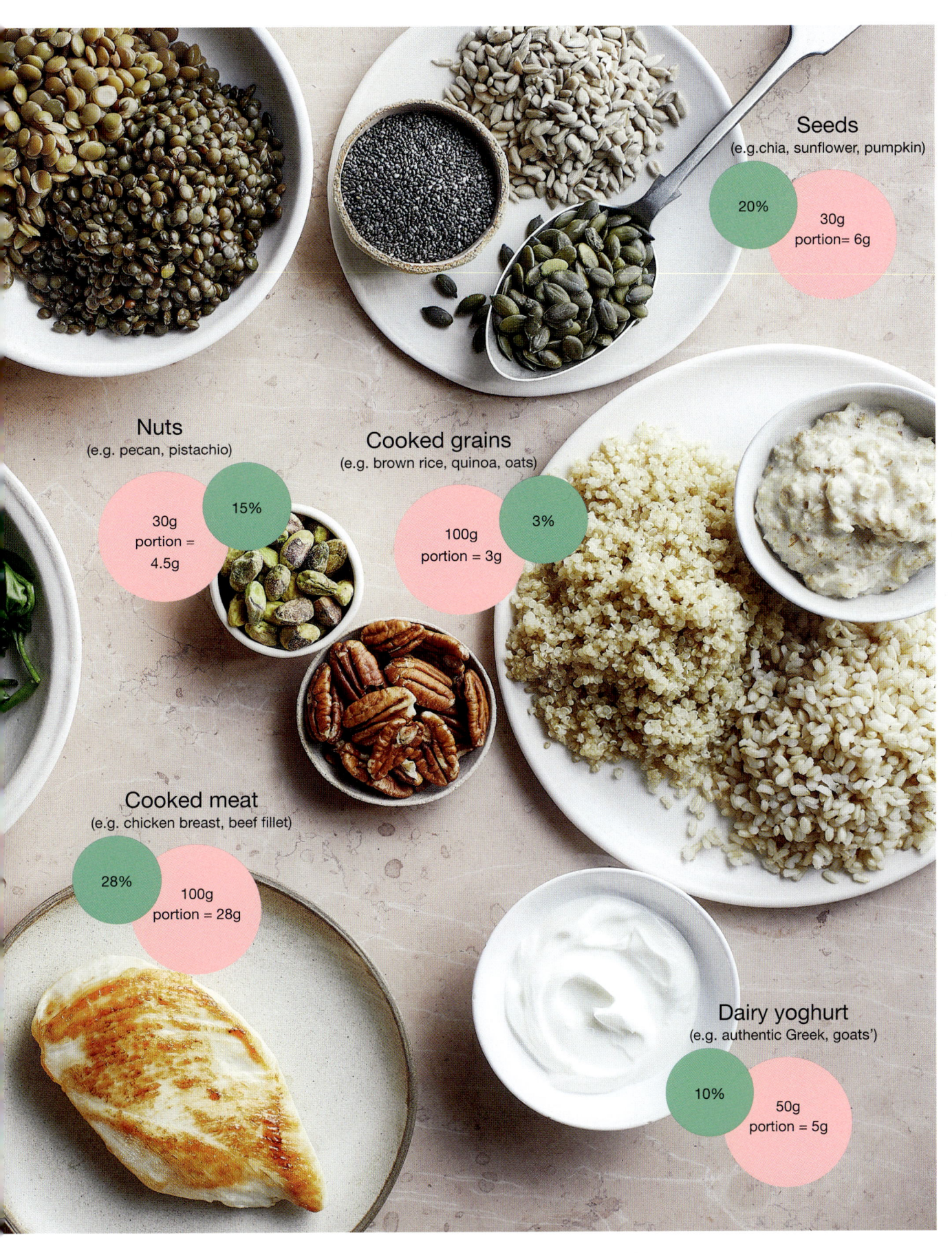

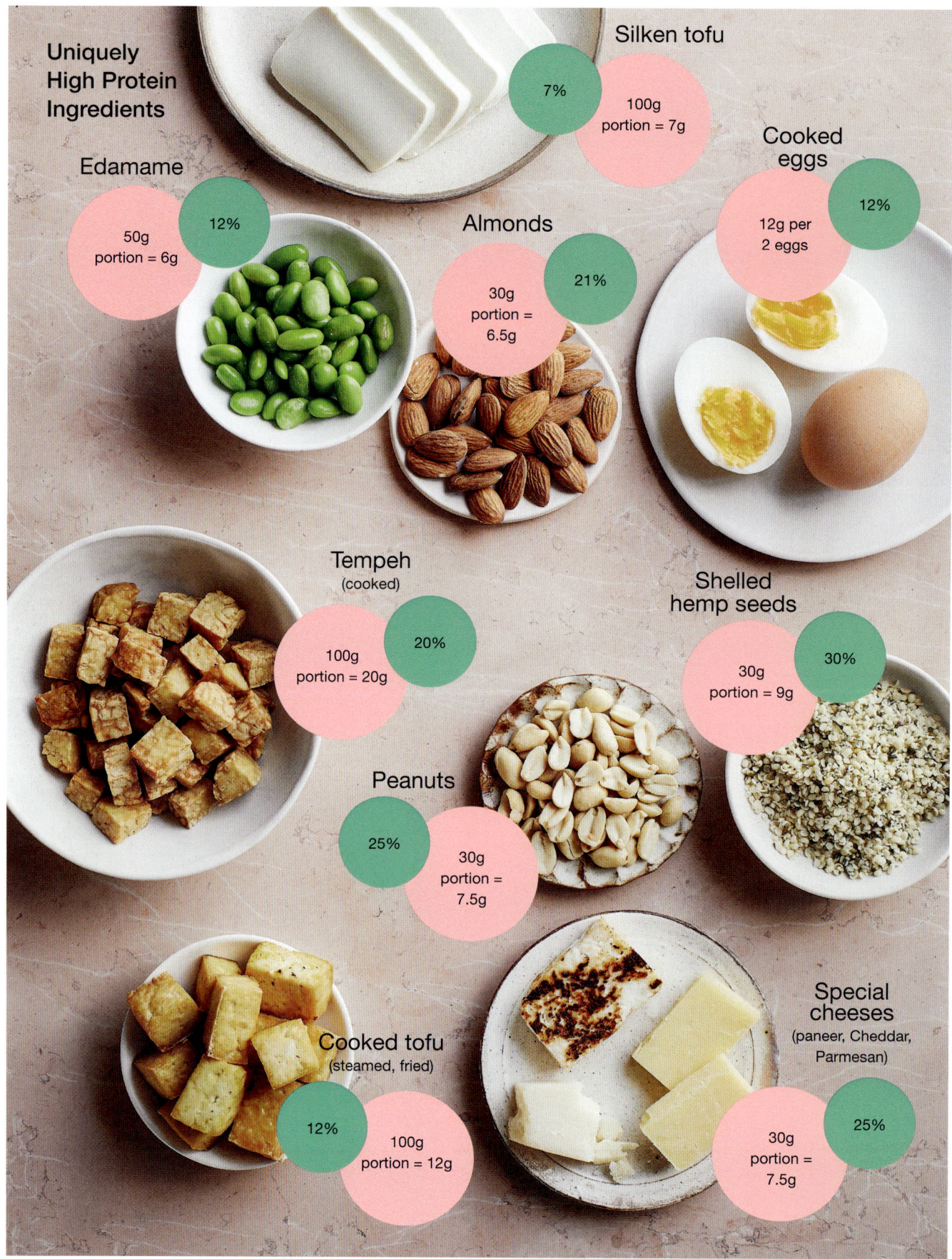

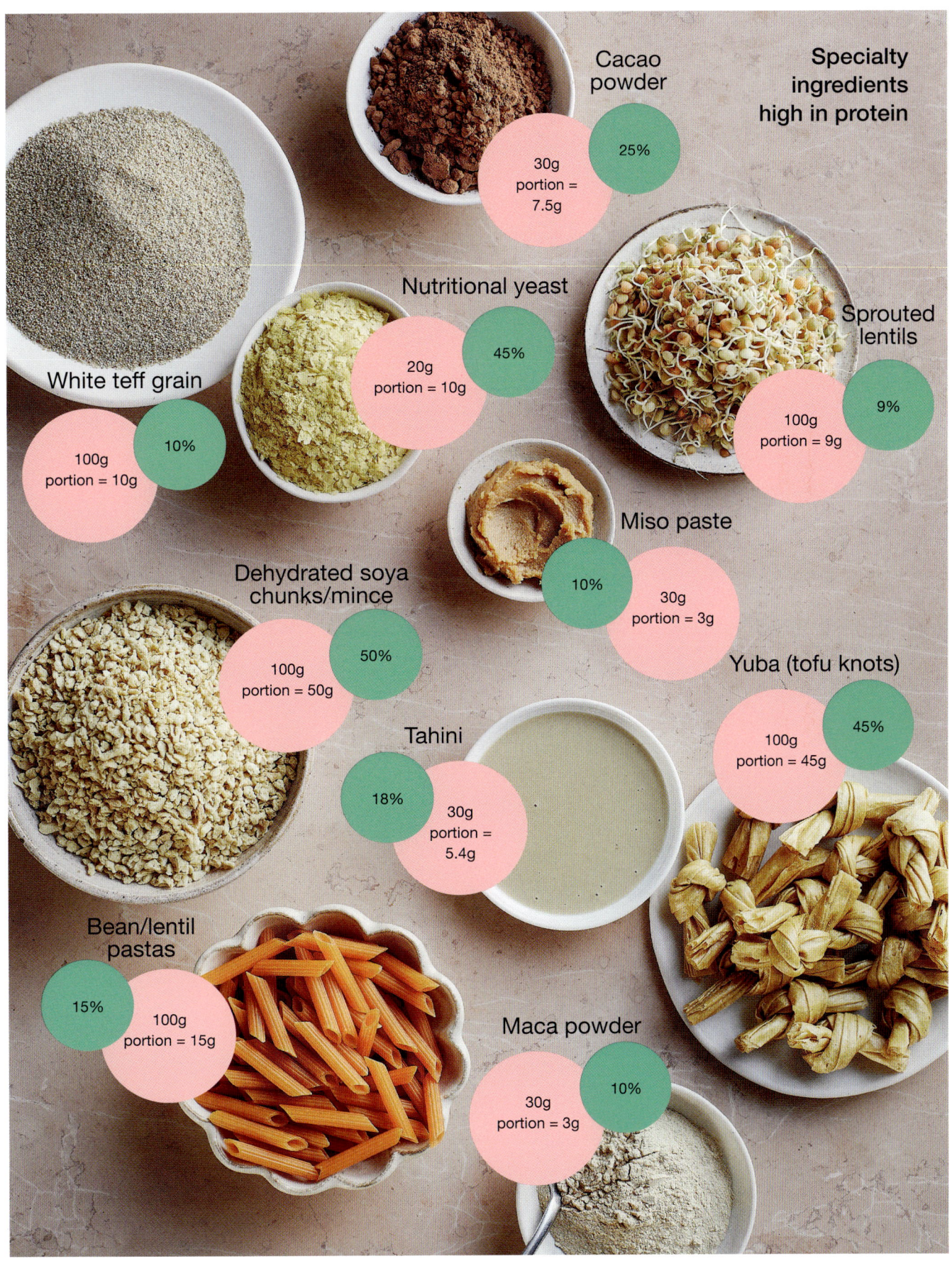

Getting more from plant protein

Speaking honestly and from experience, if you don't like soya (such as edamame, tofu or tempeh), I think you will struggle to meet your protein needs on a 100% plant-based diet. If you have an intolerance to soya, I will go so far as to say that it may be inadvisable to go on a strict plant-only diet unless you can consume the vast quantities of beans and grains required for your needs. Please take this into consideration.

And putting aside the fact that I've helpfully laid out a collection of ingredients and their corresponding protein content, I actually don't want you to focus on individual isolated foods or nutrients. We eat food as part of a 'food matrix'. That is to say, the way nutrients are packaged together in the complex structures of whole foods, and as part of a meal with other foods, will ultimately effect how your body processes them. In addition, how we combine foods, the use of herbs and spices, and the cooking methods we employ all have an influence on the overall digestibility of proteins. These are all likely to be complementary, thus increasing how much protein we can absorb from ingredients.

To ensure you consume enough protein from plants, you still have to consume a greater quantity of these ingredients to meet your nutritional needs. But there are some strategies to increase the amount of protein you can absorb from these ingredients and heighten their nutritional value. And you don't have to venture far from your home kitchen to figure out how to do so.

I always look at traditional methods of cooking and food preparation, handed down through families over centuries of experimentation, with the simple question: why?

Why would our ancestors have chosen such laborious methods of preparing food, if it wasn't for significant practical, survival or nutritional purposes? There is a tradition of food preparation techniques, such as soaking, sprouting and fermenting, across multiple cultures globally. In addition, there are parallels in food combinations, pairings and cooking methods across vastly different cuisines.

These practices make nutrients, such as protein from grains, seeds, nuts and legumes, more available, they preserve their shelf-life and decrease the amount of harmful plant chemicals that hinder our ability to digest nutrients in food.

These practices include:

Soaking

Soaking beans, lentils, nuts and seeds overnight reduces the components that can cause bloating. In legumes these include sugars such as verbascose, raffinose and stachyose which are chemicals that can lead to discomfort, but also interfere with protein digestion. Soaking can increase the amount of protein your body can extract from these ingredients.

Combining

In most meals, protein is not consumed in isolation. Combining food groups is a common pattern you find across cultures. Beans and barley, lentils and rice, tahini and chickpeas. Legacy recipes appear to have a combination of grain and legume proteins to ensure you meet your requirements. By combining these ingredients you'll consume all nine essential amino acids in good quantities, which will satisfy your body's protein requirements.

Fermenting

Products such as tempeh (fermented soya beans) actually have higher bioavailability of proteins than the original bean and are naturally high in nutrients because of this processing method. The application of microbes to 'pre-digest' food not only reduces antinutrients, like oxalates, tannins and phytic acid, which can interfere with protein absorption, but it increases the digestibility of proteins from legumes, seeds and even grains. Employed in traditional cooking methods such as sourdough bread-making with wheat grain or koji fungal cultures with rice, these practices yield far more bang for your buck and have been shown to massively increase levels of protein availability.

Germinating/sprouting

Antinutritional factors (ANFs), such as phytates and lectins are part of the intrinsic composition of plant foods. By soaking and germinating (also known as sprouting) foods, such as lentils, alfalfa, broccoli seeds and pumpkin seeds, you naturally reduce the presence of these antinutritional factors that interfere with absorption and hence increase the digestibility of nutrients such as protein, vitamins and minerals.

There are centuries of wisdom in these tried-and-tested techniques and they are something we should all practise more of in our own homes. Optimising amino-acid bioavailability through processing and specific preparation methods is a common practice across many cuisines that we should be leaning into.

The science is fascinating, but I don't expect you to carefully craft meals with specific protein combinations to ensure all your amino acid requirements are met. That's where I come in. All the recipes have been created with these combinations in mind to ensure you're getting a good collection of proteins, as well as gut- and inflammation-supporting nutrients.

Summary

EVIDENCE-BASED STRATEGIES TO INCREASE PROTEIN

SAVOURY BREAKFASTS
My breakfasts have a lot of variety, they tend to be savoury and in practice I usually have leftovers from my dinner … for breakfast!

TOPPERS
Using high-protein wholefoods like nuts and seeds to top your meals adds more quality fats, micronutrients and significant amounts of protein.

WHEN IN DOUBT, BEAN IT OUT
Lean into plant-based proteins like beans and lentils. Add them to most of your meals to bulk up the fibre content.

SOYA BROS
Tempeh, tofu and soya in general are your friends. Multiple studies have shown these to be gut and heart healthy, with great-quality amino acids. I opt for organic where possible.

In addition, try unusual, cheaper animal-based proteins such as shellfish, cod cheeks, mussels, offcuts of meat. Tinned fish is also a great way of adding protein that's delicious and easy.

From now on, whenever you think about dietary protein and what it's used for, remember it's not just muscle mass. It is critical for every macro- and micro-structure in your body.

- We generally need more protein as we age, particularly women post-menopause.

- As long as you're not overconsuming saturated fat, cholesterol or excess calories from food you should not fear eating more protein, particularly from plant-based sources. Any extra protein is easily excreted from the body via urine and does not cause harm.

- Breakfast protein is important for maintaining steady energy levels and keeping you full during the day which can prevent over eating.

- Choose plant-based proteins, as these are associated with better health outcomes, and make sure you have protein at each meal.

- It is important to recognise that protein intake alone will not reduce the rate at which you lose muscle mass as you age. You have to exercise as well, otherwise the practice is futile.

Should you use a protein supplement?

I think most people can hit their protein requirements with wholefood-based sources and, in fact, there is evidence that wholefoods provide more readily absorbable nutrients than powders. But I recognise that sometimes it can be a convenient option to have a protein shake.

For vegans aiming to maximise their protein intake, pea-, soy- and rice-based protein shakes are typically the best options for muscle growth and conditioning. Whey and other milk-based protein shakes have the best absorption of all protein powders and therefore the biggest impact on building muscle. However, it is crucial to remain vigilant about the presence of fillers and sweeteners, even in plant-based brands.

Products like collagen, casein and whey can all be highly processed and the quality of these protein supplements can vary greatly. It is essential to choose products that are free from unnecessary additives that could negatively impact your gut health.

Collagen is a very absorbable source of amino acids called proline and glycine. I think this can explain the anecdotal improvements in skin health, wrinkles and nails, although the studies are of mixed quality. It might be something you want to experiment with but remember that your diet represents the biggest lever for health and it is much more important to get that right before supplementation.

If you do choose to supplement with a protein shake these are my criteria:

- Pea-, soy-, rice-based protein or organic, grass-fed whey.
- No sweeteners, fillers or other additives.
- Choose unflavoured if possible and blend with your own desired sweetener, such as ripe banana or small amounts of honey, maple syrup or sugar.

Common side-effects of protein powders, both plant and animal based, include digestive discomfort, flatulence, bloating and constipation.

My advice is always to go slow. Whenever adding a new protein supplement: halve the recommended dose and gradually increase according to your tolerance. And, of course, prioritise whole unprocessed foods as much as possible. The studies reviewing protein consumption and health improvements are examining wholefoods, not supplements.

YOUR DIET REPRESENTS THE BIGGEST LEVER FOR HEALTH

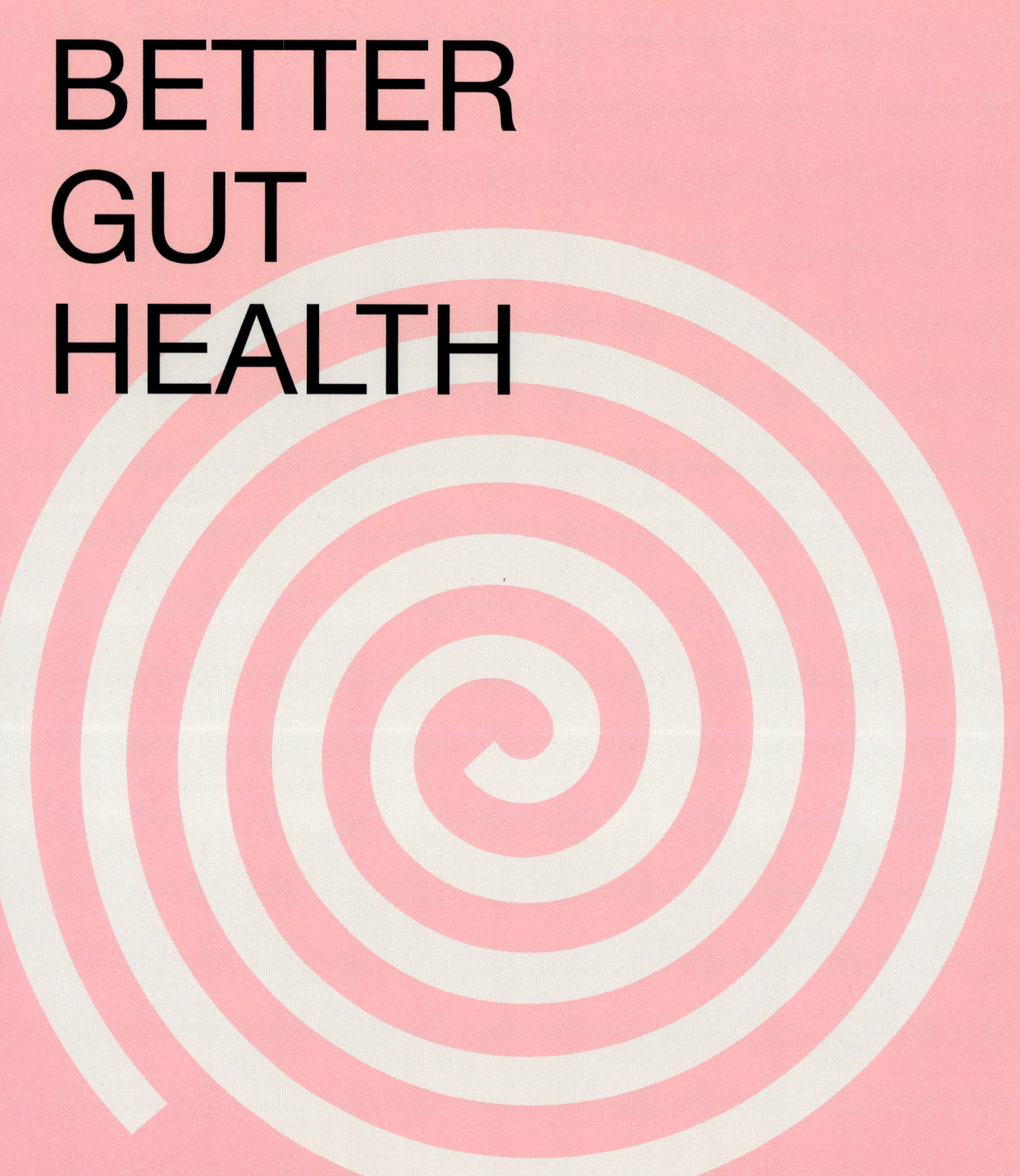
BETTER GUT HEALTH

Around the age of nine, I used to make a weekly trip to Mr Patel's sweet shop on the local high street which also conveniently doubled up as a pharmacy.

While I perused the shelves of brightly coloured chocolate bars for my Saturday morning treat, I would overhear the conversations with Mr Patel at the counter. People would ask him for treatments for a whole host of issues. Chest infections, tummy upsets, skin rashes, diarrhoea, cold sores and more.

After listening intently to their complaints, Mr Patel would ask them to wait a moment, turn around and rummage in his well-stocked cabinet out of sight. He would dutifully return clutching a small brown-coloured bottle of viscous liquid with some scratchy handwritten notes on the front. On other occasions, he might appear with a glass bottle of pills clinking against the sides, an inhaler or even a small, delicate oil dropper.

The curiosity for medicine began to brim around this time of my life and I started to discover the applications for all these wonderful remedies. I learnt that the liquids, capsules, aerosols and creams housed in Mr Patel's cabinets had magnificent efficacy for treating a host of conditions. The purified chemicals, blended into ointments or locked into precious capsules, that were so gratefully received by all of his patients, provided potent relief for their various complaints.

The spark that ignited my desire to practise medicine and join a revered profession dedicated to healing people first came to life in this little shop.

At medical school, I approached pharmacology, the study of drugs and their interactions with living systems, with wonder, recognising its critical role in patient care. The synthesis of pharmaceuticals and how they interact with the human ecosystem, affecting specific targets in the body, such as enzymes or receptors that could reduce symptoms and cure disease was fascinating.

However, as many medical practitioners have seen first-hand, these pharmaceuticals can also affect other systems within the body, sometimes leading to unforeseen side-effects and complications.

No matter how sophisticated the development of pharmaceuticals becomes, they are not without their drawbacks, and we cannot become reliant on them. For this reason, I believe it's essential to integrate holistic approaches that support the body's natural ability to thrive and maintain health.

Fast-forward 30 years and I'm now exploring the gut microbiota with the same wonder and marvel as that nine-year-old eavesdropping on conversations in a hybrid sweet shop/high street pharmacy.

And, as it turns out, there is a medicine cabinet living inside all of us.

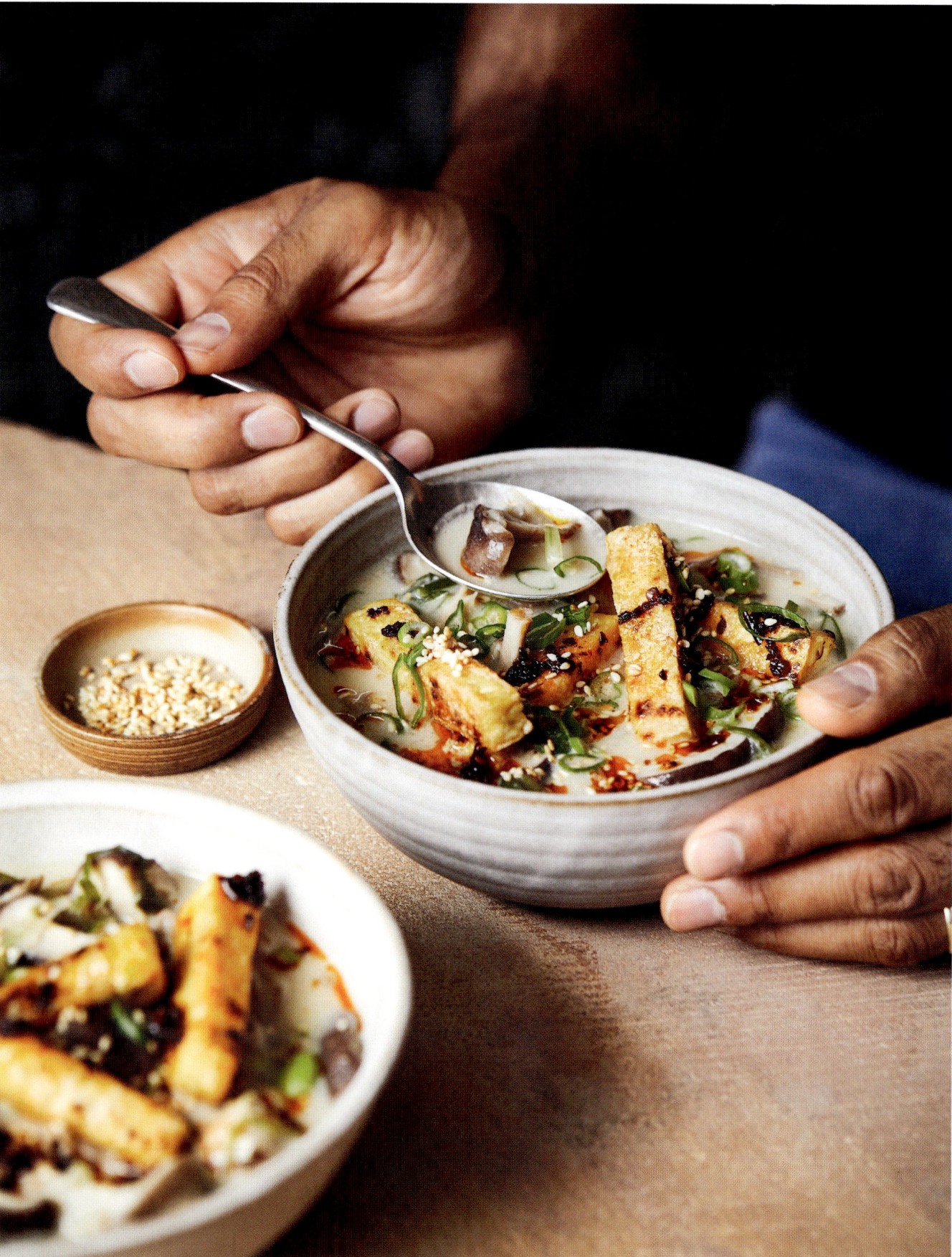

Your body already has the power

Trillions of microbes reside within us, predominantly inhabiting the large intestinal tract. They range from bacteria to fungi and even viruses, and are capable of producing chemicals with medicine-like effects.

A healthy microbe population can produce substances that act like antibiotics, which kill disease-causing microbes such as invading bacteria that could cause watery stools or inflammation in your gut. These microbes can also release chemicals that signal to your immune system to fight certain bugs and ignore others, like the chief in command of an army unit ensuring that friendlies are kept safe while the enemy is detected and neutralised.

Your microbes are even involved in increasing your dopamine levels. How you experience, or don't experience, pleasure is in part influenced by your microbes. They tweak and prod pathways in your brain to light up specific regions which help encourage you to bathe in those wonderful feelings of happiness, pleasure, enjoyment and comfort.

But, microbes are essentially foreigners inhabiting our digestive system. They have completely different DNA to our own and come in a variety of types including bacteria, viruses and fungi. This relationship has developed over millions of years as humans have adapted to different diets and environments. During this time, we have gradually become more reliant on our microbiota to perform tasks such as digestion and nutrient extraction.

These microbes perform critical roles for us, such as metabolising nutrients that our own bodies cannot process efficiently on their own, such as fibre, thereby extracting additional energy, vitamins and minerals from our diet.

Think of your body like a huge, sophisticated blue-chip company with thousands of employees. Over time, this business might choose to outsource routine functions like customer service, sales and accounting. These tasks, while essential, are delegated to external companies that can handle them more efficiently and cost-effectively. As a result, the corporation gradually loses the ability to manage these tasks internally due to its reliance on these specialised, outsourced services.

Using this analogy, we are the blue chip company and our microbes are the specialised, outsourced services. And these microbial external partners take on the critical yet 'dirty' work necessary for maintaining our foundational health. This is partly why our human genes don't encode proteins to digest fibre. We've developed a relationship with microbes to do this for us.

This co-evolution extends to our microbiota's ability to synthesise essential vitamins, influence metabolic pathways to keep our blood sugar levels in check and fight off infections. We have a deep evolutionary bond between us and our microbial partners and in essence, we all have a personal 'Mr Patel's' pharmacy inside of us all.

They're ready and willing to fetch the necessary tablets and tinctures required for a range of ailments and stocked with antidepressants, motility medications, constipation therapies, antibiotics, immune boosters, adaptogens and anti-inflammatories. You name it, your microbes have got it. It's no wonder that these microbes impact a vast number of functions such as appetite regulation, immune health, sugar metabolism and more.

Of course, I'm not suggesting that we don't need pharmaceuticals of any kind, but I want you to realise how much you already have. Conveniently housed in your own digestive tract, this inner medicine is within us all. Hence why a health-supporting recipe is one that extends beyond just protein and other macronutrients, to include a focus on helping our microbes do their critical work.

What are the benefits of a healthy gut?

Much like the importance of consuming sufficient protein, the tangible benefits of maintaining a healthy gut are extensive and pivotal for a strong, healthy body. A healthy gut can improve:

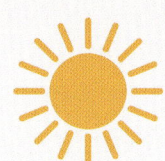

Mental health

Your gut microbes are capable of producing substances with antidepressant effects, sending signals to your brain to promote calmness. These chemicals relax the gut wall and communicate via the vagus nerve (a long, winding nerve that extends from your gut, past your diaphragm and heart, all the way to your brain) to reassure and relax your mind.

Appetite control

Microbes influence the production of appetite hormones, such as ghrelin (stimulating hunger) and leptin (signalling that you're full). Some metabolites that are released as a result of our microbes digesting fibre are called short-chain fatty acids (SCFAs). These metabolites release specific signals that communicate to our brain (via the gut–brain axis) that we're full. Keeping our microbes well fed could improve our intuitive sense of when we're full. This can reduce unnecessary cravings and improve weight control without the need to count calories or other rigid dieting practices.

Hormones

Poor gut health doesn't just manifest itself in uncomfortable symptoms such as bloating and indigestion. It can also exacerbate or cause hormone imbalances in the body leading to thyroid disease, worsening polycystic ovary syndrome (PCOS) symptoms, painful periods, premenstrual syndrome (PMS) and insulin resistance. There's emerging evidence that supporting your gut health could improve the management of these conditions. For example, a specific enzyme (beta-glucuronidase) produced by the gut microbes helps break down hormones, like oestrogen, for removal via stool and prevents excess accumulation in the body that can cause symptoms and worsen conditions.

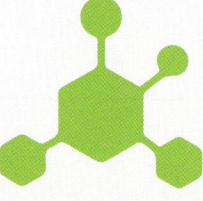

Heart health

The same SCFAs involved in appetite regulation may also have a role in controlling blood pressure and protecting us from coronary heart disease. Studies have shown that poor gut health has a role in vascular dysfunction that can lead to rises in blood pressure, as well as inflammation that leads to atherosclerosis (scarring and narrowing of the arteries). This gut–heart axis could yield novel approaches to heart disease prevention, and for now, using diet to create a healthy gut is a pragmatic tactic.

Skin health

Common skin disorders such as eczema, acne and even psoriasis could be better managed by improving the health of our guts. The 'gut–skin axis' refers to the relationship we have with gut microbes that help regulate inflammation and immune responses, which can affect skin health. Even symptoms such as skin dryness, wrinkles and pigmentation could be improved with a healthier gut microbe population.

Menopause

The diversity of gut microbiota often decreases during menopause, which can lead to weight gain and a higher risk of metabolic diseases such as type 2 diabetes, and heart disease. Because our gut microbes are so intertwined with various bodily systems, they play a significant role in menopause. The microbes' influence on oestrogen can also indirectly impact bone density, mood, insulin resistance and where fat is deposited in the body. A healthier microbe population, that could be improved with diet, could mitigate a variety of menopause-related symptoms.

As I'm sure you've gathered by now, optimal health goes beyond just maintaining energy balance, consuming enough protein and achieving a trim, toned physique.

It's essential that our dietary approaches honour the vital role played by our internal microbial community. Considering the extensive work they do to support our physical and mental wellbeing, it's crucial that we nurture them.

WE ALL HAVE A PERSONAL PHARMACY INSIDE US

THE 3 Ps OF SUPPORTING YOUR MICROBES

There's so much that can be said about strategies to improve your gut health. But, it's commonplace for people to become fixated on individual ingredients with the highest amount of probiotics, for example, or a vegetable that has a particularly high amount of gut microbe-loving fibre.

Instead, I like to keep it super simple.

Numerous ingredients can promote gut health, and by consistently incorporating these key elements into each meal, you will be effortlessly nurturing your beneficial microbes. I guarantee you'll reap the benefits if you can stick with these three core principles of eating for gut health that yield the greatest benefits and are woven into each recipe in this book. Prebiotics, polyphenols and plants.

1 Prebiotics

Prebiotics are specialised types of indigestible fibre that possess unique properties which bolster our microbial population and deliver significant health advantages.

Even small quantities, as little as 5g daily, can foster the proliferation of specific gut bacteria like bifidobacteria and lactobacilli, and the production of short-chain fatty acids (SCFAs) that enhance your health, as described on page 36.

If you're not used to including these types of foods in your diet, I always advise people to go super slow. Introduce small amounts of these ingredients and gradually increase the dose over weeks and months, not days. Your microbes have to develop the ability to break down these ingredients.

Imagine if you were new to pushing weights in the gym, you wouldn't confidently stride over to the squat racks and try and deadlift your own bodyweight. A reasonable approach would be to start slow, and gradually move up in intensity, allowing your muscles to develop strength and tolerance of increasing weight.

Using the same reasoning, start slow with your fibre content and gradually push up the dose that your microbes can tolerate. They're like our children. Give them time and they'll naturally grow in confidence to digest more fibre for their own good and, of course, ours.

The table opposite identifies ingredients with excellent amounts of prebiotic fibres, vital for nourishing the beneficial bacteria in your gut, but it's not an exclusive or exhaustive list. (For nutritional breakdowns using the latest data set, see Appendix on pages 276–279.)

Ingredients	Prebiotics (per 100g)
Jerusalem artichokes	21g
Garlic	19g
Common beans	15g
Leeks	12g
Onions	10g

Other prebiotic-rich foods to eat more of include:

- **Pulses:** black-eyed peas, red kidney beans, lentils, butter beans, chickpeas
- **Other fruit and veg:** asparagus, dandelion, green leaves, apples, bananas
- **Whole grains:** barley, rye, wheat bran, oats
- **Nuts and seeds:** almonds, flax and chia seeds
- **Special ingredients:** cacao, seaweed, jicama (Mexican turnip)

Please remember that variety is also super important. Every ingredient will contain a different profile of prebiotics, and you actually don't need much to reap the benefits. In fact, to get the recommended 5g of inulin prebiotics per day, you would need to eat … half a small onion.

The exact amounts of fibres can also vary based on ingredient maturity. For example, ripe versus unripe bananas can massively differ in their prebiotic fibre content, with the unripe banana having a lot more resistant starch (see page 41).

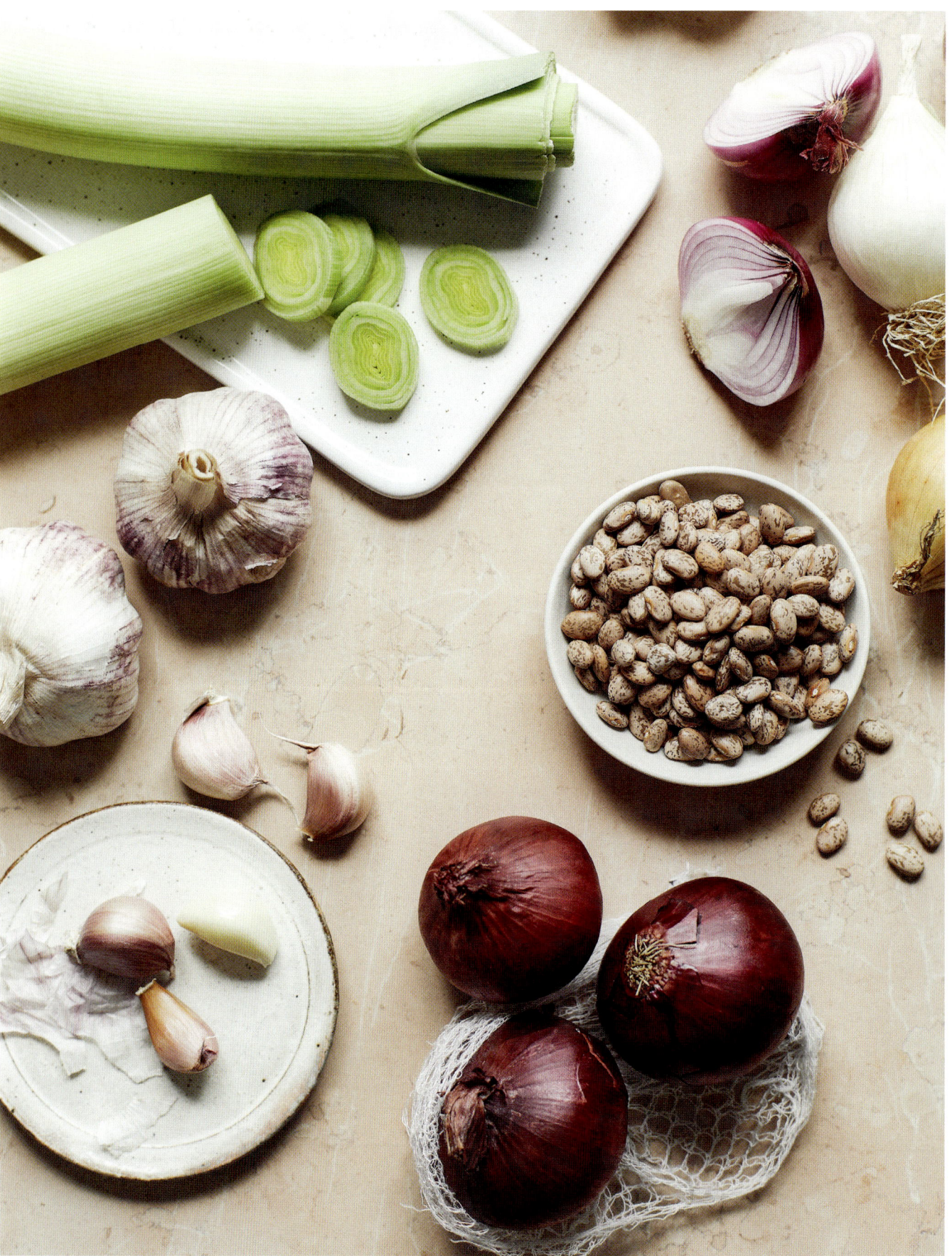

Prep makes a difference

Preparation method can also significantly affect an ingredient's prebiotic content, mainly due to the effects of heat, processing and the physical breakdown of the food's structure.

For example, cooking can reduce the resistant starch in foods like potatoes and bananas by making the starch more digestible. However, cooling these foods after cooking can increase their resistant starch content to a higher level than their raw state through a process known as retrogradation. Other starchy foods that benefit from this process include pasta (for salads), sushi rice and corn. So cold pasta, corn or potatoes, eaten in a salad the day after cooking, could boost your gut bugs more than when eaten freshly cooked!

The well-established technique of drying in the sun, which is present across many cuisines, can potentially better preserve the fibre content of foods than cooking. Drying fruits like berries and vegetables like beetroot maintains a high level of dietary fibres. Freezing also preserves fibres, but the defrosting process may lead to some loss of water-soluble components, so make sure you don't throw away that water when defrosting!

Fermenting, another technique of preserving food that has been present in human civilisation for millennia, can also increase the prebiotic content of your food. The bacteria, fungi or yeasts (depending on your method of fermenting) used break down the ingredients, often turn them into more potent prebiotics. Foods like sauerkraut, kimchi and kefir are good examples of where fermentation increases the availability of prebiotic fibres, as well as providing probiotics (see page 52).

Peels often contain much of the fibre in your food. Whether it's courgette, cucumber, squash or turnips, try and keep the skins on your ingredients to reap more of their microbe-supporting benefits. Just remember to give them a good scrub, especially if they're not organic.

Including these prebiotic-rich foods in your diet can help improve your overall digestive health and contribute to a healthier gut microbiome. You'll find them in recipes throughout this book.

2 Polyphenols

Polyphenols are diverse compounds found in fruits, vegetables, nuts and seeds that extend beyond the 22 vitamins and minerals that are typically used to characterise the nutrient value of food. These substances are not classified as essential, yet research highlights their critical role in enhancing health, and your gut microbes love them.

Polyphenols are a notable group of plant chemicals (also referred to as phytochemicals) that you'll predominantly find in colourful foods. But that's not to say that you won't find them in white and beige foods like grains, onions, mushrooms and cabbages.

In fact, polyphenols can be found in a range of foods and are most densely concentrated in herbs and spices like oregano, cloves and star anise, as well as nuts and seeds including walnuts, pumpkin and sesame seeds. They exert strong antioxidant and anti-inflammatory properties that safeguard cellular health and because they reach the large intestine intact, they help your gut microbes flourish.

Additionally, polyphenols can suppress harmful bacteria and support the growth of beneficial microbes which nurture the gut walls, leading to less gut inflammation and a healthier digestive system.

The charts on these pages show some of the ingredients with the highest quantity of polyphenols, expressed as milligrams of polyphenols per 100g. We have rounded these values, for the exact numbers please refer to the Appendix on page 278-9.

Vegetables	Polyphenol content (mg/100g)
Red Swiss chard leaves	>1300
Globe artichoke, heads	>1100
White Swiss chard leaves	830
Red cabbage	>450
Spinach	250
Red pepper	230
Brussels sprouts	220
Broccoli	200
Pak choy	190
Green pepper	180
Kale	180
Red beetroot	160

It's worth adding a gentle reminder not to judge vegetables by one characteristic alone. Even though some may appear low in polyphenols, they contain other plant chemicals with health benefits.

For example, Brussels sprouts and broccoli may not contain much in the way of polyphenols, but they have unique sulphur-containing phytochemicals called glucosinolates, which are responsible for the distinctive bitter flavour and super health benefits that we'll discuss in the inflammation section.

Some of the fruits and berries I use are very high in polyphenols, which is why fruits are so important in the diet and I regularly include them as part of my high-protein diversity bowls (see pages 142–167).

Fruits	Polyphenol content (mg/100g)
Prune	>1100
Black raspberry	980
Fig, dried	960
Blackcurrant	820
Blackberry	>560
Plum	>400
Strawberry	>280
Orange	280
Peach	>270

Spices, herbs and oils	Polyphenol content (mg/100g)
Clove	>1600
Ceylon cinnamon	9700
Caper	3600
Oregano, dried (wild marjoram)	>3100
Sage, dried	>2900
Rosemary, dried	>2500
Common thyme, dried	>1800
Star anise	>1800
Cacao, raw powder	>2000
Coffee	>200
Extra virgin olive oil	>50

Notable mentions for nuts, seeds and other products with high polyphenol counts include:

Nuts and seeds	Polyphenol content (mg/100g)
Chestnut	>2700
Walnuts	>1500
Flaxseeds, ground	>1500
Pistachios	>1400
Sunflower seeds	1400
Pecans	>1200
Hazelnuts	670
Peanuts	400
Almonds	>280
Brazil nuts	240
Cashew nuts	230
Pumpkin seeds	140

As well as polyphenols contributing to the complexity of flavours in food, which gives rise to them being so delicious, they're also thought to have benefits beyond supporting your microbes.

These range from being neuroprotective and anti-ageing to even having anti-diabetic effects by influencing the secretion of insulin and how the body processes sugar in the bloodstream. Including a rich diversity of polyphenols may also help reduce cholesterol and protect your heart from atherosclerosis (a process of scarring and narrowing of the arteries around the heart). So, load up on these ingredients.

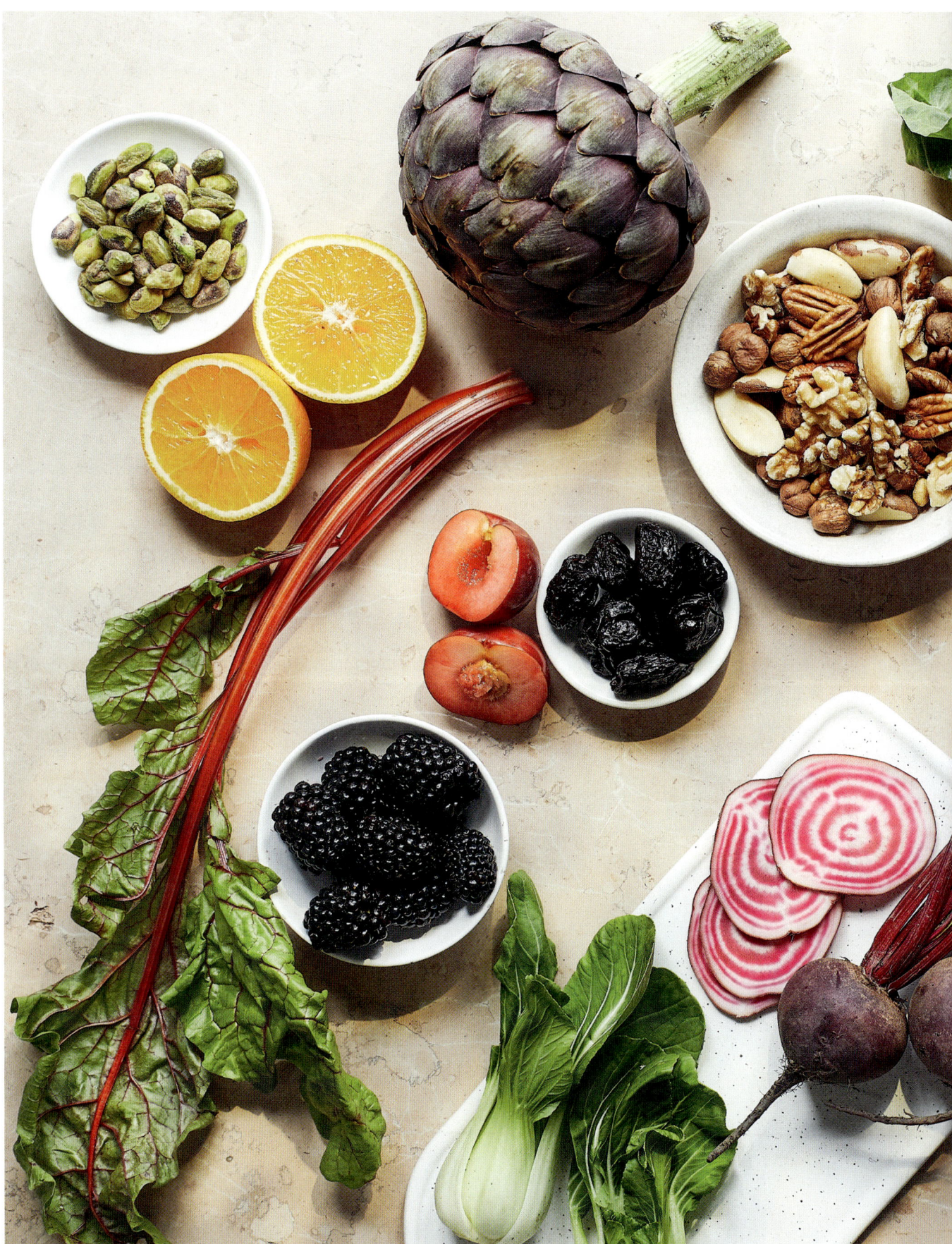

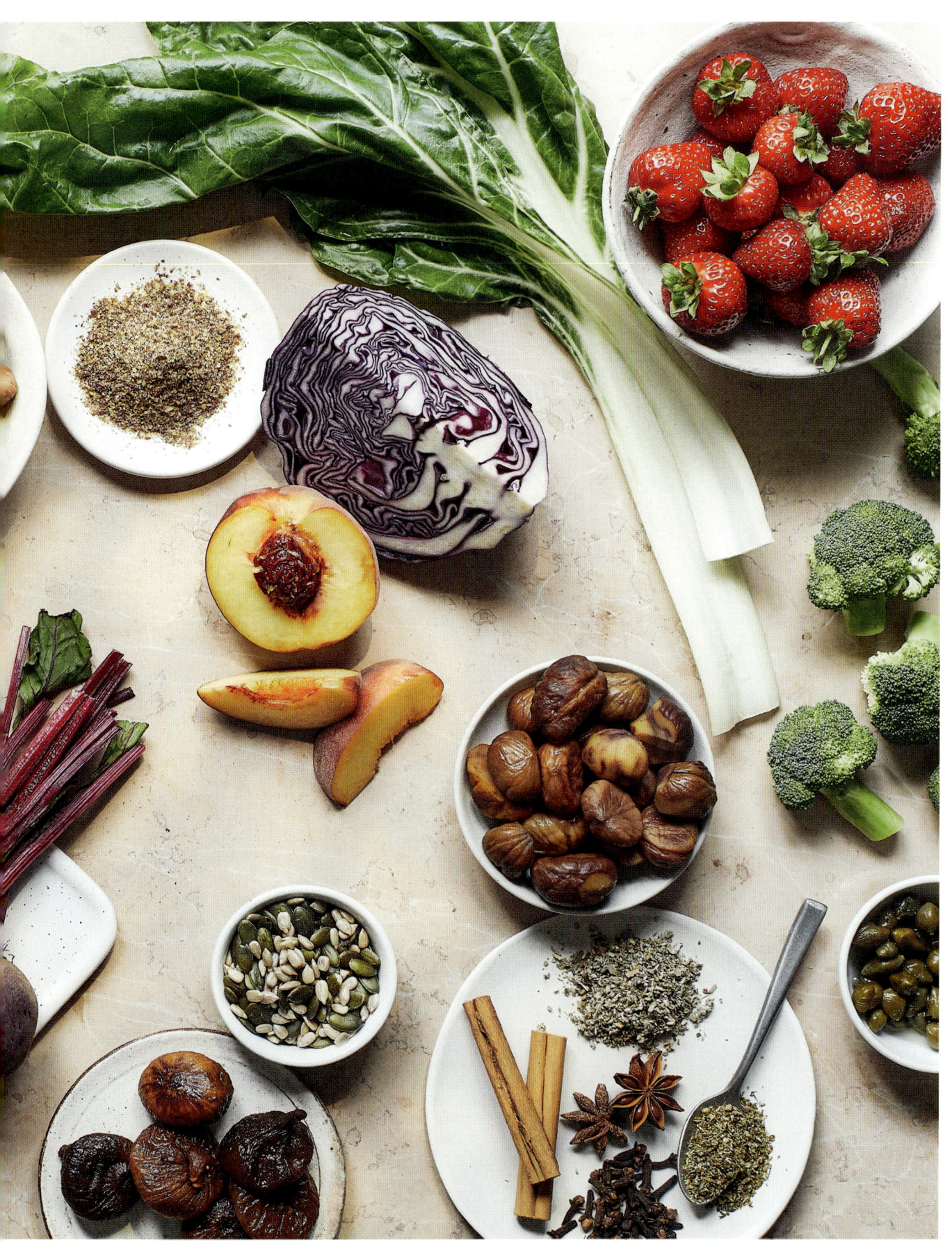

3 Plants

A plant-centric diet is a microbe-centric diet. Plants are what your microbes want, and having a variety of interesting polyphenol-rich ingredients in your diet will please them, as is reflected by the research we have available.

Diets that include a variety of plants, such as wholefood plant-based and Mediterranean diets, show positive impacts on gut health due to the synergistic effects of nutrients you find in whole fruits, vegetables, grains, nuts and seeds. These diets are linked with healthier gut microbiomes, reduced intestinal inflammation and overall improved health outcomes, which is why I'm such a fan of eating more plants.

We have to balance our excitement for plant-centric diets with a reasonable focus and attention on protein as well, but it shouldn't dampen your enthusiasm for putting plants first on your plates.

Increasing daily plant intake promotes the growth of beneficial bacteria and studies have shown that enhancing wholefood plant consumption can significantly boost both the diversity and function of your gut microbiota. Foods such as nuts and seeds are rich in bioactive compounds and, when combined with other fibre- and nutrient-dense foods, such as beans, greens and berries, they further enhance the function of your gut microbes.

Research consistently shows that higher intakes of these plants correlate with better health outcomes. This relationship is also characterised by a 'dose-response' effect, which means the more of these foods you eat, the greater the health benefits. This is a signal that they're genuinely having a positive impact on your health.

In fact, within just a few days of adding more plants to your diet, studies have shown a rapid shift in the microbe populations measured in the gut.

Within 48 hours of starting to eat a Mediterranean-style diet, researchers have found significant changes in the gut microbiota that have even led to reductions in blood cholesterol. Research underscores how quick and responsive your bugs are to dietary changes and the potential health impact you can have with your fork at each meal.

Studies suggest that consuming up to 800g of fruits and vegetables per day (equivalent to ten portions) is optimal for maximising health protection. This is why I try and get at least three portions of vegetables per serving at each mealtime. My recipes will show you how to do this.

In addition to plant quantity, plant diversity is also important. Studies have demonstrated that consuming more than 30 different plants per week, promotes beneficial gut microbe diversity that could lead to significant reductions in disease risk. Plant points are a practical measure encouraging diverse plant consumption to optimise your gut health. Each plant point represents a unique plant type consumed and the aim is to collect as many points as possible per meal. Look out for plant points on each recipe.

While the recipes in this book are primarily plant-based, they'll also emphasise the other important attributes of high protein content and lowering inflammation, making them well-rounded, health-promoting meals.

I also still believe that the ideal human diet does incorporate animal products, but more as occasional indulgences rather than everyday essentials. Consequently, this book includes some recipes that feature high-quality fish and poultry, reflecting their use as luxury items rather than dietary mainstays.

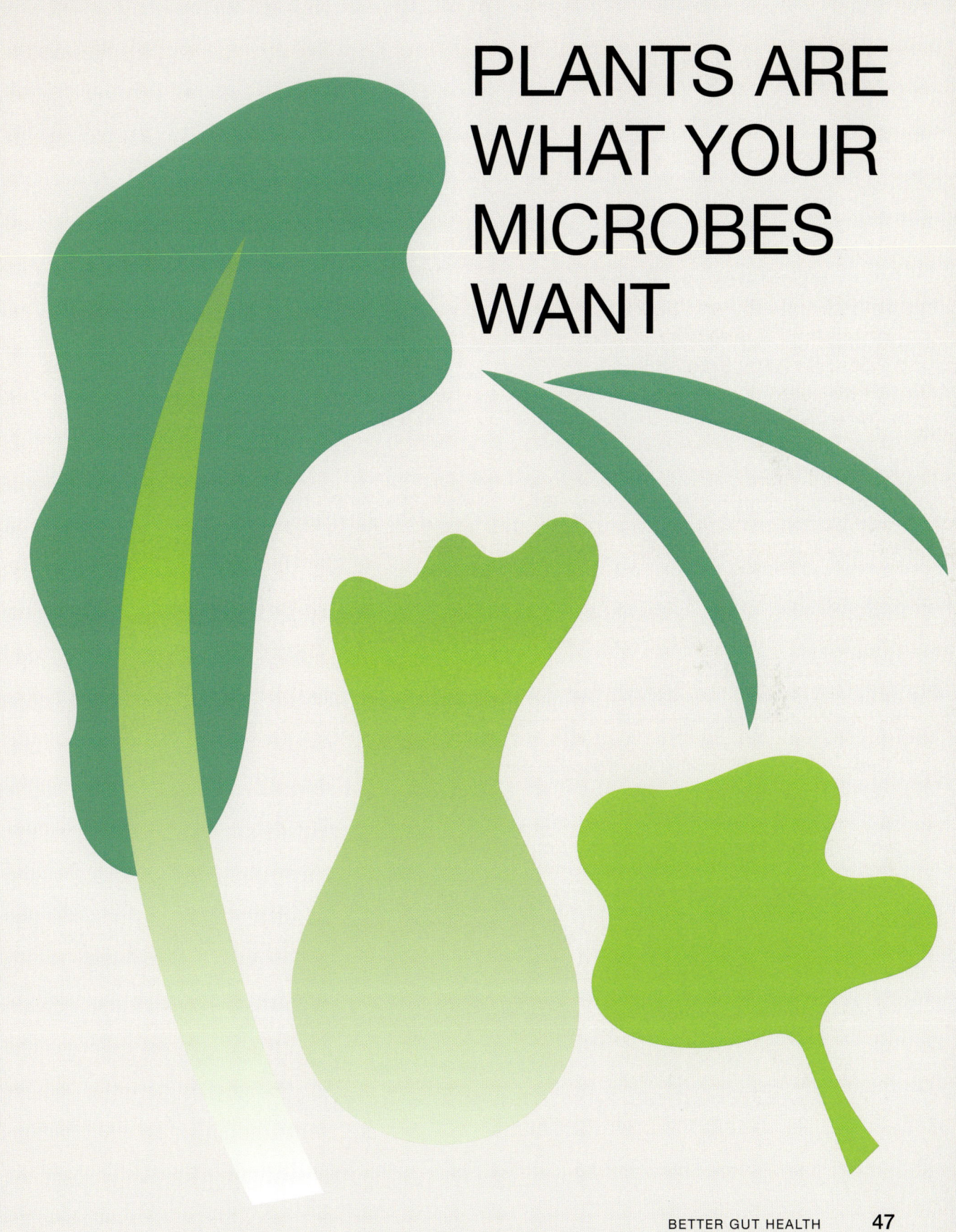

PLANTS ARE WHAT YOUR MICROBES WANT

BETTER GUT HEALTH 47

What if my gut is leaky?

Every time you eat, your digestive process kicks in. From the moment you mash the food in your mouth with your teeth, you expose more surface area to the enzymes in your mouth and stomach that can begin to break down the food into smaller components for absorption.

Past the stomach and along the intestines, it's then combined with various salts and emulsifiers from your gallbladder and delivered to the microbes along your digestive tract. Your food will soon become a collection of the very basic building blocks of sugars, fats and proteins plus the many other byproducts of microbe metabolism.

These building blocks then need to be absorbed into your body by passing through the very thin gut wall lining. On the otherside of the lining, they're transported around the body via the bloodstream to where they can be utilised.

Technically, this will be the first time your food transitions from being external to your body (in the digestive tract) to internal (in your bloodstream). Essentially, your food is perceived as a 'foreigner' by your body, and is consequently treated with a high degree of suspicion.

Just like your skin barrier has to be ready and waiting for any cuts or opportune pathogens trying to invade your body, your intestinal barrier (comprised of mucus, immune defences and a thin layer of gut cells) is similarly primed for any foreign invaders, friendly gut microbes or products of digestion that shouldn't be there.

The nutrients from food are squeezed into tight junctions between your gut cells in the intestinal barrier and absorbed in the bloodstream for use in the body. In essence, your gut *should* be 'leaky', or at least permeable to nutrients, but not so leaky that it causes issues.

There is a balance to be struck here.

On the one hand we want a normal state of leakiness to absorb food, but it should be tight enough to prevent microbes and larger particles from escaping the digestive tract and seeping into the bloodstream.

This entire process of allowing nutrients in, but keeping bugs out, is all taking place under the watchful eye of your immune system. They are ready and waiting to kick into gear if anything that shouldn't be there tries to get in.

If the leakiness of your gut was increased (formally described as 'intestinal hyperpermeability' in the academic literature), your immune cells are quickly going to trigger a response. Naturally, they'll start to recruit more immune cells to the areas of hyperpermeability, generating inflammation that can spill over and cause damage to the digestive tract.

If microbes and their components breach the walls of your intestines, they can trigger a heightened response from your immune system. A classic character called lipopolysaccharide (also known as LPS), which is a component of bacterial walls, is something that turbo-charges your immune system causing even more deleterious effects.

Numerous studies have linked higher amounts of LPS in the bloodstream with chronic inflammation that can manifest in a constellation of vague symptoms, such as brain fog and abdominal

What are the symptoms of leaky gut?

discomfort, as well as autoimmune conditions, colitis and skin allergies.

Your intestinal barrier is a mighty powerful defence force. It's capable of secreting a whole arsenal of defences including antibiotic-like chemicals, inflammatory proteins and even chemical signals that increase the motility of your gut, speeding along the transit of products through the digestive system to be rapidly expelled.

Why might you need such a heavy-handed immune response in your gut, I hear you ask?

Well, think back to a time in your youth (or adulthood) when you misjudged the cleanliness of a restaurant and carelessly ordered an item that you later regretted.

Your gut would have kicked into action to minimise the infective potential of that dodgy kebab by spraying the contents with as many antimicrobial chemicals as it could produce to neutralise any bacteria. Your immune cells would have doused them with fiery inflammatory products to kill them off and signalled to your gut to move them along as quickly as possible.

Any time you get a stomach bug or food poisoning, despite the bloating, pain, indigestion and disastrous aftermath, think of it as an evolutionary masterpiece designed to protect you from a hostile world.

If your gut is hyperpermeable or 'excessively leaky' the symptoms are vast and vague ranging from bloating, cramps, fatigue and low mood to skin complaints, sensitivity to multiple foods, headaches and excessive gas.

But more worryingly, this increased gut permeability is linked to heart disease, cancers and autoimmune conditions. Whether or not the permeability is in part causing or at least worsening those conditions is yet to be determined, but a worrying trend is emerging.

It's hard to diagnose leaky gut because the symptoms are so vague, plus there are no validated clinical diagnostic tests.

And quite commonly, as I'm sure many of you are doing right now, people will recognise one or more of these vague symptoms and start identifying as leaky gut sufferers. Duly they will head straight to Google where an abundance of blogs, protocols and transformation stories await them.

With this newfound knowledge, they'll begin to self-assess and head down the path of DIY fixes that invariably involve restricting multiple foods and, if they can afford it, food sensitivity testing.

Commonly this can lead to persistent restrictions on multiple ingredients, food anxiety (which is definitely not great for your gut health) and ultimately a very limited diet that your microbes won't enjoy.

So, tread carefully in this area.

BETTER GUT HEALTH

How do I prevent or treat a leaky gut?

First, I think it's important to reiterate here that your gut is very resilient, and just like a rugged pair of denim jeans, your gut barrier is designed to be worn. When people hear the term 'leaky gut', it gives the false impression that our digestive tracts are easily damaged and weathered. It's quite the opposite. This robust perimeter is constantly exposed to microbes, inflammatory proteins, debris, toxins and noxious chemicals. Like a well-seasoned fishing boat with a hardy skipper, you can throw a lot at it. In fact, it's lined with stem cells, specialised cells that can regenerate into multiple types of cells and quickly replenish damaged ones in need of repair.

It's also important to note that while dietary factors may be able to reverse excessive intestinal leakiness and mucosal damage, it's yet to be definitively proven that rectifying a leaky gut can fix the conditions associated with it, such as inflammatory bowel disease (Crohn's disease and colitis), irritable bowel syndrome (IBS), food intolerances and other functional gut disorders.

A pragmatic approach would be to at least maintain good gut health by encouraging a diet that supports gut intestinal barrier integrity and lessens the likelihood of excessive 'leakiness'.

Things in your diet that could increase leakiness or permeability include:

Ultra-processed food

Common ingredients in ultra-processed foods (UPFs) such as polysorbate 80, emulsifiers and gums can all disrupt the balance of your intestinal barrier. This can lead to more permeability, a heightened immune response and the inflammation that ensues. Remove UPFs from your diet as much as possible.

High-fat diets

High-fat diets, specifically diets high in saturated fat and trans fats (from fatty cuts of meats, deep-fried foods and processed meats), are linked with increasing intestinal permeability by inflaming the gut lining.

Alcohol

Even in small amounts, this unfortunately is a major culprit of poor digestive health for a lot of people.

Sugar

An increase in blood sugar has been shown to reduce the integrity of the intestinal barrier. High-sugar diets may be related to worsening leaky gut, but this is yet to be proven in humans. For now, I would fastidiously limit added sugar in your diet.

Not having enough fibre

Our gut microbes love fibre and it encourages a healthy amount of mucus that provides a sort of cushion to the thin gut lining. A lack of fibre in the diet is linked to more leakiness.

However, it's not just food that can affect the leakiness of your gut. Certain conditions that can be genetic in origin or disease states can increase it. These include inflammatory bowel disease, intolerance to certain foods like gluten and even excessive exercise, can all increase permeability. Others include:

Poor sleep

Mice studies have shown that disrupting their circadian rhythm (the 24-hour sleep–wake cycle that governs all living cells) can cause disturbances in the gut that increase leakiness.

Stress

In a small study in which participants were threatened with public speaking or electric shocks, leading to rises in stress hormones such as cortisol, the psychological stress increased their intestinal permeability.

Drugs

Excessive use of drugs such as nonsteroidal anti-inflammatories like ibuprofen can also damage the gut wall, leading to symptoms and even worse side-effects such as gastric bleeding.

Speak to a nutrition expert

Aside from supporting good gut health with prebiotics, polyphenols and plants, for treatment of 'leaky gut' symptoms, I always recommend consulting a nutrition professional.

An expert can responsibly guide you through a treatment protocol that involves recording symptoms and sometimes careful removal of specific foods, reassessing symptoms, reinoculation of the gut with specific nutrients and sometimes specific probiotics and gentle reintroduction of foods. This reintroduction is critical, and a practitioner can help you address which specific foods and what quantities to test your tolerance.

Sometimes this is referred to as Remove, Reassess, Reinoculate, Reintroduce and Repair. Or some other collection of words all starting with 'R'.

It's an ocean of information out there. Learn to swim with a professional before you confidently paddle out alone. If you can't tell the difference between foods with mannitol, fructan or sorbitol, don't try a solo protocol. It's worth the investment of working one on one with a health professional.

BETTER GUT HEALTH

Fortify with ferments and probiotics

With the increased interest in gut health comes the popularity of supplements and quick daily doses, designed to satisfy our desire for ultimate health despite our inherent laziness. Our yearning for a quick gut fix has ballooned into a multibillion-dollar probiotic industry built on pretty poor data.

I do believe that consuming the correct strain of microbes in adequate amounts could improve an individuals microbe community. However, we only have animal studies and some human trials that display weak effectiveness with nutraceuticals and probiotic supplements to treat gut symptoms or at least promote a healthy gut. Anecdotally, however, many people believe that probiotics have helped them restore balance at least symptomatically.

The proposition of taking a daily probiotic to rejuvenate the trillions of microbes that live in your digestive tract is an attractive one that holds a glimmer of promise.

However, very much like the friends you made during secondary school and university days, most of the microbes that reside within you are the ones you grew up with. These guys tend to stick around and are hard to displace.

Just as there has to be space in your social calendar for new friends, probiotics are like new buddies trying to fit into your already packed schedule. Unless they're super persistent, it's not going to happen.

Where I reserve judgment, however, is in the case of fermented foods. These are like the new friends that bring snacks to the party. We like these new friends.

These products, such as krauts, kimchi and fermented pickles, not only provide diverse microbial strains to introduce into your existing gut population, they also provide fibre. A 'packed lunch' for the microbial journey through the digestive tract if you will.

Prior to pasteurisation and sterilisation techniques used in modern food manufacturing (which on balance is a good thing for health), we wouldn't have struggled to get up close and cosy with microbes. Most of our food would have been teeming with bugs, both good and bad.

Other lesser-known probiotic foods from around the world include tempeh (Indonesia), tepache (Mexico), marula (South Africa), khalpi (Nepal) and gari (West Africa). In fact, all Indigenous cultures would have created a ferment of some sort as a method of preserving food and inadvertently improving their gut health.

Try to fortify your gut with the delicious ferments on pages 238–9 that you can make easily and far cheaper than storebought versions.

FAKE FERMENTS?

Several recent studies show that ferments have a positive impact on gut inflammation and microbial diversity. But with so many health claims on products these days, how do you tell a real ferment from a fake? Here are some pointers:

Fermented foods will be found in the refrigerated section only, not on the shelves.

Most fermented foods will say 'live and active cultures' on the ingredients label.

Brines and pickles are not fermented foods. If you see vinegar or acetic acid on the ingredients label, chances are it's not an active fermented food and any live microbes will have been neutralised by the acid.

Is it all in the diet?

With more available testing and at-home investigations (of which I'm a fan) more questions are being asked about how to improve and change our gut microbiome. But while the obvious answer might be what's on our plates, there's more to our microbes than just what we put into our stomachs.

It's simplistic to suggest that gut health is all about diet. In reality, the impact of poor sleep, lack of sunlight, long haul-travel, little exercise and high stress can all adversely affect your bugs. I've met many patients who have a wonderful diet, but their gut microbe tests tell a different picture. One that reflects a lack of mental self-care, rather than a shortage of Doctor's Kitchen meals.

Daily gut feel

An evidence-based strategy to support gut health has to be inclusive of all the elements that set the foundations for a strong gut community. For many of us, the hardest nut to crack is psychological stress. We can motivate ourselves to go to the gym, get ourselves tucked up in bed earlier, eat gut-supporting foods, but dealing with the complexity of the mind can be difficult. For that reason I encourage people to have a 'Daily Gut Feel', to mitigate the mental stress that hugely impacts the gut.

Take as little as 60 seconds every day to check in with yourself and ask three questions:

What is your gut telling you?

How's your mind?

What are you grateful for?

In addition, take a moment to breathe deeply as often as you can during the day. You will find the time to do this no matter how busy you are, I guarantee. In fact, I remember fitting this into my schedule while working full-time in A&E. In between patients, while washing my hands, I would focus on deep inhalation through my nose, pushing the diaphragm down and forcing my belly out, with corresponding slow exhalation through the mouth. Practise it regularly for the sake of your gut and microbes. I can hear you taking a deep breath now, great stuff!

Below is my ultra-simplified go-to list for gut health. Try it for 30 days and see if you feel the benefits. The specific 'doses' I've presented here match those found in the academic literature for health benefits. It's more than probable that the reason why these ingredients are so beneficial for our bodies, are because they're so beneficial for our bugs.

EVIDENCE-BASED DIETARY STRATEGIES TO IMPROVE GUT HEALTH

So you don't forget, my reminder for you is to hit your daily **BBGS**. Try and eat at least one daily serving of:

☐ **BEANS**
80g of tofu, black beans, chickpeas, lentils, etc (canned or from a jar is fine).

☐ **BERRIES**
80g of blackberries, blueberries, etc (frozen is fine).

☐ **GREENS**
80g of chard, kale, spinach, dandelion, etc (frozen is fine).

☐ **SEEDS AND NUTS**
30g of sesame, walnuts, pistachios, etc (just a handful).

LOWERING INFLAMMATION

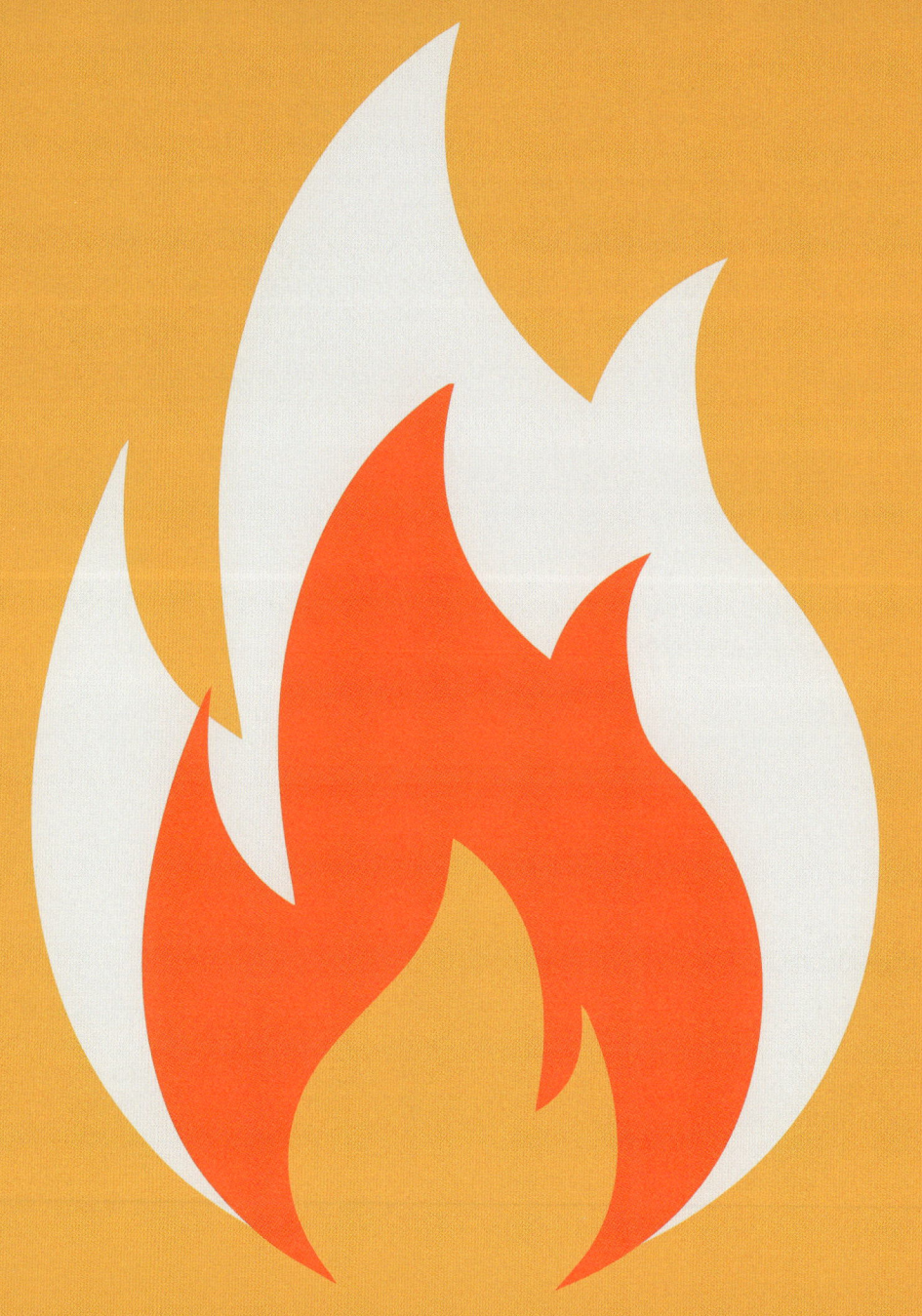

Imagine you're in the woods on holiday with a big group of friends and family. It's springtime, and the air in the early evening is cool. You've discovered a nice open area in the woodland to set up camp for the night. You pitch your tents, and you begin to build what every great camping holiday needs. A nice fire.

A campfire is a very special thing. It provides warmth in the cold canopy of the night, a beautiful glow to illuminate your site, a tool for cooking and even a deterrent to fend off any opportunistic predators and animals. But it also poses a risk.

If you don't keep an eye on your fire, it could quite easily get out of control. The fire presents an obvious burn hazard, it could create so much smoke you can't see or breathe, and if it were to get very unruly it could set your tent alight and burn down the entire site. Inflammation is like your internal campfire.

INFLAMMATION IS LIKE YOUR INTERNAL CAMPFIRE

On the one hand, controlled inflammation is a godsend. It's the tool that your immune system uses to protect you from invading pathogens. Your immune cells can identify and kill cancer cells that circulate your body every day, because inflammation is used as a signalling tool as well as a weapon of defence. Like the campfire, it's keeping you safe and protected.

Inflammation is quite simply remarkable, and one of the most important outcomes of our biological evolution that has enabled us to survive as a species. But the machinery that has facilitated our existence in a hostile world can become a hindrance in a developed modern environment.

A number of minor and seemingly insignificant stressors in our new world can accumulate into a smouldering cauldron of inflammation. These include stress, toxins in our environment, chronic infections, excess weight, loneliness and prolonged use of medications which can lead to countless symptoms.

Uncontrolled, persistent, low-grade inflammation, also referred to as 'meta-inflammation', can manifest as low mood, fatigue, pain and brain fog. This type of chronic inflammation 'simmering' away in the background is also in part related to many diseases of modern living including obesity, heart disease, cancer, dementia, even psychiatric and autoimmune conditions. Like a campfire out of control, the effects are far-ranging around the body and potentially catastrophic.

Food can be both pro- and anti-inflammatory. Using our analogy, it represents both lighter fuel for the campfire, as well as an extinguisher to tame it. It's a tool that we can use to regain control of chronic inflammation and bring this powerful and necessary process into balance.

But what actually is inflammation?

Inflammation is the language of your immune system.

It's a natural process that involves the release of specific proteins that can signal immune cells to respond to damage and assist in repair, and inflammatory proteins that can physically injure microbes and cells. We measure inflammation in the body by looking at specific markers in the blood.

Typically, inflammation is a *temporary*, protective response that helps in the coordination of a complex network of signals and organs that represent your immune system. An inflammatory response should be a short-lived process and resolve over hours, days or, at worst, weeks.

However, what we are witnessing in diseases of modernity is a persistent pro-inflammatory signal.

The inflammatory response can be obvious, such as a swollen and painful limb after a mosquito bite has punctured the skin and caused a severe infection that spreads. Or it can be subtle, at the cellular level, and without any obvious physical signs.

An excess of inflammatory proteins coursing through your bloodstream can damage artery walls causing them to gradually enlarge, which narrows the space for blood to flow through, and can culminate in heart attacks and heart disease. Excessive inflammation in the blood can also impair hormone function, such as insulin, which affects the efficiency of sugar transport from your bloodstream into muscle and liver cells for storage. This disruption can increase the risk of developing type 2 diabetes.

These conditions will also have other contributing factors, but the story of heart disease, cancer, metabolic diseases such as type 2 diabetes, and even mood disorders like depression, can all be told through the lens of inflammation imbalance. You can regard inflammation as the driving force behind many diseases of modern living. It also tends to increase with age, which in part can explain the increasing prevalence of conditions like heart disease, cancers and dementia the longer we live. You could argue that inflammation is the master regulator of ageing; the higher your inflammation, the faster you will age.

Remember, inflammation is absolutely necessary for life. Without it your immune system would not have the tools to fight infections, kill cancer cells and protect your body from toxins. We don't want to rid ourselves of inflammation completely, but the balance between driving inflammation and reducing it needs to be addressed. Luckily, there are things that we can do to mitigate the inevitability of excess inflammation.

REMEMBER, INFLAMMATION IS ABSOLUTELY NECESSARY FOR LIFE

INFLAMMATION-FIGHTING FOODS

Something that we utilise on my Doctor's Kitchen app is the Dietary Inflammation Index (DII), a research tool used to measure the inflammation potential of a person's diet.

Each wholefood has the potential to be pro- or anti-inflammatory, and researchers have developed a scoring system to rank each food according to its potential impact on inflammatory proteins such as interleukins, tumour necrosis factor-alpha and C-reactive protein that can be measured in the blood.

This system has been shown to link certain diets with illnesses that are influenced by inflammation. The higher the score, the worse the inflammation and the higher the risk of disease. Conversely, foods that have lower inflammation scores, as well as dietary patterns like the Mediterranean diet, which has an overall anti-inflammatory score, are associated with disease protection.

The more anti-inflammatory foods in your diet, the better protection you have from heart disease, strokes, dementia, mental health conditions, cancer and all the other diseases of ageing.

As a general rule of thumb, all wholefood plant-based ingredients tend to be anti-inflammatory. Whether it's a carrot, pea or a bean, they all seem to reduce inflammation in the body.

Ingredients that raise inflammation include fatty cuts of red meat and poultry, processed meats (like salami), excessive amounts of refined sugar and carbohydrates, ultra-processed foods (including plant-based faux meats) and deep-fried foods.

However, despite the inflammation potential of individual foods, there is evidence that combining certain foods that raise inflammation, like beef for example, with anti-inflammatory foods, such as greens, herbs and spices, can bring the net effect of inflammation into balance. This is important to remember. We should not judge individual foods on specific anti-inflammatory attributes, but rather consider the holistic perspective of our plates.

With this in mind, here are some foods you want to focus your diet around to reduce inflammation.

Berries

Blackcurrants, blueberries, strawberries, raspberries and blackberries all contain vitamins and fibre, as well as anti-inflammatory chemicals such as anthocyanins and flavanols. These are specific types of polyphenol, the chemical class we discussed in the previous section, that give foods their red, blue and purple colours.

Polyphenols have been shown to cross the blood-brain-barrier where they can potentially improve inflammation in the brain which could enhance cognitive health. Berries are some of the richest sources of these colourful plant chemicals which is why they're such potent antioxidants in the diet.

According to measures of anti-inflammatory activity, blackberry, blackcurrant and cranberry have some of the highest levels.

Eat them fresh or frozen, rather than in jams and juices where some of the compounds are removed, the fibre has been reduced and lots of sugar is added. Just a handful daily has been shown to reduce the risk of dementia and heart disease and even improve memory by boosting the health of your brain cells.

Interestingly they also contain anti-ageing compounds (also called senolytics), one of which, fisetin, has been studied extensively as a nutraceutical. The jury is still out on the benefits of supplementing with individual compounds, like fisetin, resveratrol and anthocyanins from berries. So, to ensure you don't miss out on the numerous other beneficial compounds, it's always better to consume berries whole rather than in a purified supplement.

Greens

Kale, Swiss chard, broccoli, rocket, watercress and Brussels sprouts are all rich in micronutrients and fibre. But the plant chemicals they contain are also powerfully anti-inflammatory which may explain why people who have just one daily serving of greens in their diet have a significantly slower rate of brain decline.

Flavonoids like quercetin, found in kale and spinach, are powerful antioxidants with strong anti-inflammatory effects. Glucosinolates in cruciferous vegetables break down into biologically active compounds that have been shown to have anti-inflammatory and detoxifying properties.

Go for darker vegetables that may have a higher density of these chemicals such as cavolo nero, and sprouted greens such as broccoli sprouts, which have higher amounts of glucosinolates.

Aim for at least a daily portion of cooked greens, and ideally I have a green side at lunch and dinner most days. Lesser known and used varieties of greens such as moringa, jute leaves, bitter greens, dandelion and nettle have equally promising attributes. These are novel foods that we should be cultivating (and eating) to increase the diversity of plant chemicals we can use to prevent inflammation.

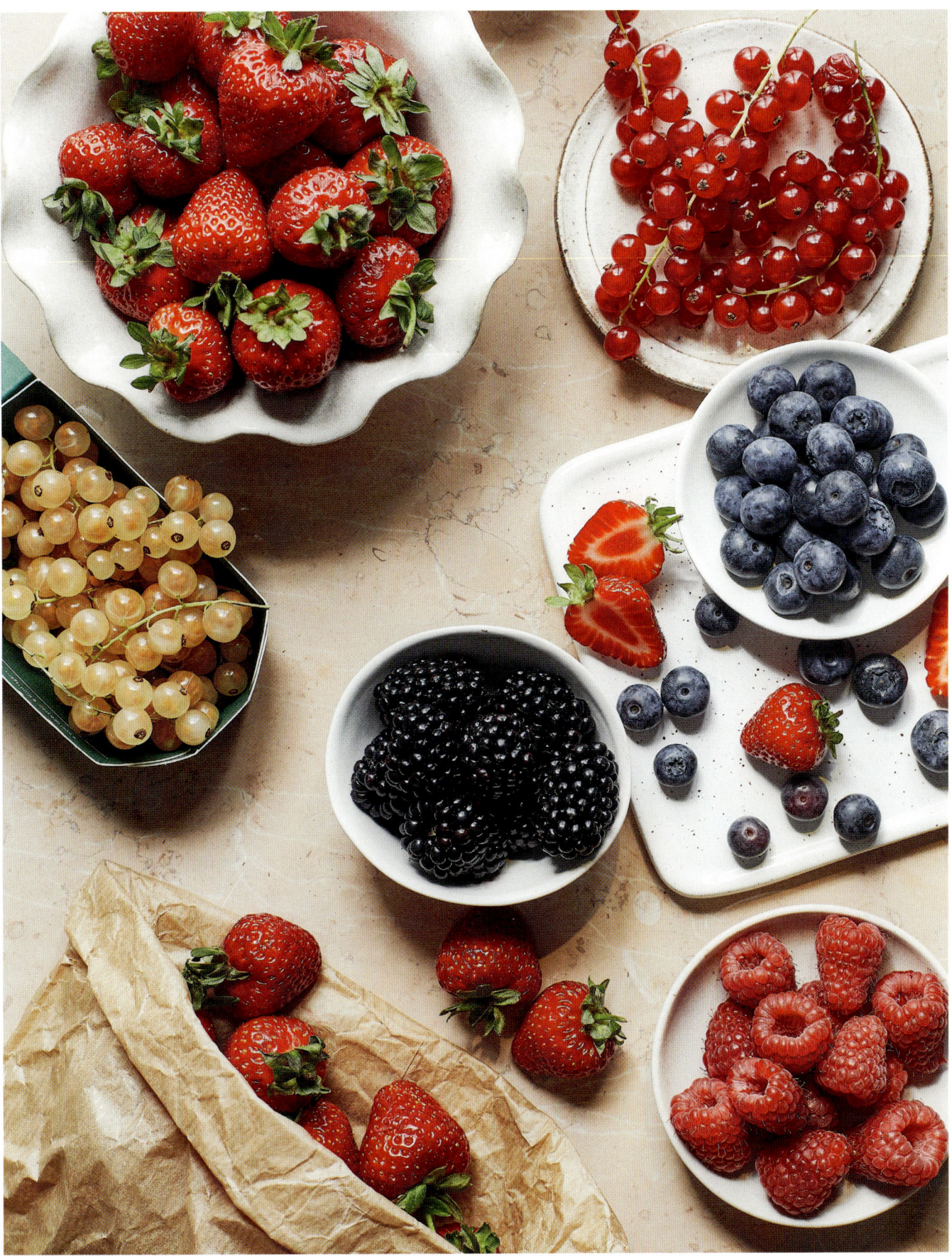

Nuts and seeds

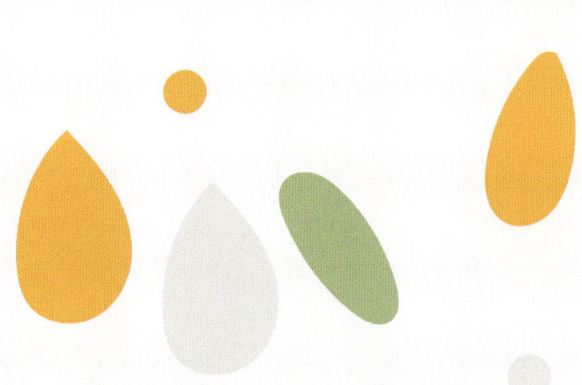

Walnuts, pine nuts, almonds, sunflower seeds and more are a treasure trove of anti-inflammatory and health-boosting nutrients.

Some are rich in omega-3 fatty acids and alpha-linoleic acid (or ALA), found concentrated in walnuts, chia, hemp, flax and pumpkin seeds. While these aren't as anti-inflammatory as long-chain omega-3s found in fish and algae, they still provide heart and cognitive health benefits by nourishing blood vessels and promoting the generation of brain cells.

As sources of omega-3 fatty acids, they also help produce a special type of fat-derived molecules called lipoxins. These are responsible for reducing the inflammation response after an injury or infection to promote rapid healing.

Nuts and seeds are also high in flavonoids. For example, walnuts contain ellagitannins, which can help fight inflammation, along with phytosterols that lower blood cholesterol. Additionally, they tend to be high in vitamin E, the anti-inflammatory micronutrient. In fact, just a 30g handful of sunflower seeds or almonds contains 50% of your daily requirements of vitamin E.

Nuts and seeds are also a natural source of arginine, an amino acid that can help alleviate inflammation. Walnuts, pumpkin, hemp and sesame seeds are some of the best sources of arginine, which the body converts to nitric oxide, a compound that improves blood flow and protects your heart.

There is some emerging evidence that nuts and seeds could also help with healthy ageing, metabolism and energy levels by boosting the production of nicotinamide adenine dinucleotide (NAD+). This plays a critical role in our mitochondria, the powerhouses of our cells. Peanuts, hemp, chia and sesame seeds are particularly rich in vitamin B3 (niacin), a precursor to NAD+, which may explain the potential impact on longevity.

To get the maximum benefits of nuts and seeds, soaking and sprouting them releases more of the proteins and phytonutrients. It also reduces certain antinutrients, which increases their digestibility. See page 29 for more about this.

Herbs and spices

Turmeric, clove, cinnamon and ginger are the four spices with the biggest anti-inflammatory potential according to various measures, including the Oxygen Radical Absorbance Capacity (ORAC) scoring system. They also appear to have the greatest impact on inflammatory proteins (such as cytokines), as well as the ability to reduce the activity of pro-inflammatory enzymes.

Interestingly, some well-known herbs are equally powerful, which may explain why they were prized by ancient Greek and Roman civilisations. These include oregano, rosemary, sage and thyme, all of which have very high ORAC scores and measure up against turmeric pretty well. For example, rosemary contains the unique bioactive compounds rosmarinic acid and carnosic acid, and human studies have shown a reduction in blood markers of inflammation when ingested as a wholefood supplement.

There is also a misconception that fresh is always better than dried, but this is not necessarily the case. In the example of ginger, what's interesting is that dried and fresh ginger contain different quantities of the same compounds. The main compounds in fresh ginger are gingerols, while dried (ground) ginger mainly contains shogaols – which are dehydrated products of gingerols. Mixing up both dried and fresh spices and herbs could be a worthwhile strategy to get a variety of the different beneficial plant compounds.

WORTH THE INVESTMENT

A word of advice: invest in your herbs and spices. Most supermarket own brands are of poor quality, so I tend to buy online and from independent stores that trace the origin of the products and do not radiate or heat-treat their spices and herbs. I also prefer to buy whole seeds (such as coriander or fennel seeds) and crush them myself to maximise their wonderful flavours as well as their precious healthy chemicals. I've recorded a spices masterclass on my YouTube channel with a spice expert on how you should taste raw spices to determine the quality yourself.

LOWERING INFLAMMATION

Oily fish

Sardines, mackerel, herrings, anchovies and salmon are higher in specific anti-inflammatory fats called long-chain omega-3 fatty acids, specifically eicosapentaenoic acid (EPA) and docosahexaenoic acid (DHA).

These EPA and DHA fats are precursors for a very special group of fat-derived molecules called specialised pro-resolving mediators, some of which include resolvins, protectins and maresins. These play a crucial role in resolving inflammation and cleaning up after the activity of your immune system.

Imagine your body is like a major European city and the immune system is the emergency services. After a car traffic incident on the motorway, the ambulance service arrives to treat any wounded victims, the police are present to keep order and secure the area, and the fire fighters are used to break into vehicles and release trapped passengers if needed. This is your immune system in action.

However, after the incident has resolved and the emergency services have left the scene, it's a bit of a mess. You need cleaners to remove any glass, clear the area of debris and fix any broken road signs. It's a very particular and specialised set of jobs and without them, the chaos caused by a traffic incident would continue to be felt by commuters.

These specialised pro-resolving mediators in your body manage the inevitable aftermath of inflammation and the activity of your immune system. They will ensure that the destructive potential of inflammation isn't unnecessarily prolonged which could contribute to low-grade meta-inflammation and the health consequences I described earlier. Consuming sufficient EPA and DHA from food or supplements such as fish oil and algae oil is important to support the functioning of this critical unit.

Olive oil

Another phenomenal product that I use liberally in both cooking and dressing is good-quality, high-polyphenol, extra-virgin olive oil. It's safe to cook with at low to medium temperatures, good producers will provide a harvest or production date, and it should be sourced from a single area instead of being blended from multiple countries.

It should taste grassy and peppery and produce a slight cough tickle when consumed. Depending on the source, you also can experience all sorts of wonderful tasting notes, including floral and fruity flavours.

Polyphenols like oleocanthal and oleuropein, monounsaturated fats like oleic acid and the high vitamin E content all contribute to the anti-inflammatory effect of extra-virgin olive oil. It's been shown to inhibit the activity of pro-inflammatory enzymes such as cyclooxygenase (COX), similar to the action of anti-inflammatory drugs like ibuprofen. It down-regulates genes involved in inflammation and even improves the function of arterial vessels by increasing the production of nitric oxide, which dampens inflammation. No wonder it's linked to better heart health and longevity, and higher intakes may be associated with a reduced risk of death related to dementia.

I invest in olive oil; it's expensive but worth the extra spend. An olive oil with these heart and brain health benefits should be lab tested to show more than 250mg of polyphenols per kilo of oil. This information can be found on the bottle or the manufacturer's website.

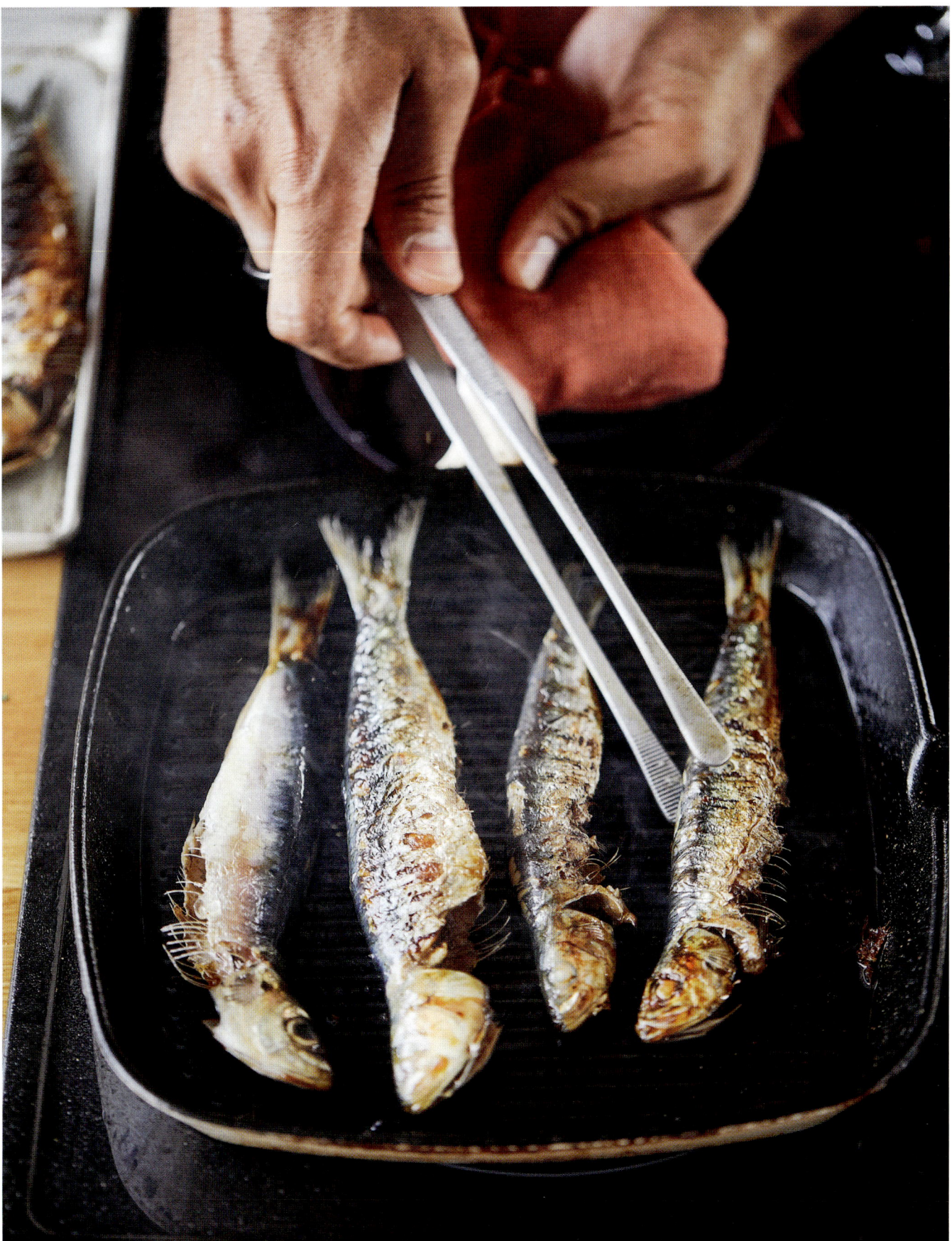

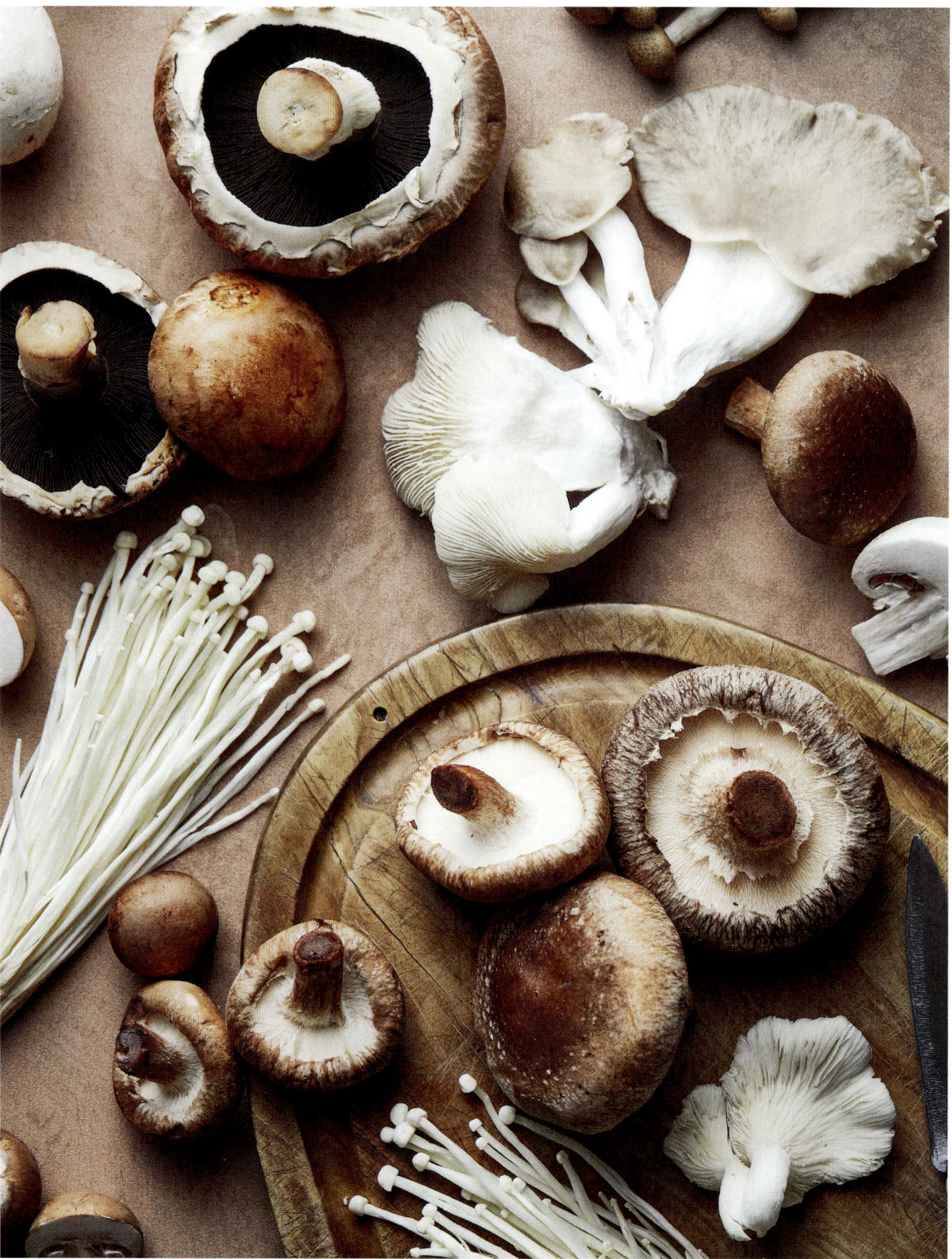

Special shout out for shrooms

Culinary mushrooms such as shiitake, button, field, portobello, enoki and oyster are marvellous ingredients that contain unique antioxidants and fibres that reduce inflammation.

Mushrooms are rich in polysaccharides, like beta-glucans, that act as prebiotics which your gut microbes love to feed on, plus plant chemicals called phenolics that possess strong antioxidant activity. In addition, triterpenoids unique to mushrooms reduce the activity of pro-inflammatory enzymes such as cyclooxygenase (COX) and lipoxygenase (LOX).

Simultaneously, mushrooms can enhance the effectiveness of your immune response by boosting cells such as natural killer cells and macrophages, while reducing pro-inflammatory proteins. This paradoxical double act seems to create a more balanced immune response, which is why medicinal mushrooms (reishi, chaga, turkey tail and lion's mane) have a long history of use in traditional Chinese medicine. More recently, they have also been used to fight cancer, in combination with conventional therapies, by stimulating the immune system to recognise and attack cancer cells, but more trials are needed to demonstrate how effective this strategy might be.

A WORD OF WARNING

However, a word of warning to heed the excitement around mushrooms, particularly in the wellness arena. I caution people using medicinal mushrooms erroneously in drinks and especially mushroom blends in all sorts of products, such as energy balls, protein shakes, cookies and so on. They should not be consumed in this way. People should educate themselves on the specific uses of medicinal mushrooms and whether the mushrooms are appropriate for their needs before consuming them regularly. You wouldn't combine a random concoction of pharmaceuticals into a drink and swig that with your overnight oats every morning. And in the same way, we need to treat these medicinal mushrooms with more respect.

Is inflammation all in the diet?

Inflammation can present itself in numerous ways in response to our lifestyle, environmental exposures, and even our thoughts. Furthermore, these simple and accessible activities can help restore your body's inflammation balance and promote health:

Reduce stress

Psychological stress can manifest as inflammation in the body in ways that involve hormones and your immune system. Whether it's danger from a potentially fatal situation, your annoying colleague at work loading your to-do list or seeing something that angers you while scrolling social media, your body perceives stress in the same way.

These very different scenarios produce identical stress hormones from the hypothalamus and pituitary gland in your brain and your adrenals, which are located on your kidneys. Your body doesn't differentiate between these stressors. It's important to remind yourself of this when you find yourself getting stressed over something minor in the grand scheme of life.

During the stress responses there is a double act between two key hormones:

Cortisol, the primary stress hormone, actually has anti-inflammatory actions when it's released in the short term. It suppresses your immune system, which inhibits the production of pro-inflammatory molecules. However, persistent and chronic elevations of cortisol from stress can over-suppress your immune system and lead to cells becoming less responsive or 'resistant' to cortisol which diminishes its anti-inflammatory effect.

DHEA (dehydroepiandrosterone) is a precursor to the sex hormones oestrogen and testosterone. DHEA counters the effects of cortisol and also has an anti-inflammatory role. Again, in the context of persistently high levels of cortisol, DHEA levels are suppressed which can lower sex hormone levels and the overall effect of this scenario is excessive inflammation and a poorly functioning immune system.

Having strategies to reduce everyday stress is critical to manage physical inflammation. Whether that's reframing practices, meditation or simply not listening to the news first thing in the morning, a daily dose of stress relief is an important antidote to modern life. Find out what your stressors are and ruthlessly build environments and develop strategies to mitigate them for the sake of your health.

THE BIGGEST DOSE OF ANTI-INFLAMMATORY MEDICINE YOU CAN TAKE EVERY DAY IS EXERCISE

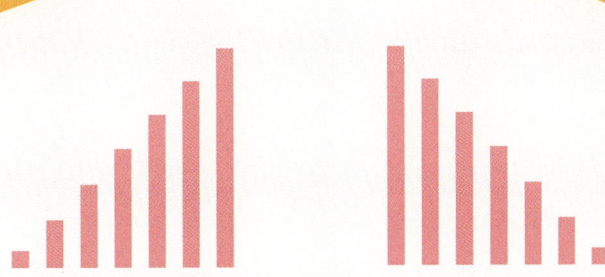

Exercise

The biggest dose of anti-inflammatory medicine you can take every day is exercise.

This might seem surprising, because during exercise your cortisol levels rise, your blood pressure soars and you create micro tears in your muscles that, when viewed under a microscope, will clearly display a mountain of inflammation.

Exercise itself is pro-inflammatory, but the consistent practice of it will encourage your body to become resilient and thus the net effect of exercise will be anti-inflammatory.

Movement boosts brain cell health, improves the function of your blood vessels, increases the resilience and strength of your muscles and boosts your mitochondria, which improves your energy. It also lowers your cortisol levels and helps release endocannabinoids that improve your mood.

From an inflammation perspective, myokines in your muscle cells are released when exercising. These are key proteins that enter the bloodstream and 'train' your immune cells, like macrophages, to calm and relax which ultimately reduces inflammation. Exercise can also burn up excess fat that produces inflammatory proteins, which again serves to rebalance the inflammation in your body.

In addition to dancing, walking, cycling, strength training, high-intensity interval training (HIIT), or whatever your daily exercise is, make sure you're not sitting for extended periods during the day. Our muscles thrive on regular use, and excessive periods of stillness (apart from during sleep) can build inflammation in your body. Micro stretching, walking meetings and standing desks are things that I do to increase my daily movement for those anti-inflammatory benefits.

Fasting

Whether you're doing it intentionally or not, everyone fasts. Fasting is simply the period of time when you're not eating. Some of us eat until late at night and have breakfast first thing in the morning, in which case our 'fasting window' is short. A longer fasting window is simply finishing dinner earlier and pushing back breakfast into mid-morning or sometimes all the way to lunch.

I do this because extending your fasting window may have anti-inflammatory benefits. Fasting can suppress something called the inflammasome, a component of our immune system that triggers a cascade of inflammation responses. Fasting also encourages fat cells to release adiponectins, which have been shown to reduce inflammation within the walls of heart vessels.

However, because it's so hard to measure the biological effects of fasting in individuals, it's impossible for me to tell you whether 10 or 18 hours of fasting per day is best. Nevertheless, as a general rule of thumb, I think everyone could benefit from a fasting window of at least 12 hours. Practically, this could mean having your last meal at 7pm and not having breakfast until at least 7am.

In addition, you don't necessarily need to fast to achieve some of these anti-inflammatory benefits. You can mimic these effects by simply eating less food, skipping meals every so often, plus dietary strategies such as 5:2 (eating normally for five days in the week, and very low calories for two). Choose the tool most convenient for you.

EVIDENCE-BASED DAILY DIETARY STRATEGIES TO LOWER INFLAMMATION

This is my super-simplified list of daily dietary-based interventions to control inflammation. Try ticking one off at a time until all four become habitual.

SPICE IT UP
Add a spice or herb of choice at each meal.

USE OLIVE OIL
Use good-quality extra-virgin olive oil daily to cook or dress your food with.

ANTI-INFLAMMATORY DRINKS
Enjoy a daily anti-inflammatory drink (see pages 270–1).

CHOOSE WHEN TO EAT
Define your eating window to a maximum of 12 hours every day.

A diet geared for health needs to be protein-sufficient, gut-health supporting and anti-inflammatory. Luckily, it's straightforward to cater for these three core pillars. These recipes will show you how delicious and easy it can be, as well as providing ideas for snacks and simple, flavourful, additions to your meals.

Your personal kitchen pharmacy is where, in my opinion, the enjoyable, fun and achievable journey to health starts. So let's get cooking!

Each recipe will have the values for protein, fibre and plant points **PER SERVING**.

- Protein in grams
- Fibre in grams
- Number of Plant Points

In addition, each recipe will show you how to **boost your protein if you wanted more.**

PROTEIN BOOST

Make sure to look out for unique QR codes on each recipe. Scan them to check out a library of similar meals on The Doctor's Kitchen that the code will take you to.

BREAK-FAST

&
BRUNCH

The Doctor's Daily Bread

PISTACHIO, CURRANT AND LINSEED BREAD

Prep 10 minutes, plus soaking
Cook 1 hour 15 minutes

Makes 12 slices

- 3 tbsp olive oil, plus extra for greasing (or you can use butter or coconut oil)
- 20g whole chia seeds
- 35g psyllium husks (powdered)
- 150g jumbo rolled oats
- 50g brown linseeds
- 50g currants
- 100g pistachio nuts
- 100g pumpkin seeds
- 1½ tsp salt

I'm using the same technique as 'life-changing bread', a bread recipe online that I've been obsessed with since 2016 and one that I regularly make for my wife who is gluten free. It's high protein, high fibre and a staple in my freezer. I serve this as a savoury option, toasted, with ricotta, lemon, black pepper and a drizzle of oil, or as an indulgent sweet snack, again toasted, with nut butter, fresh berries and a tiny drizzle of raw honey.

Grease a 900g loaf tin with olive oil, butter or coconut oil.

Combine all the dry ingredients in a mixing bowl and give it a good stir with a wooden spoon. Pour in the olive oil and 400ml water. Give it a good mix, adding a splash of water if needed – it should be thick and slightly sticky in texture.

Spoon the mixture into the loaf tin, pressing it down into the corners of the tin with the back of a spoon or the flat of your hand. The mixture shouldn't stick to your fingers. Leave the mixture to rest in the tin for about 30 minutes. You can leave it in the fridge overnight if you wish.

Preheat the oven to 170°C fan.

Bake the loaf for 1 hour until firm and starting to colour. Carefully remove the tin from the oven, tip the loaf out onto a wooden chopping board, then place the loaf directly on the oven rack. Bake for another 15 minutes to cook through. It should have a nice golden crust on the outside.

Leave the loaf to cool completely before slicing, then store in an airtight container in the fridge or pre-sliced in the freezer. I always toast the bread before using it.

Note
If you prefer this without currants, replace with an extra 50g linseeds or pumpkin seeds. Some people find it easier to line the loaf tin with baking paper, so it's easier to take the loaf out. I just make sure the tin is well greased.

Protein 8.6g | Fibre 8.3g | Plant Points 6.5

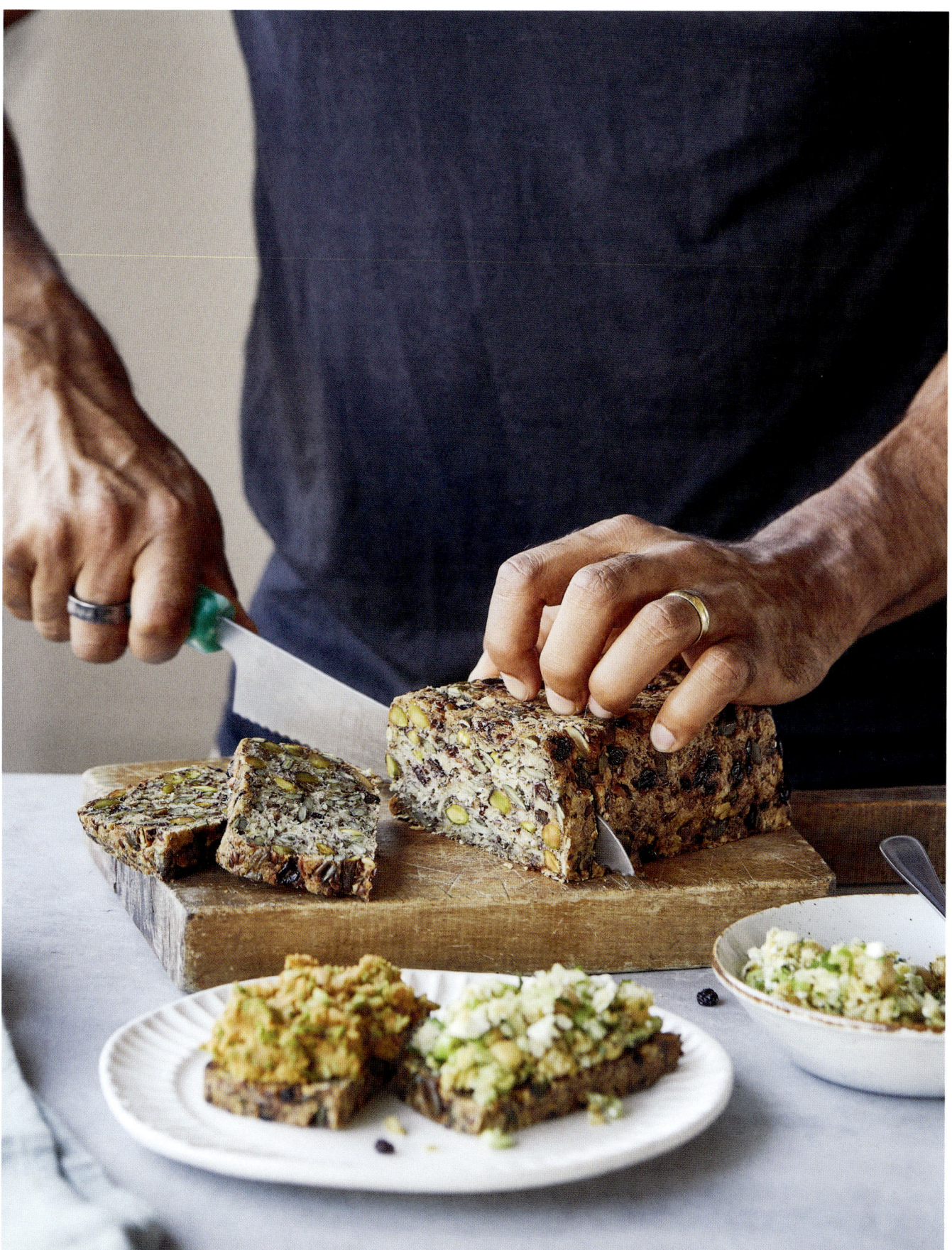

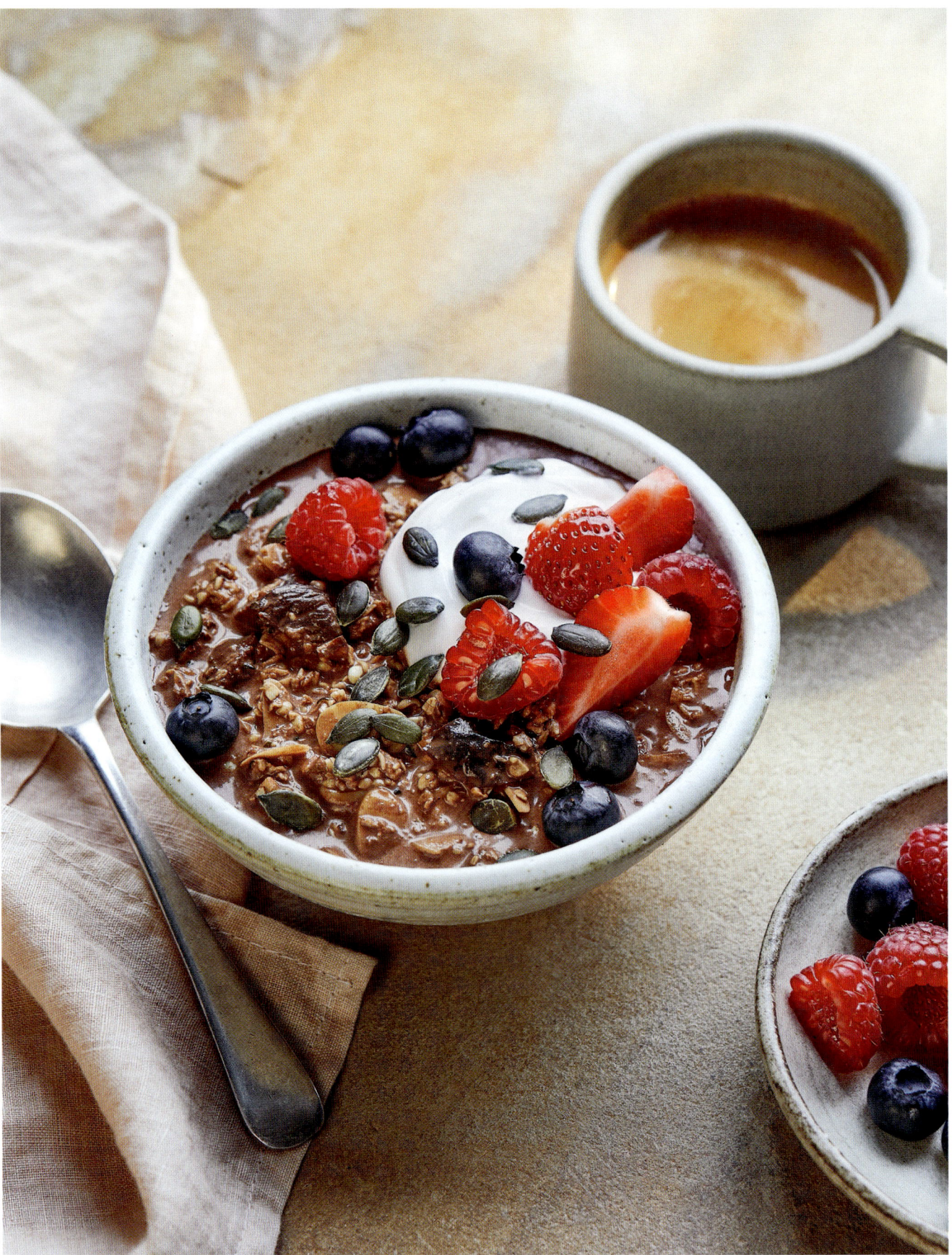

Overnight Protein Porridge with Cinnamon, Turmeric and Cacao

Prep 5 minutes, plus soaking overnight

Serves 1

30g shelled hemp seeds
20g jumbo rolled oats
20g cacao powder
½ tsp ground cinnamon
¼ tsp ground turmeric
15g flaked almonds
15g walnuts, crumbled
10g desiccated coconut
100ml whole milk or plant-based alternative
2 prunes, roughly chopped

To serve
80g mixed berries
20g pumpkin seeds or nut butter of choice
1 tbsp thick natural yoghurt

I pack my overnight oats with two key anti-inflammatory spices, cinnamon and turmeric. Soaking increases the digestibility of the oats and the cacao and hemp seeds provide a nice dose of protein. To add even more protein, you could use an unflavoured protein powder or even collagen, but I prefer to boost it with a healthy dose of pumpkin seeds or crunchy peanut butter. Have fun with this one. You can make a few jars at a time and they'll keep nicely in the fridge for a high-fibre, high-protein grab-and-go breakfast. A dollop of natural yoghurt or kefir is a beautiful contrast to the rich chocolatey-ness.

Add all the dry ingredients together to a large glass jar. Screw the lid on and shake vigorously to mix all the components together.

Remove the lid and stir in the milk, 50ml water and the prunes. Replace the lid and place in the fridge overnight.

In the morning, add a splash more milk if needed, and serve topped with the berries, pumpkin seeds or nut butter and yoghurt.

PROTEIN BOOST
Add more cacao powder, nut butter. You can also use an unflavoured protein powder.

Protein 36g
Fibre 13.1g
Plant Points 9.5

Avocado Lentil Cakes with Smoked Salmon and Kimchi

Prep 5 minutes
Cook 5 minutes

Serves 2

2 tbsp sesame seeds
4 lentil cakes (corn, rice or wholewheat crackers will also work well here)
1 avocado, halved, stone removed and thinly sliced
100g kimchi
150g smoked salmon
80g sprouted lentils
1 tbsp toasted sesame oil

I used to roll my eyes at these basic corn cakes. They initially reminded me of my mum's old weight-loss catalogues. But for a 'no frills, no fuss' midweek morning situation … they're actually amazing. Sub out the kimchi for a milder fermented food like sauerkraut or pickled cucumber if you're not a fan of the spice levels, but these go so well with the smoked salmon! You're getting three portions of vegetables in this dish plus over 20g protein per person. A fantastic start to the day.

Toast the sesame seeds in a dry pan over a medium heat for 1 minute until you can smell their aroma.

Build each lentil cake, starting with avocado slices, followed by the kimchi, smoked salmon and sprouted lentils.

Drizzle the lentil cakes with the toasted sesame oil and top with the toasted sesame seeds.

PROTEIN BOOST

Add more salmon or sprouted lentils. Some lentil cakes have more protein in them too, look out for those in shops.

Protein 26.9g
Fibre 8.1g
Plant Points 5.25

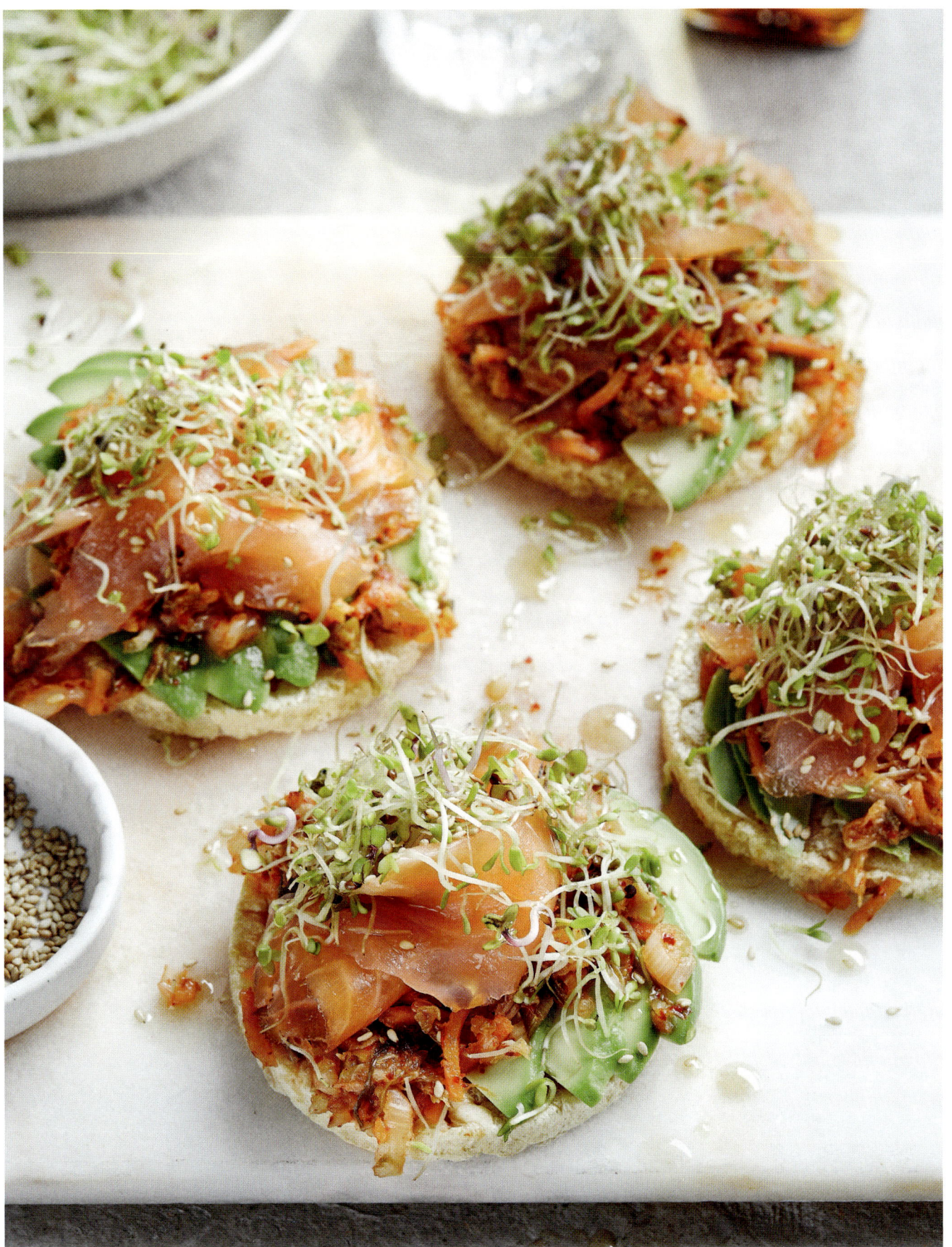

Crispy Chickpeas on Green Toast

Prep 5 minutes
Cook 25 minutes

Serves 2

- 1 x 400g can chickpeas, drained and rinsed
- 1 tbsp za'atar, plus extra to serve
- 1 tbsp olive oil
- 150g peas (fresh or defrosted from frozen)
- 4 tbsp tahini
- 2 tbsp nutritional yeast
- Zest and juice of 1 lemon
- 4 slices of spelt sourdough (or regular), toasted
- 10g parsley, finely chopped
- 20g pea shoots, roughly chopped (optional)

You get a double legume hit with this easy breakfast recipe, that counts as your beans, greens and seeds for the day. Tahini is a wonderfully rich source of calcium and protein, that will keep you satiated and nourished. This is a glorious combination that works exceptionally well to change up beans on toast. Any soft herbs will work and the za'atar gives herbaceous, spicy flavour to the chickpeas.

Preheat the oven to 200°C fan and line a baking tray with baking paper.

Spread out the chickpeas onto the lined baking tray and dry thoroughly with kitchen paper. Add the za'atar, olive oil and some seasoning. Mix thoroughly with your hands and bake for 20 minutes until crispy.

Meanwhile, blend the peas, 2 tablespoons of the tahini, the nutritional yeast, lemon juice, a pinch of salt and a splash of hot water in a bullet blender into a smooth green paste. Add more water if needed to help it blend properly.

Spread onto the toasted sourdough, top with the crispy chickpeas, remaining tahini, a sprinkle of za'atar and the lemon zest and finish with the chopped parsley and pea shoots, if using.

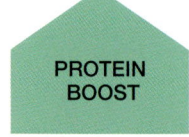

PROTEIN BOOST

Add more nutritional yeast, tahini or chickpeas.

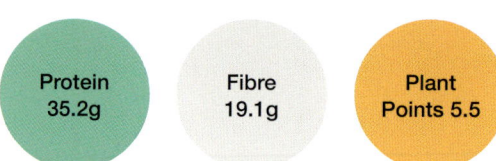

Protein 35.2g
Fibre 19.1g
Plant Points 5.5

BREAKFAST & BRUNCH

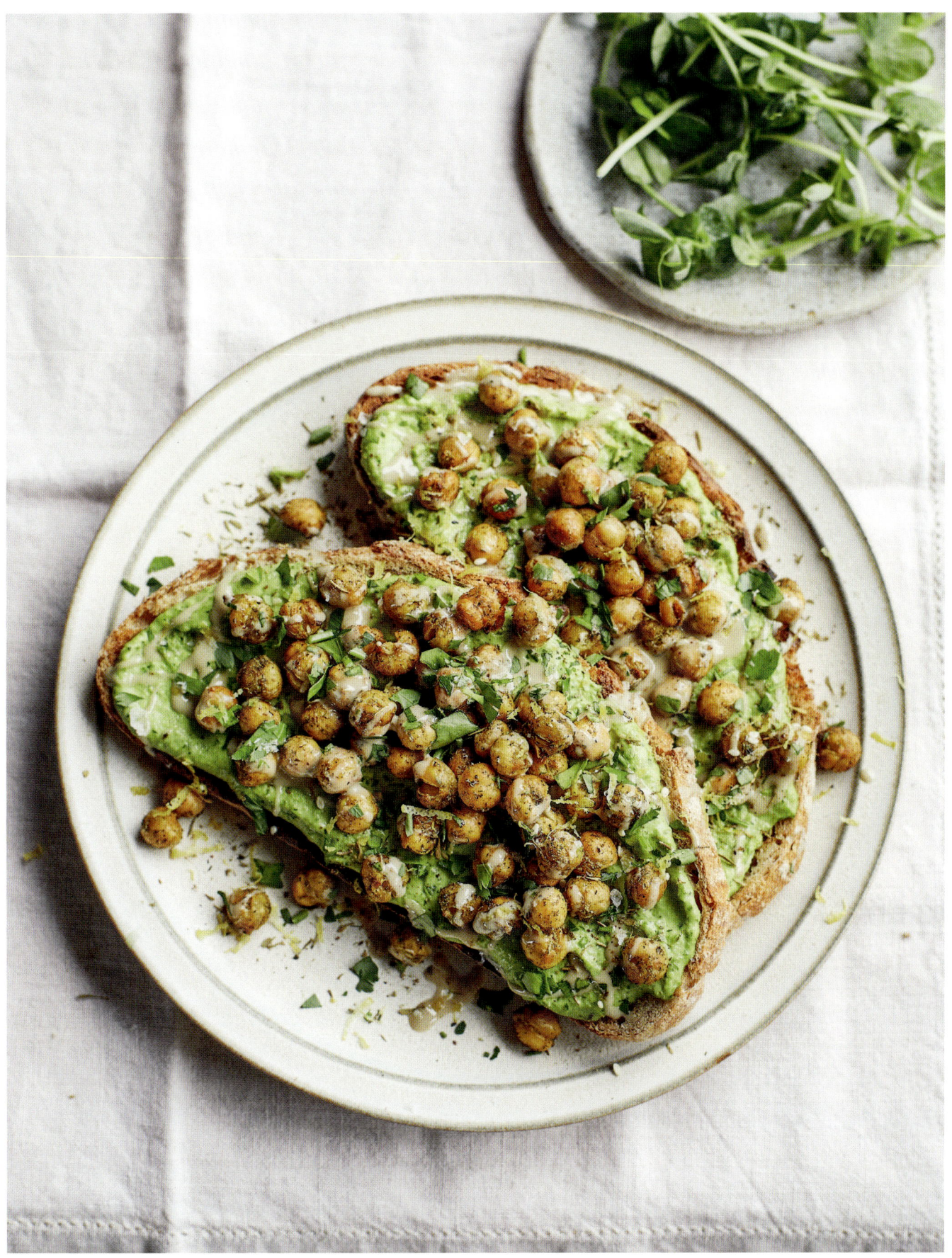

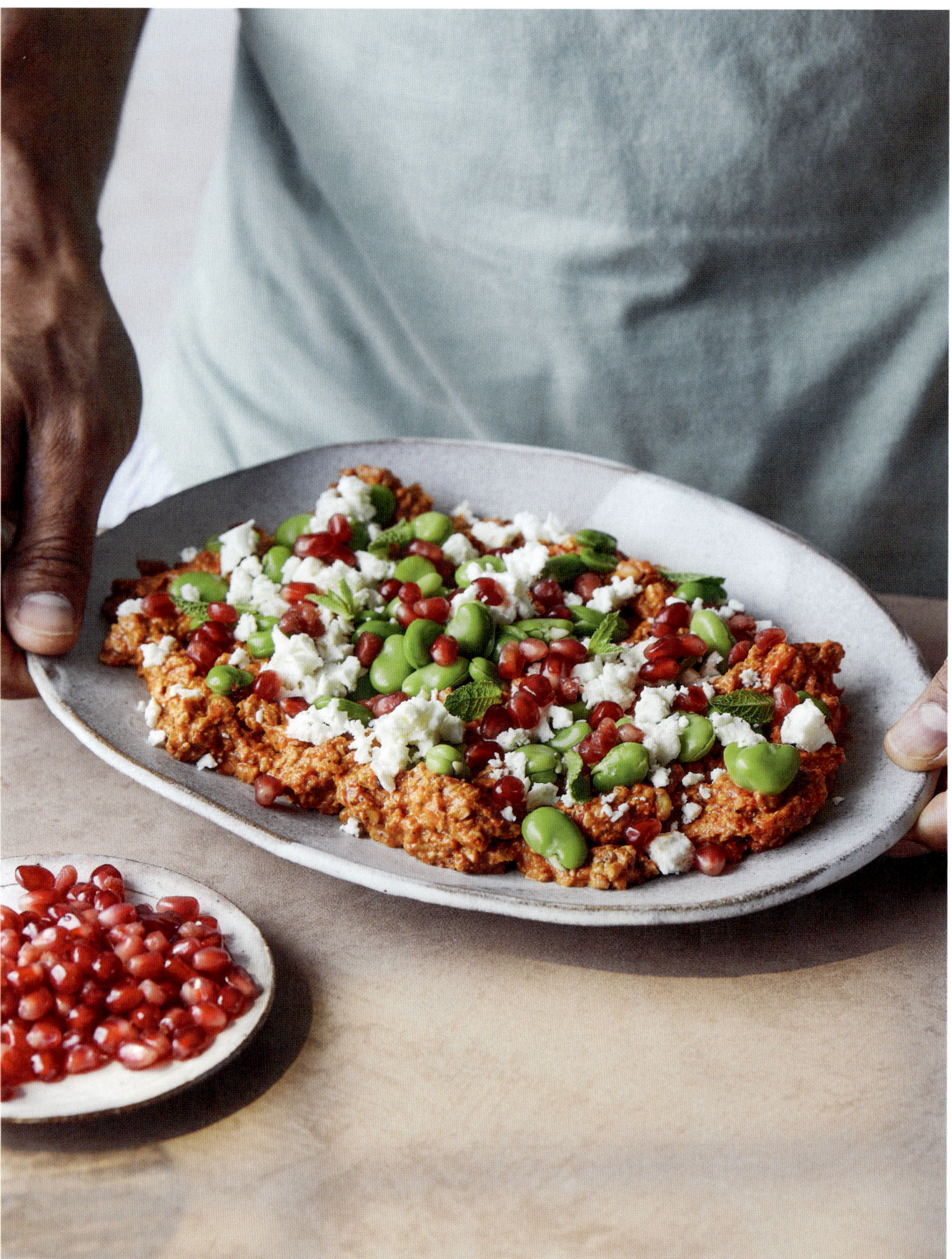

Feta, Red Pepper and Pomegranate

Prep 5 minutes
Cook 10 minutes

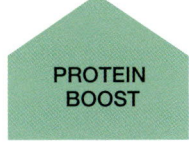

Serves 2

100g walnuts, roughly chopped
200g red peppers from a jar, drained
2 tsp cumin seeds, lightly toasted and crushed
2 tbsp olive oil, plus extra to serve
25ml just boiled water
½ tsp sea salt
1 tsp sumac
Juice of 1 lemon
1 garlic clove, grated
150g fava beans, cooked
100g feta
2 sprigs of mint
30g pomegranate seeds
2 tbsp pomegranate molasses (optional)

Based loosely on a muhammara paste, this nutty, tart and sweet base is a great pairing for the salty feta, fibre-rich beans and pop of fresh mint. The walnuts are surprisingly high in protein as well as those anti-inflammatory phytonutrients that many nuts contain, plus they deliver a lovely texture to contrast the smooth fava beans. Perfect for a different kind of brunch at the weekend but you can also batch this to prep ahead for the week. It all comes together seamlessly!

Blend the walnuts, red peppers, cumin seeds, olive oil, hot water, salt, sumac, lemon juice and garlic in a high-speed food processor until a rough red paste is formed. Add some more hot water if needed to loosen the mixture. You may need to scrape down the sides of the food processor a few times.

If you're using fava beans from a can, drain the liquid and warm them gently in a saucepan over a medium heat.

Slather the red paste onto a platter, and build up your platter with the warm beans, feta, mint, pomegranate seeds and pomegranate molasses, if using. Finish with a drizzle of olive oil to serve.

PROTEIN BOOST

Add more feta, fava beans or walnuts. Use cooked chickpeas instead of fava if you prefer.

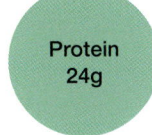 Protein 24g

Fibre 8.7g

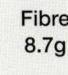 Plant Points 5.5

BREAKFAST & BRUNCH

Miso Beans on Toasted Rye

Prep 5 minutes
Cook 10 minutes

Serves 2

1 x 400g can white beans
160g edamame beans
1 tbsp white miso paste
1 tsp smoked paprika
2–3 slices of rye bread, toasted
2 tbsp olive oil

While rummaging through my fridge and cupboards, I came up with this slightly out of the ordinary combination of beans, edamame and miso. The umami flavour pairs wonderfully with the rye bread and a smoky hint of paprika rounds out the sweet edamame too. It's a combination that boosts your protein and fibre and delivers on those anti-inflammatory benefits with the edamame.

Add the white beans with their liquid to a small lidded saucepan over a medium heat and bring to a gentle simmer. Add the edamame beans, miso paste and smoked paprika and gently stir into the mixture. Cover with the lid and gently heat for 5 minutes until piping hot.

Drizzle the rye bread toast with olive oil. Spoon the beans on top of the toast, season with freshly ground black pepper and serve.

PROTEIN BOOST

Some crumbled sautéed tempeh would work well with this or a hard- or soft-boiled egg served on top.

Protein 20.8g
Fibre 15.2g
Plant Points 4.5

82 BREAKFAST & BRUNCH

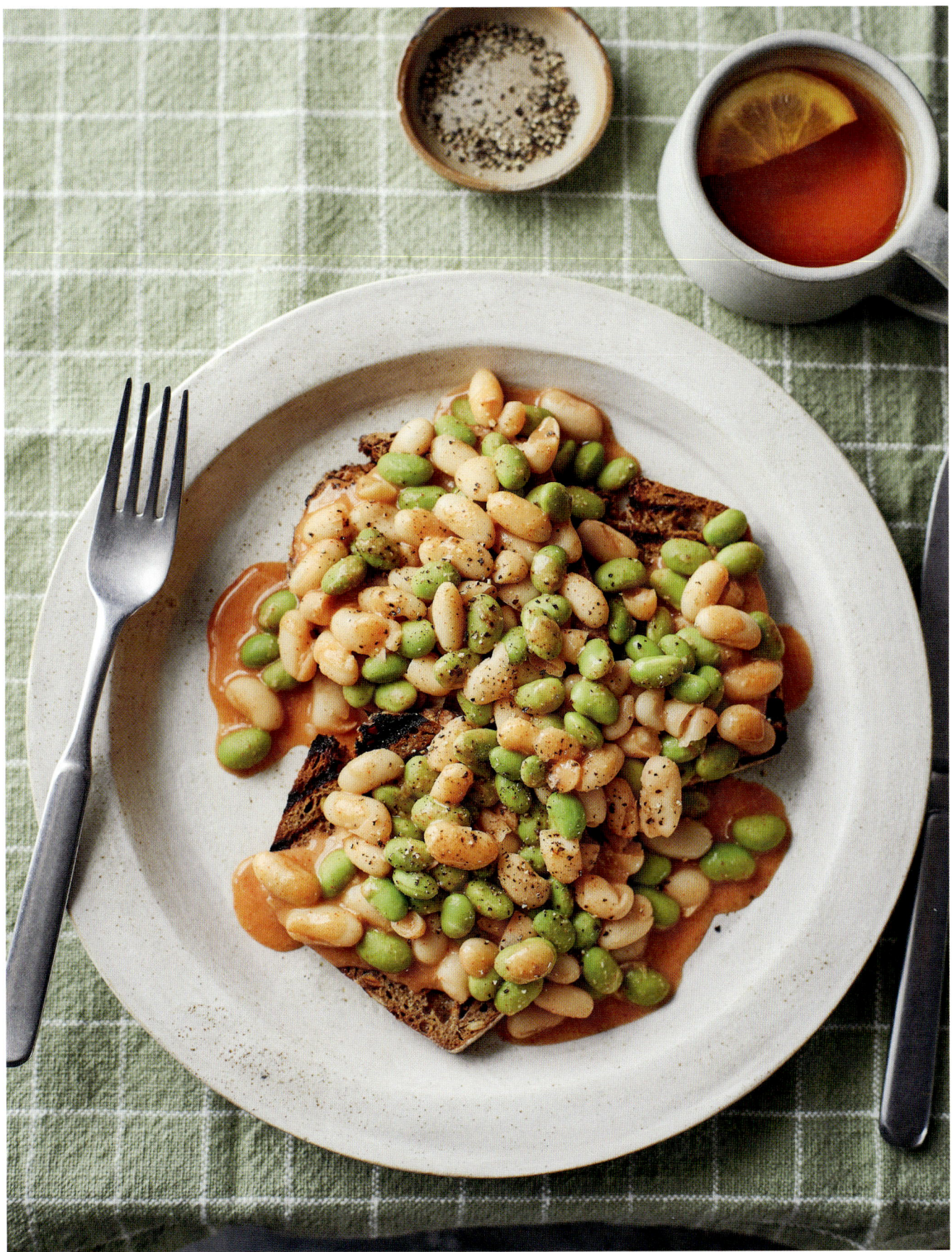

SPEEDY BREAKFAST STRATEGIES

When you just want something in a rush without faff for the mornings, you need to have some basics. These are like the white tees or black socks of your wardrobe. Everyone needs these essentials and you'd be surprised how many ways in which you can use them in various combinations.

One-pan Scrambles

Take a pan, any pan, and throw your ingredients into it over a medium heat. I use this strategy most days when I'm at the studio or at home with only 10 minutes for breakfast. A high-protein breakfast will keep you satiated, and these scrambles tick the box.

Serves 1

PEPPER AND TURMERIC TOFU WITH KRAUT AND RYE

Prep 5 minutes
Cook 10 minutes

100g firm tofu, crumbled
1 tbsp olive oil, plus extra to drizzle
½ tsp ground cumin
¼ tsp ground turmeric
½ tsp freshly ground black pepper
1 tbsp tomato purée
100g fennel, diced
50g sauerkraut
50g baby tomatoes, halved
1 slice of rye bread, toasted

Add the crumbled tofu, olive oil, spices and tomato purée to a bowl and toss to mix.

Add the tofu mixture to a small sauté pan over a medium heat and cook for 4–5 minutes, then push the contents to one half of the pan, add a drizzle of oil and the diced fennel.

Cook in separate halves of the pan for another 5 minutes until the fennel is slightly coloured and the tofu is nicely cooked.

Add everything to a serving bowl with the sauerkraut, baby tomatoes and toasted rye bread drizzled with olive oil.

Protein 18.4g | Fibre 8.7g | Plant Points 6.25

84 BREAKFAST & BRUNCH

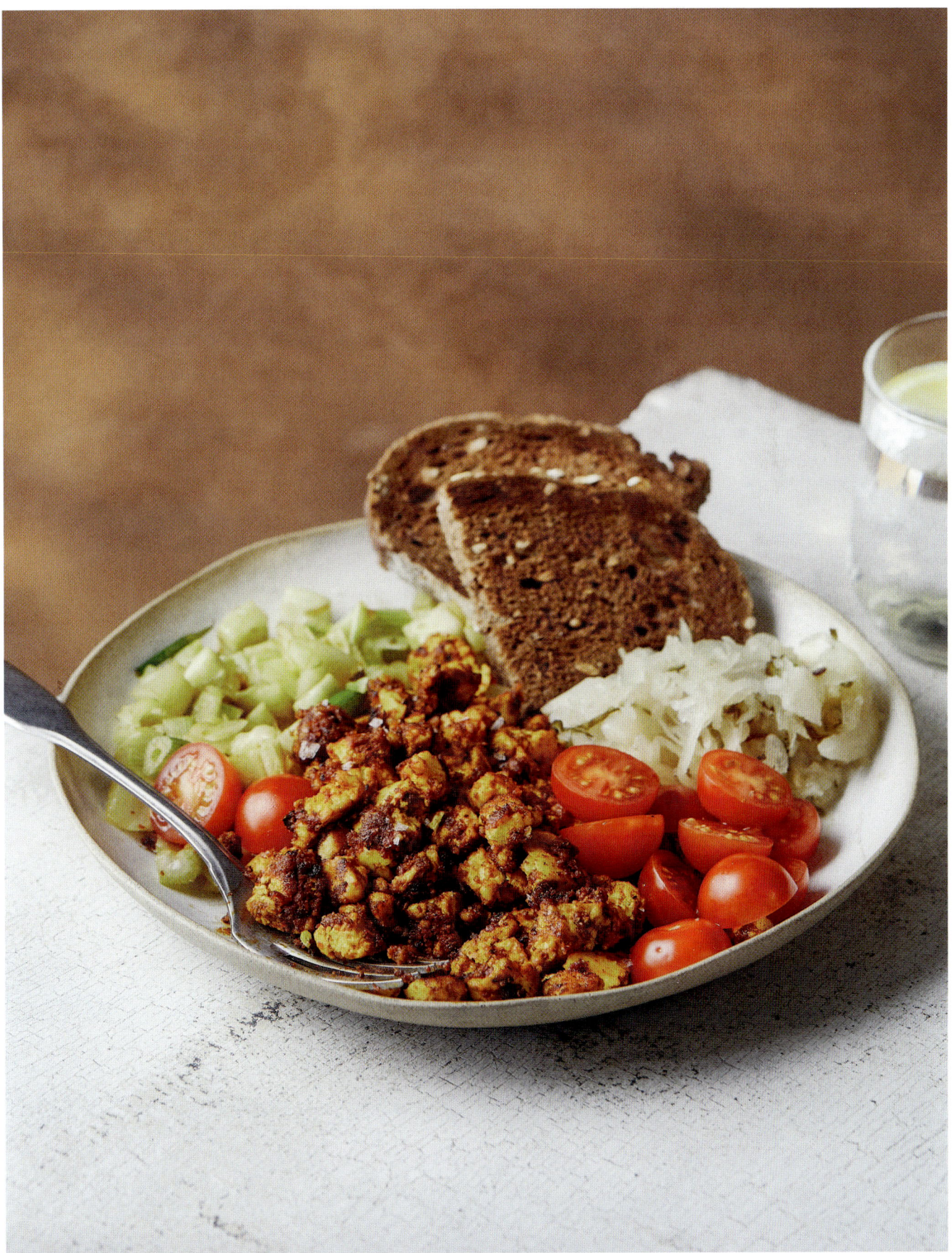

Serves 1

GREEN PESTO BEANS WITH EGGS AND HAZELNUTS

Prep 5 minutes
Cook 10 minutes

1 tbsp green pesto
½ x 400g can white beans, drained and rinsed
1 tbsp olive oil, plus extra to drizzle
100g shiitake mushrooms
1 tsp dried oregano
1–2 eggs, whisked
50g rocket leaves
20g hazelnuts, chopped

Note
You will be left with half the pesto beans to use for another day. I make variations of this dish with all sorts of mushrooms, different beans like black beans or chickpeas and a different marinade like harissa, red pesto or sundried tomato paste.

Mix the pesto with the white beans in a bowl and set aside.

Add the oil and shiitake mushrooms to a small sauté pan over a medium heat and cook for 6–8 minutes until golden. Try not to disturb them in the pan, let them caramelise.

Add the oregano, seasoning and push the ingredients to one half of the pan. Add another drizzle of oil and pour in the eggs, whisking with a fork as you do. The eggs should scramble in about 1 minute.

Take off the heat, move the eggs to one side and add half the pesto beans and the rocket leaves. Top with the chopped hazelnuts to serve.

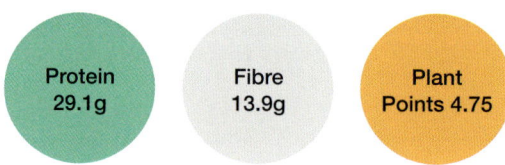

Protein 29.1g | Fibre 13.9g | Plant Points 4.75

Serves 1

LENTILS, EGGS AND KIMCHI

Prep 5 minutes
Cook 10 minutes

1 tbsp olive oil, plus extra to drizzle
80g asparagus or broccoli, roughly chopped
60g cooked beluga lentils
1 tsp sundried tomato paste
2 eggs, whisked

To serve
50g kimchi
1 tbsp pumpkin seeds
Fennel, Oregano, Chia and Pumpkin Seed Crackers (page 262) or sourdough bread

To a lidded sauté pan over a medium heat, add the olive oil and asparagus or broccoli and stir for a minute.

Move them to one side and add the lentils. Stir the sundried tomato paste into the lentils. Cover with the lid to cook through the ingredients for 3–4 minutes.

Remove the lid, move the contents to one half and add another drizzle of oil and pour in the eggs, whisking with a fork as you do. The eggs should scramble in about 1 minute.

Take the pan off the heat and serve in the pan with the kimchi, pumpkin seeds and seeded crackers or sourdough.

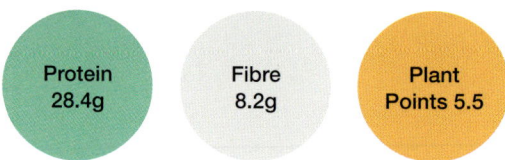

Protein 28.4g | Fibre 8.2g | Plant Points 5.5

BREAKFAST & BRUNCH

Toast Toppers

Quick and nutritious meal options can be game-changers for sticking to your healthy eating habits. This is where an easy 'toast topper' comes in handy (pictured on page 73). These recipes are not only convenient but also packed with essential nutrients and proteins for whatever your choice of bread. When it comes to toast, I tend to opt for rye, seeded bread or the Doctor's Daily Bread on page 72 that I've packed tons of fibre into. I keep them sliced in the freezer for extra convenience, ready for toasting whenever I need.

SMASHED CHICKPEAS

Prep 10 minutes

Serves 2

1 x 400g can chickpeas, drained and rinsed
25g feta
1 tbsp olive oil
50g spring onion, finely chopped
50g celery, finely chopped
1 tsp dried oregano
10g parsley, finely chopped

Place all the ingredients into a mixing bowl with salt and pepper and smash with the back of a fork.

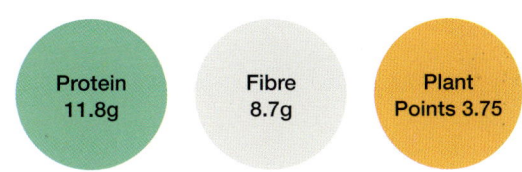

Protein 11.8g | Fibre 8.7g | Plant Points 3.75

PAPRIKA PEA TOPPER

Prep 5 minutes

Serves 2

100g peas (fresh or defrosted from frozen)
1 x 400g can cannellini beans, drained and rinsed
100g edamame beans
1 tbsp olive oil
1 tsp sweet paprika
½ tsp ground cumin

Blend all the ingredients together in a processor with seasoning and a little hot water (off the boil) to loosen the mixture. It should be a rough mixture, not a purée.

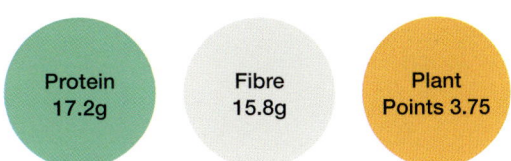

Protein 17.2g | Fibre 15.8g | Plant Points 3.75

BREAKFAST & BRUNCH

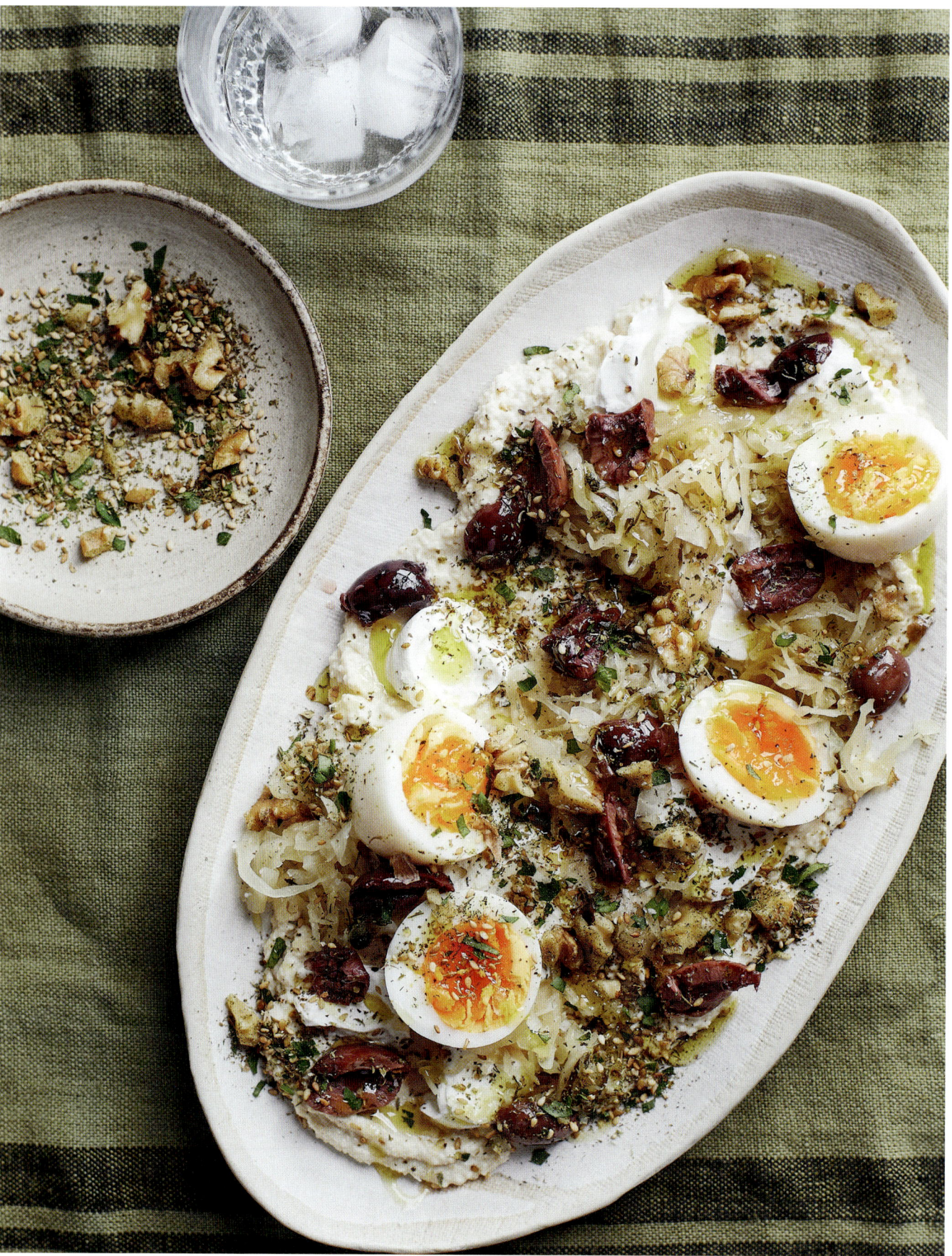

Eggs and Kraut

Prep 5 minutes
Cook 10 minutes

Serves 2

2 eggs
150g hummus
50g pitted Kalamata olives
100g labneh or cottage cheese
100g sauerkraut
2 tsp za'atar
1 tsp dried oregano
10g parsley, finely chopped
50g walnuts, roughly chopped or crushed in a pestle and mortar
2 tbsp olive oil

Fermented veg appears in my diet most days in various forms. I like to start my day with it to make sure I have it ticked off and to keep the gut microbes happy! This herbaceous combination of za'atar, oregano and parsley is a fabulous arrangement for the sharp sauerkraut and labneh. The walnuts add texture and protein to the creamy hummus and eggs.

Place the eggs in a saucepan of boiling water for 7 minutes and then remove with a slotted spoon. Plunge them into a mixing bowl filled with water and ice while you prepare the rest of your ingredients.

Smother the base of a platter with the hummus. Peel and halve the eggs and add to the platter with the olives, labneh or cottage cheese and sauerkraut.

Mix the za'atar and oregano with the parsley, walnuts and olive oil in a small mixing bowl and scatter over the ingredients on the platter to serve. Season with salt and pepper.

PROTEIN BOOST

Add more hummus; or walnuts; tuna or mackerel would also work well.

Protein 22.6g
Fibre 9.1g
Plant Points 5

BREAKFAST & BRUNCH

One-pan Greens and Goats' Cheese with Pickled Red Onions

Prep 10 minutes, plus marinating
Cook 15 minutes

Serves 2

- 1 tbsp olive oil, plus extra to serve
- 200g kale, stalks and leaves, roughly chopped
- 200g peas (fresh or defrosted from frozen)
- 50g dill, stalks and fronds separated, finely chopped
- 1 tsp ground coriander
- 1 x 400g can white beans, drained and rinsed
- 100g goats' cheese
- 50g sunflower seeds, toasted and roughly smashed in a pestle and mortar, to serve

For the pickled red onions
- 50ml apple cider vinegar
- 50ml hot water, recently boiled
- 1 tsp white sugar
- ½ tsp salt
- 50g red onion, thinly sliced

Sharp pickled onions cut through that delicious tang of goats' cheese. This combination of soft dill, beans and peas with the lushest dairy is as delicious as it is healthy. The greens and onion pack this dish with anti-inflammatory chemicals as well as specialised fibre that keeps your gut bugs happy and well functioning to support heart and brain health and balance sugar levels.

First, make the pickled red onions. Mix all of the ingredients for the pickle except the onions in a small mixing bowl. Add the sliced onions to the bowl and leave to sit for at least 30 minutes. The red onions will become a beautiful hue of pink. You can double the ingredients to make more and store in the fridge in an airtight container.

Add the olive oil, kale, peas, stalks of the dill and ground coriander with seasoning to a lidded sauté pan over a medium heat and stir. Cook for about 2–3 minutes until the greens begin to wilt.

Stir the white beans through the greens, add a splash of boiling water and cover with the lid for 4 minutes to cook through.

Remove the lid, the mixture should be bubbling away. While still over the heat, spoon chunks of the goats' cheese onto the beans and greens. They will melt into little pockets.

Scatter the pickled red onions on top of the mixture and take off the heat.

Drizzle with a slick of olive oil and scatter over the dill fronds and toasted sunflower seeds to serve.

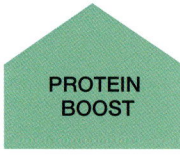

PROTEIN BOOST

Add more pumpkin seeds or goats' cheese.

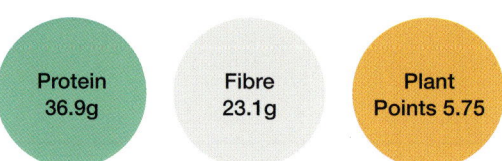

Protein 36.9g | Fibre 23.1g | Plant Points 5.75

BREAKFAST & BRUNCH

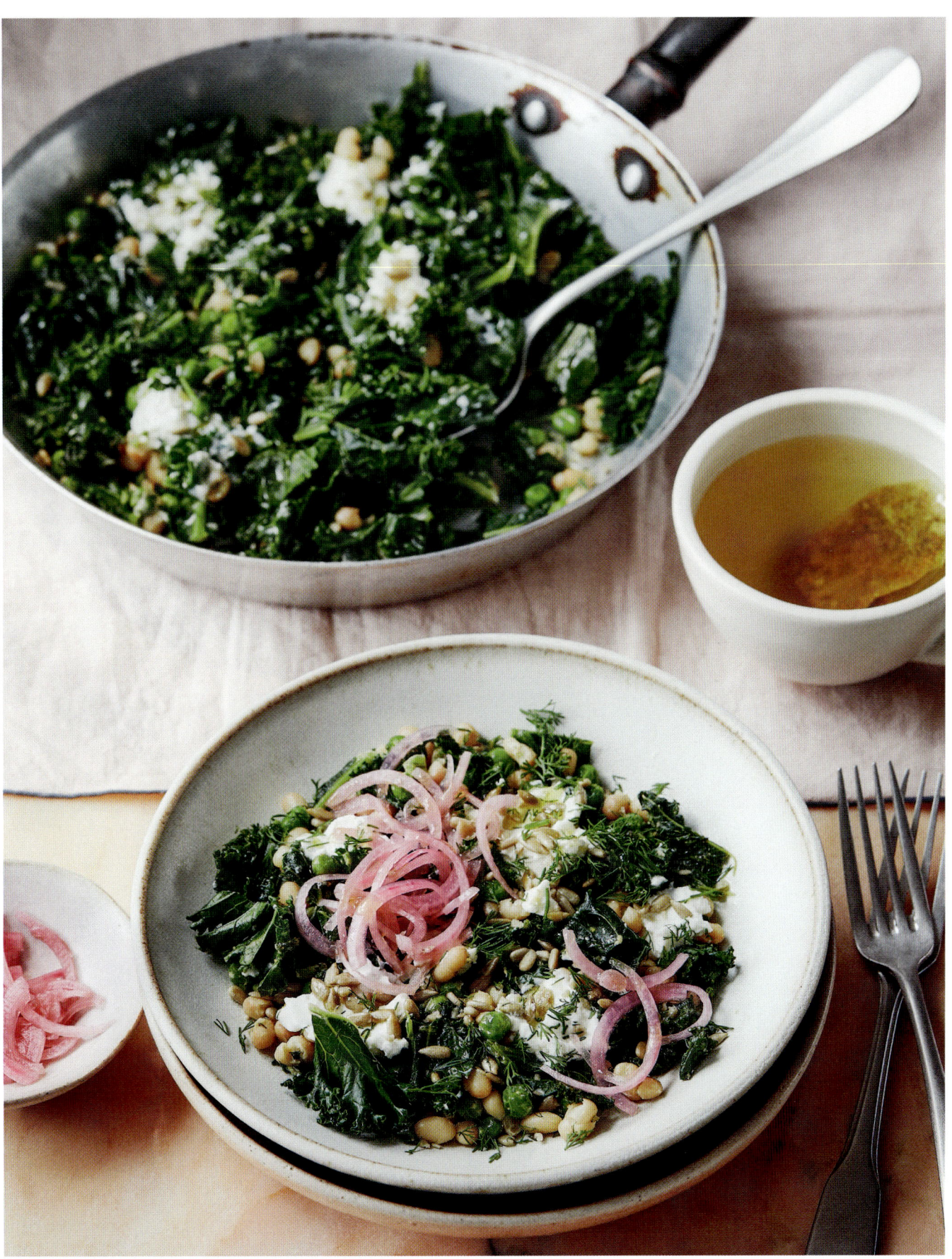

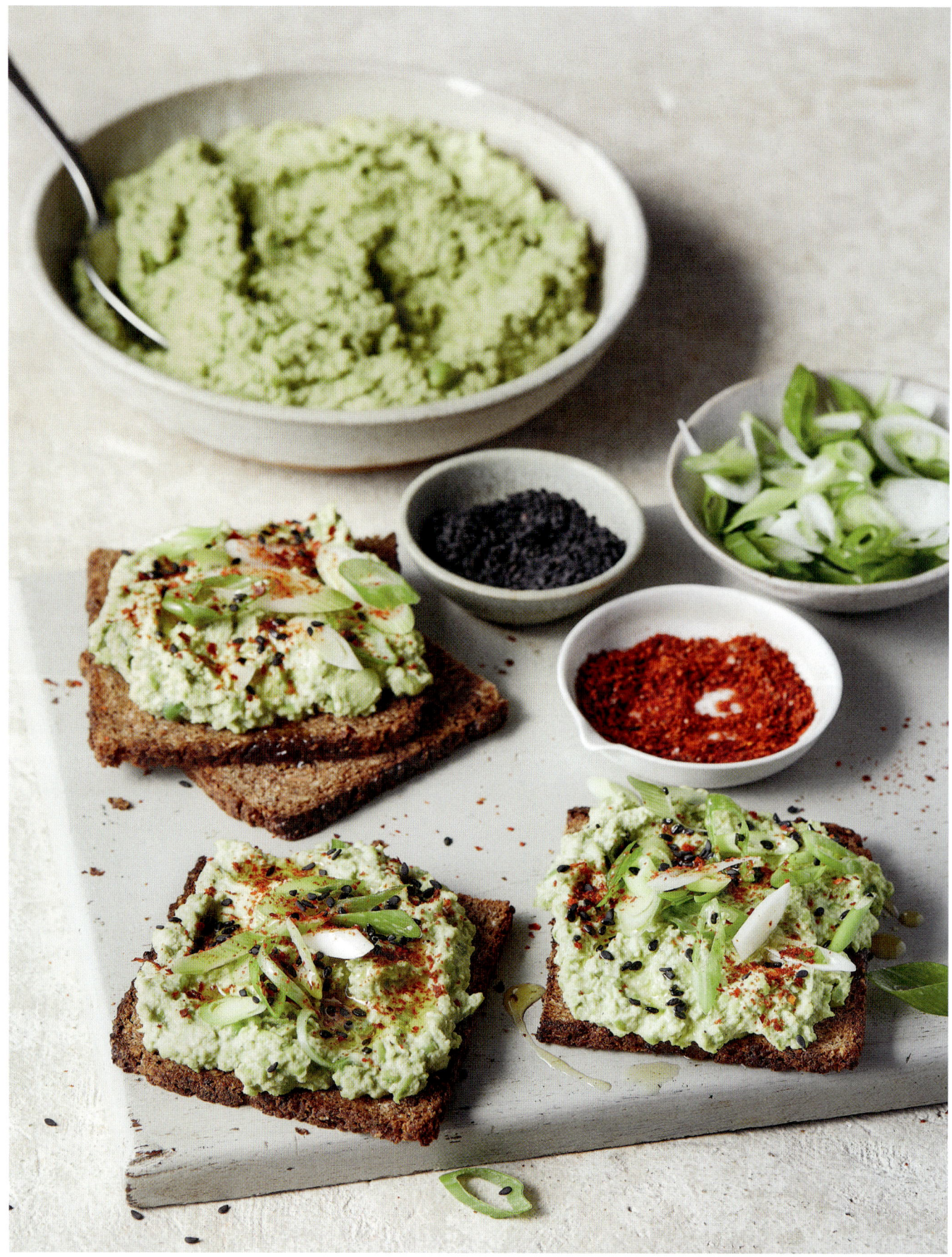

High-protein Edamame and Pea Spread on Rye Toast

Prep 5 minutes
Cook 10 minutes

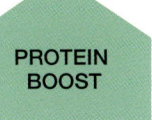

Serves 2

200g edamame beans
200g peas (fresh or frozen)
50g tahini
Juice of 1 lemon
20g nutritional yeast
1 tsp garlic powder
1 tbsp olive oil, plus extra to serve

To serve
2 slices of dark seeded rye bread, toasted
½ tsp gochugaru (Korean chilli flakes)
40g spring onions, sliced on an angle
1 tbsp black sesame seeds

Edamame is one of my favourite legumes. They're among the highest in protein, plus they have a wide selection of anti-inflammatory phytonutrients that contribute to balanced inflammation and a well-functioning immune system. Blended into a spread and smothered on toast is a great way to eat them and this is super easy to batch cook for rapid grab-and-go breakfasts that are far cheaper and higher in protein than avocado.

Add the edamame beans and peas to a saucepan of boiling water and simmer for 3 minutes to soften the legumes.

With a slotted spoon, scoop out the edamame beans and peas into a food processor and add 50ml of the cooking water, the tahini, lemon juice, nutritional yeast, garlic powder, olive oil and a good pinch of black pepper. Blend to the consistency of hummus, adding more of the cooking water to loosen the mixture if needed. Season with salt and pepper.

To serve, spoon the spread on the toasted rye bread and top with the gochugaru flakes, spring onions, black sesame seeds and a drizzle of oil.

PROTEIN BOOST

Add more edamame or tahini; serve with soft-boiled eggs; top with crispy tofu (see page 149).

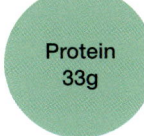

Protein 33g
Fibre 18.5g
Plant Points 7.25

BREAKFAST & BRUNCH

Whipped Feta with Dill, Grapes, Chickpeas and Smoked Mackerel

Prep 15 minutes

Serves 2

100g feta
160g celery, finely diced
100g red grapes, halved
25g dill, finely chopped
100g cucumber, diced
1 x 400g can chickpeas, drained and rinsed
1 tbsp olive oil
1 tsp red wine vinegar
200g smoked mackerel fillet

Whipping feta creates a luxurious foundation for the sharp sweet flavour of grapes and the tender caress of chopped dill. The combination is fantastic. I've used a good dose of the herbs for flavour and functional benefits too, providing polyphenols for gut health along with the chickpeas, and oily fish for protein and anti-inflammatory fats. You can gently warm the mackerel in an oven at 180°C for 10 minutes if you prefer, or half the time in an air fryer.

Crumble the feta into a mixing bowl with a whisk, add about 25ml water a little at a time and whip into a smooth mixture. You may need more or less water depending on how firm and moist the feta is.

To a separate mixing bowl, add the celery, red grapes, dill, cucumber and chickpeas with the oil and vinegar and season with salt and pepper. Mix with your hands.

Add the whipped feta to the base of a large platter and smooth across the dish with the back of a spoon.

Scatter the celery and grape mix over the whipped feta and flake over the mackerel pieces.

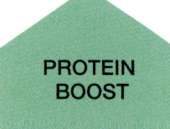

PROTEIN BOOST

Add more chickpeas, mackerel.

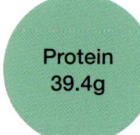

Protein 39.4g | Fibre 9.4g | Plant Points 4.5

BREAKFAST & BRUNCH

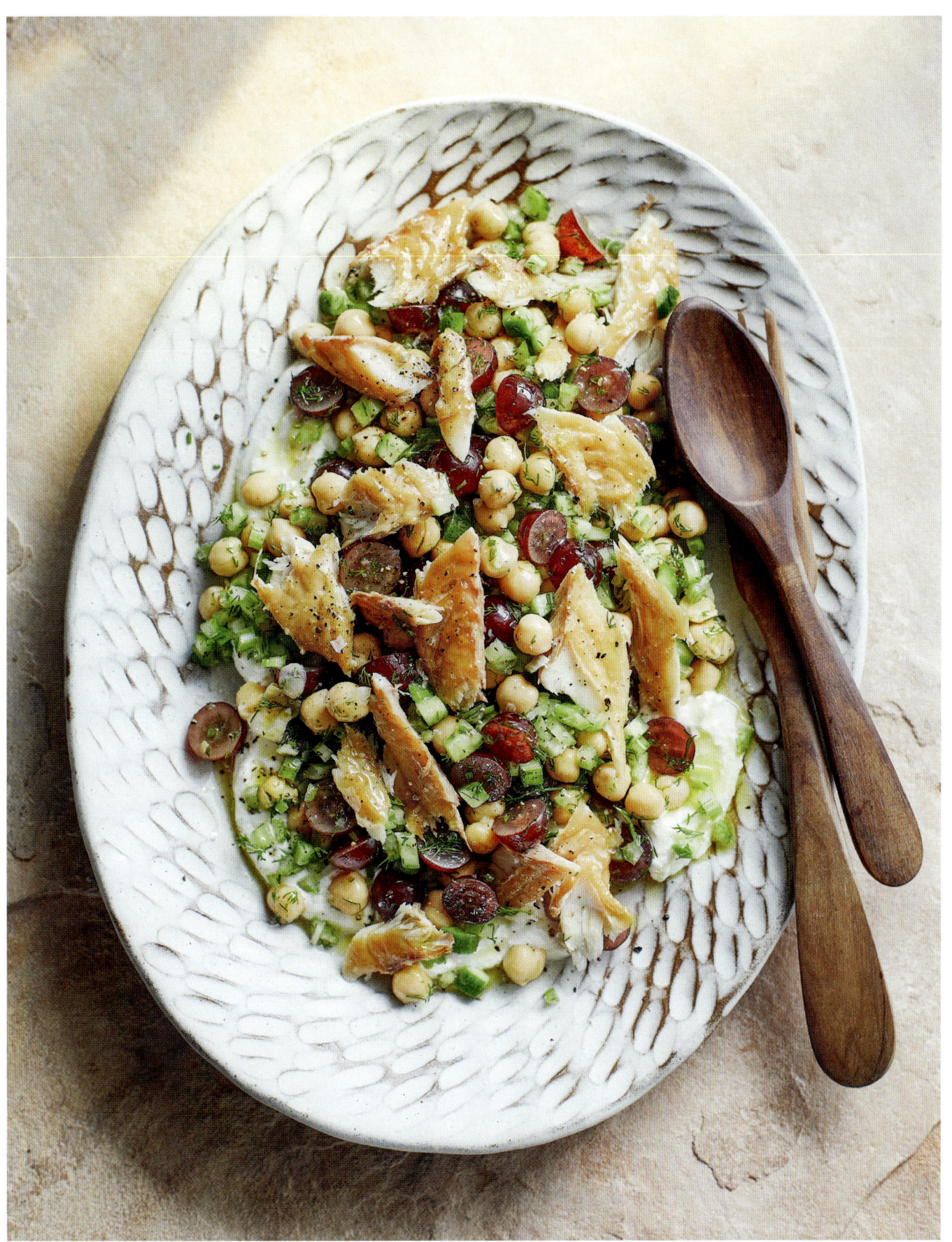

Overnight Pear and Pearl Barley Porridge with Star Anise

Prep 5 minutes, plus soaking overnight
Cook 20 minutes

Serves 2

100g pearl barley
350ml whole milk or plant-based alternative
50g shelled hemp seeds
30g chia seeds
1 star anise
½ tsp ground cinnamon, plus extra to serve
1 pear, grated, plus extra to serve
2 tbsp almond butter
Runny honey, to sweeten to your taste (optional)

This recipe combines the ease of overnight grains with the luxurious experience of hot, sweet, milky porridge in the morning. The pearl barley is nutty and delicious. Soaking overnight makes it quicker to cook and releases some of the nutrients, allowing it to be better absorbed in your gut and easier to digest. The sweetness of the pear is enough flavour for me, but use honey if you wish. The gritty texture of pear, that scrapes against your teeth when you bite into the juicy flesh, is down to specialised fibres that your gut microbes adore. This gut-friendly breakfast will set you up for a fantastic day.

Add all the ingredients, excluding the pear, almond butter and honey, if using, to a small lidded saucepan, and leave to soak, covered, overnight in the fridge.

The next morning, add a good splash of water to loosen the porridge mixture and add the grated pear.

Place the pan on the hob and bring the porridge to a simmer, then reduce the heat to low and cook, part-covered with the lid, for 15–20 minutes, gently stirring with a wooden spoon. Stir in the almond butter until combined. The barley should become soft and slightly translucent with a beautiful nutty bite when ready.

Spoon the porridge into serving bowls and finish with a dusting of extra cinnamon and extra grated pear. You could also drizzle over a little honey.

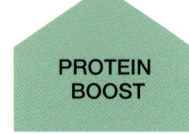

PROTEIN BOOST

Add an unflavoured protein powder, collagen or chopped pecans.

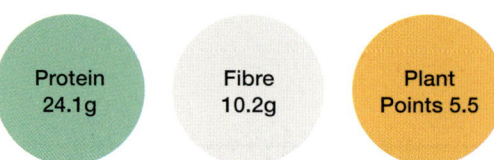

Protein 24.1g
Fibre 10.2g
Plant Points 5.5

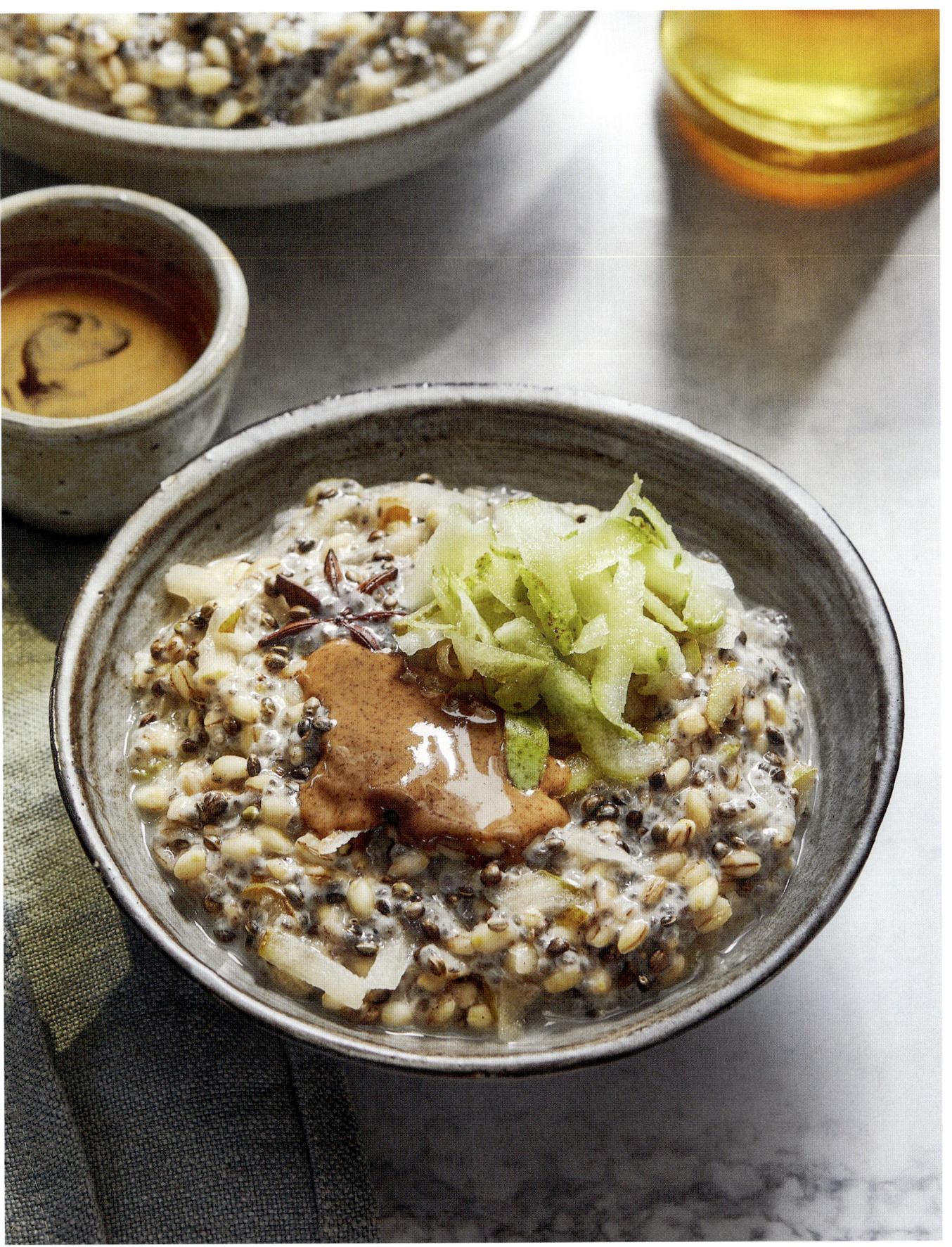

Greens and Basil Tofu Scramble

Prep 5 minutes
Cook 15 minutes

Serves 2

1 tbsp olive oil, plus extra to serve
200g leeks, roughly chopped
150g kale, stalks and leaves, roughly chopped
200g herb-flavoured extra-firm tofu, roughly crumbled
2 tsp za'atar
½ tsp dried chilli flakes
30g pistachio nuts, toasted and roughly chopped
15g basil leaves, torn
2 slices of rye bread, toasted, to serve

I like to mix up my breakfasts. While I love eggs and I think they provide a fantastic selection of nutrients, such as choline, carotenoids and readily available protein, they also contain fats that can raise cholesterol. A pragmatic approach is to vary what you have for breakfast every day and tofu is a great way to mimic the high nutrient content of eggs with different soy phytonutrients that are fantastic for inflammation and gut health. If you can't find herb-flavoured tofu, use extra-firm plain and double the basil leaves.

Heat the olive oil in a large, lidded sauté pan over a medium heat. Add the leeks and kale stalks with seasoning and cook for about 6–8 minutes until nicely softened and tender but not coloured.

Add the kale leaves and cover with the lid. Turn the heat to low and cook, stirring occasionally, for 5 minutes until the greens have wilted.

Toss in the crumbled tofu with the za'atar and chilli flakes and stir for a few minutes to combine and infuse the flavours. Take the pan off the heat and stir in the pistachios and basil leaves and season with salt and pepper.

Serve the tofu scramble on the toasted rye bread drizzled with extra olive oil.

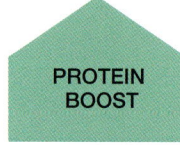

PROTEIN BOOST

Use more tofu or pistachios.

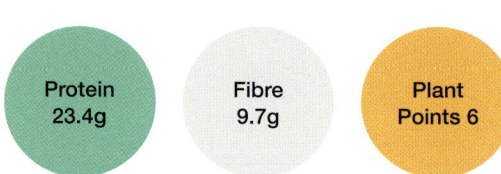

Protein 23.4g
Fibre 9.7g
Plant Points 6

BREAKFAST & BRUNCH

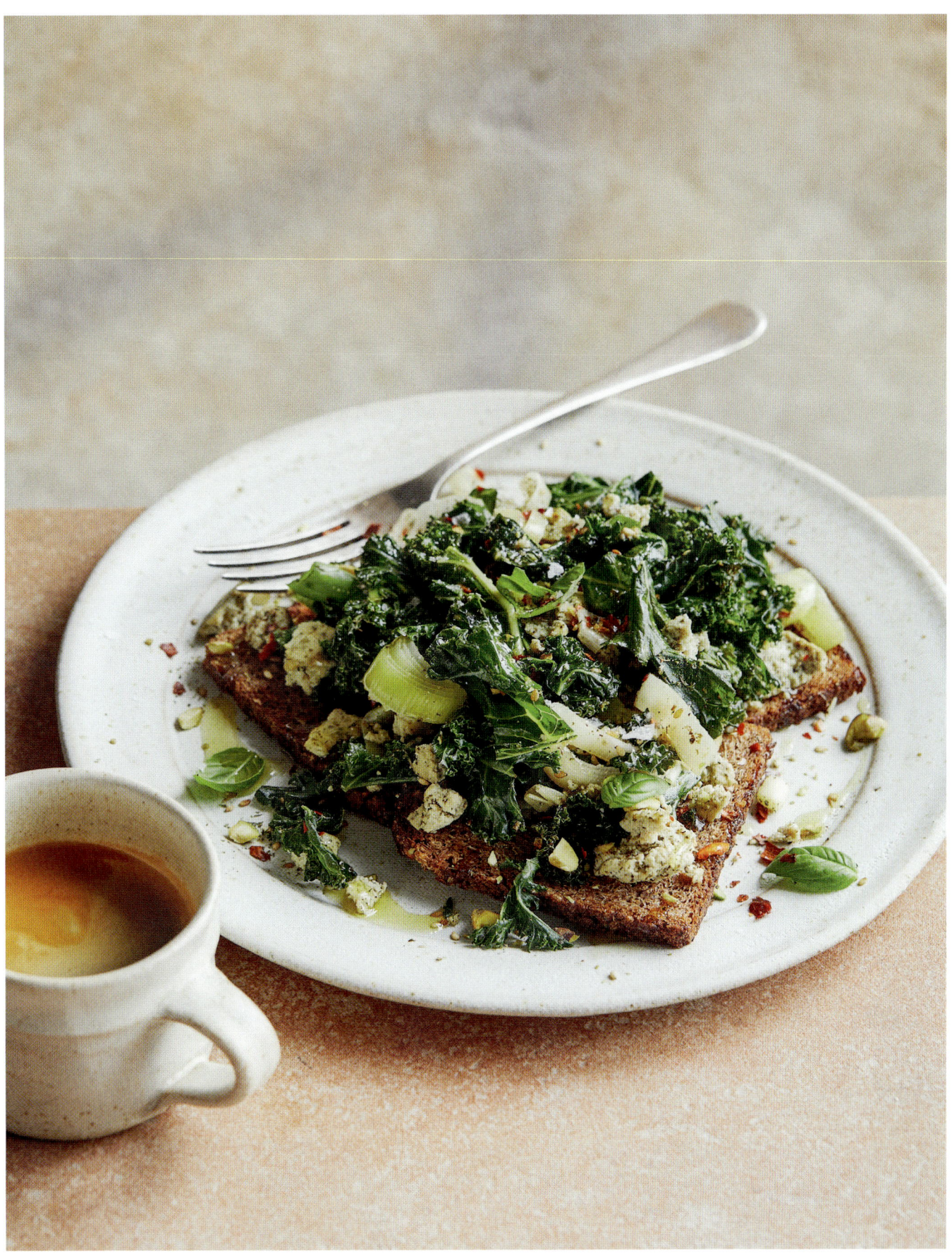

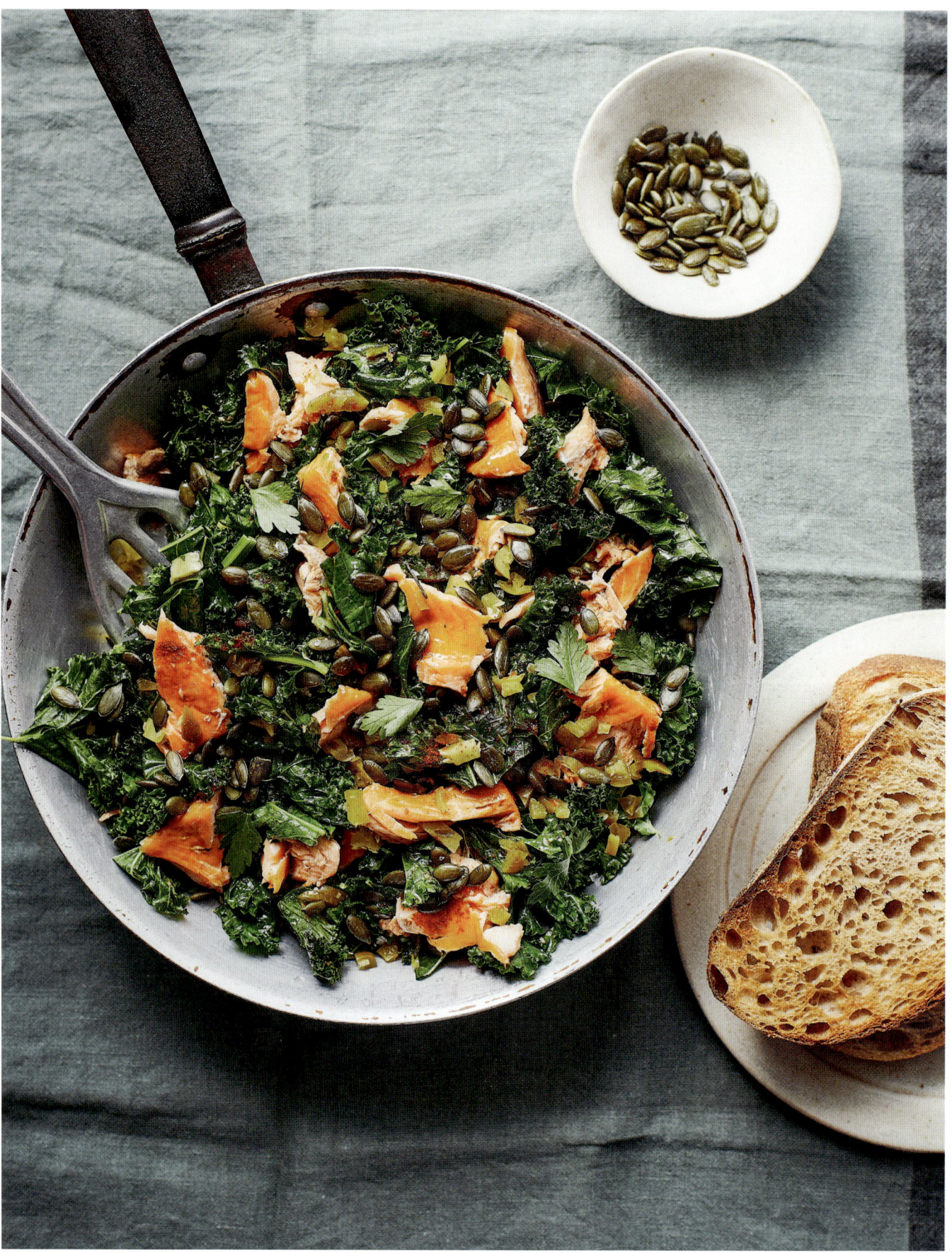

Hot-smoked Salmon and Greens

Prep 10 minutes
Cook 10 minutes

Serves 2

1 tbsp olive oil
200g kale, stalks and leaves, roughly chopped
50g parsley, leaves and stalks separated, roughly chopped
200g hot-smoked salmon, flaked into big chunks
1 tbsp just-boiled water
25g jalapeños from a jar, finely diced
Pinch of hot smoked paprika
30g pumpkin seeds, lightly toasted, to garnish
Sourdough, toasted, to serve (optional)

A classic one-pan breakfast for me whenever I'm filming in the studio. I love the delicious, punchy flavour of hot-smoked salmon. The combination with kale, parsley and pumpkin seeds is a perfect marriage of flavour and function. This high-protein start to the day, packed with anti-inflammatory omega-3 fats, will keep you fuller for longer and energised.

Add the olive oil to a lidded sauté pan over a medium heat with the kale, parsley stalks and most of the parsley leaves with plenty of seasoning and stir for 2–3 minutes until lightly wilted.

Add the chunks of salmon with the boiling water, cover with the lid and cook for about 2–3 minutes.

Remove the lid and add the jalapeños, remaining parsley leaves and paprika. Top with the pumpkin seeds for garnish and a drizzle of oil. Serve on its own or with some toasted sourdough.

PROTEIN BOOST

Add more salmon or pumpkin seeds.

Protein 37g

Fibre 8.1g

Plant Points 3.5

BREAKFAST & BRUNCH

3 WAYS WITH DAIRY

Despite the high prevalence of lactose intolerance, yoghurts and cheeses **appear to be easier to digest for people, perhaps because most of the troublesome milk sugars are 'pre-digested' by microbes and hence less problematic. Dairy can be a great source of quality protein and healthy fats, plus good quality products are a source of live microbes which can be great for your gut.**

1. Go sweet and savoury

A dollop of cottage cheese, crushed walnuts and a tiny drizzle of raw honey is a beautiful snack which has the benefits of microbe-friendly fibres in the walnuts and honey, plus the presence of live cultures in the cheese. You can also try this with feta, goats' cheese and, of course, shards of Parmesan.

To serve 2

- Top **100g cottage cheese**, with **50g walnuts**, and **2 tsp raw honey**

Protein 9g

- I also enjoy this boujee little snack if I have some extra time:

Simply add **1 tbsp olive oil** to a sauté pan over a medium heat, roughly chop **40g raw almonds** in half and add them to the oil, cooking until they turn golden and brown (about 4–5 minutes). This extra step flavours the oil. Sprinkle over a little salt and allow to cool before scattering over the top of **100g Greek yoghurt**. Sprinkle with **1 tsp dried or fresh oregano**, drizzle with **1 tbsp pomegranate molasses** and enjoy with a spoon.

Protein 14.1g

2. Seed crackers and cheese

Most crackers are poorly made, consisting of refined flours, additives and high amounts of salt. However, my Seeded Crackers (page 262) contain chia (a fantastically high-protein and high-fibre seed), pumpkin and sunflower seeds that pair beautifully with labneh, good-quality olive oil and za'atar. A wonderful starter or gut-boosting snack when you want something quick and healthy.

To serve 2, top some **seeded crackers (page 262)** with **100g labneh, 2 tsp za'atar** and **1 tbsp olive oil**.

Protein 14.1g

3. Berry and dairy

A gut- and brain-boosting combo that contains a significant portion of protein as well. I tend to choose authentic full-fat Greek yoghurt that should only have three ingredients (milk, cream and live cultures with nothing else added) and it should have a minimum of 5g of protein per 100g, but some of them contain more than 10g.

To serve 2, top **100g authentic full-fat Greek yoghurt** with **50g fresh or frozen berries, 30g flaked almonds, 20g shelled hemp seeds** and **½ tsp ground cinnamon**. Add **a drizzle of date syrup** if you need to make it sweeter.

Protein 9.5g

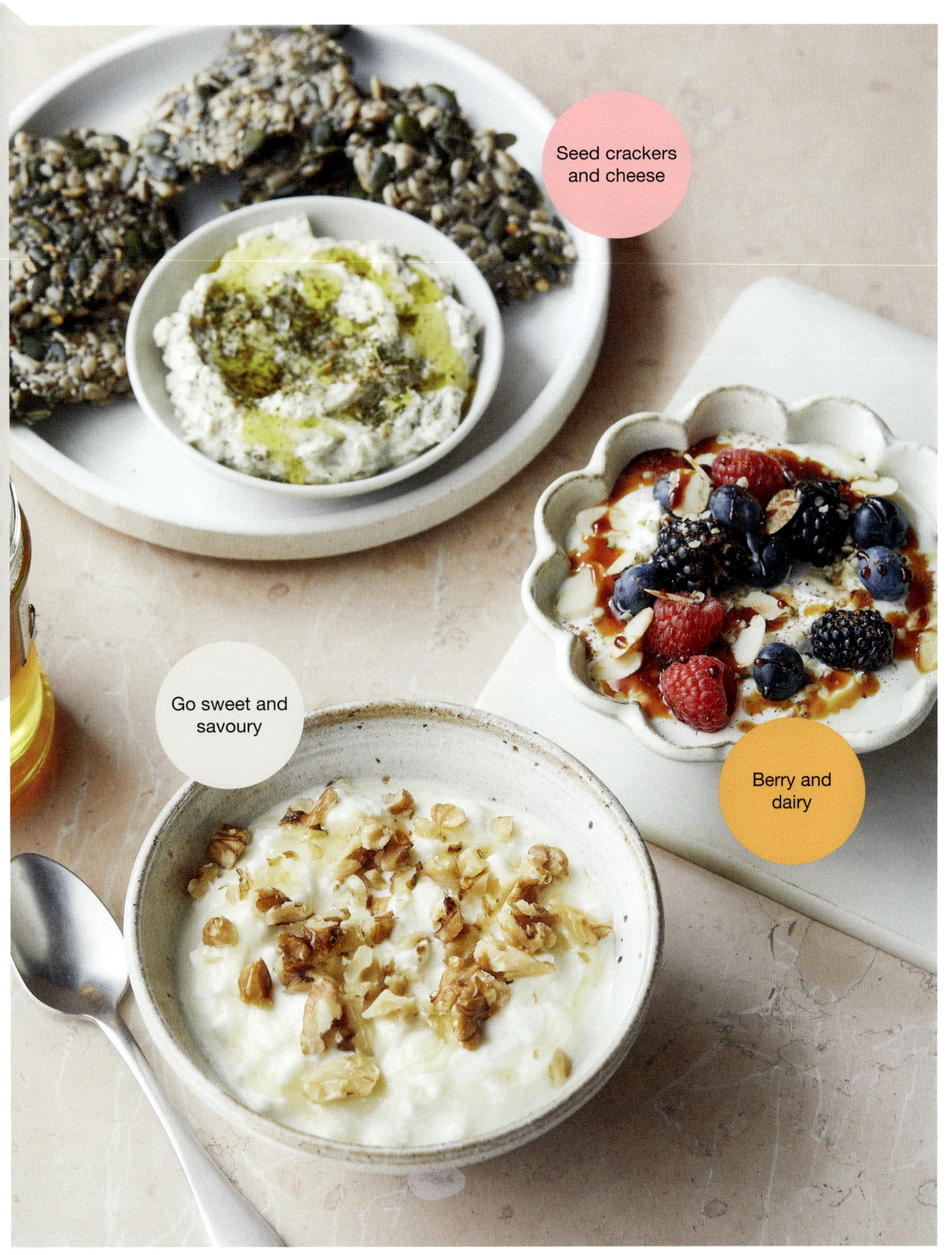

Seed crackers and cheese

Berry and dairy

Go sweet and savoury

ONE
-PAN

DINNERS

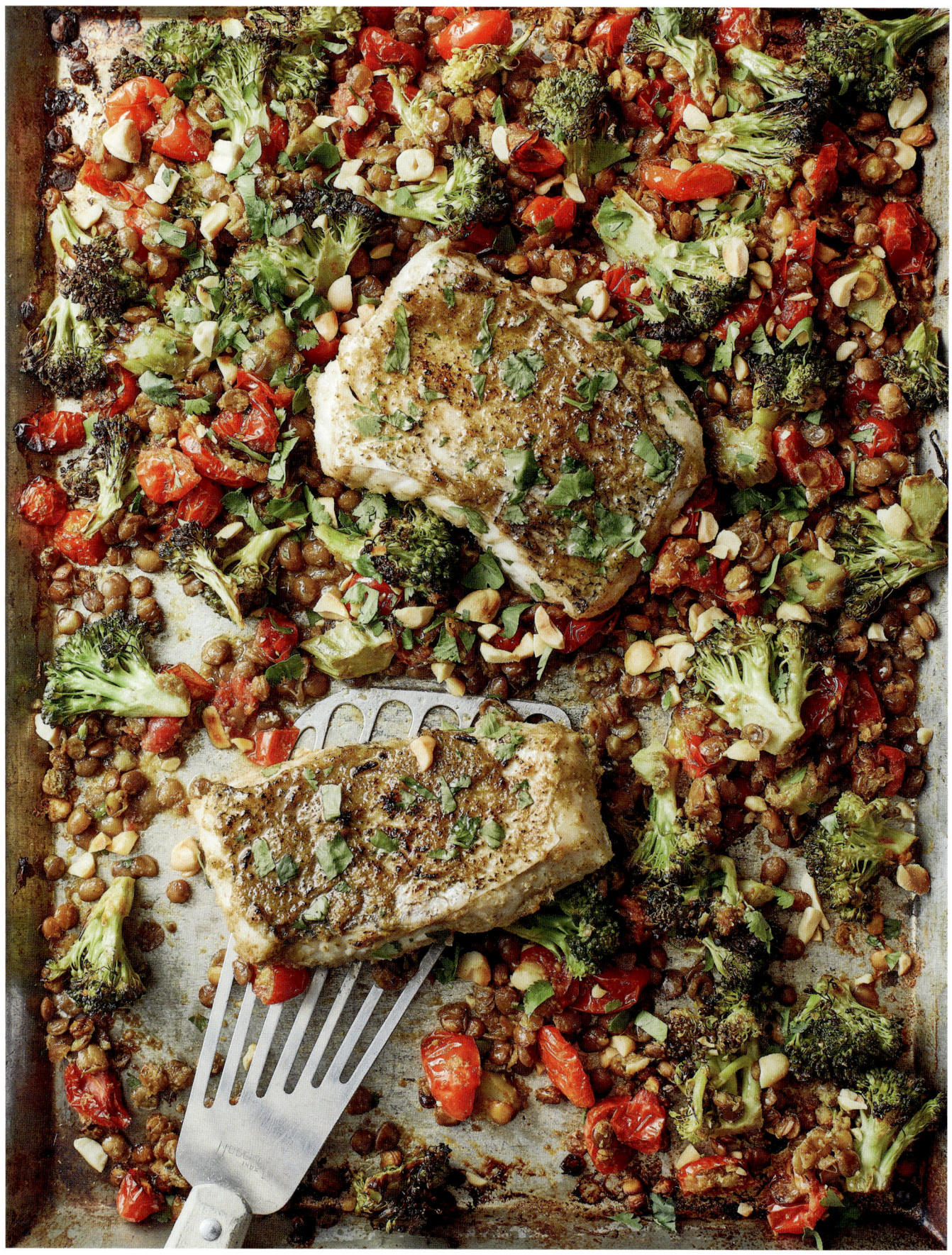

Thai Green Curry Lentil and Hake Traybake

Prep 10 minutes
Cook 30 minutes

Serves 2

300g hake fillets
4 tbsp Thai green curry paste
2 tbsp olive oil
200g baby tomatoes, halved
250g broccoli, stalks diced into 1cm pieces and florets broken into 2cm pieces
1 x 400g can green lentils, drained and rinsed

To serve
10g coriander leaves, roughly chopped
30g peanuts, toasted and crushed
Juice of 1 lime

A simple traybake where a good-quality Thai green curry paste does all the work for you. For midweek meals I rarely have the energy to make a paste from scratch, and this is where having good-quality convenience products to hand really comes into its own. The bitter phytonutrients in this brassica vegetable are what bring the anti-inflammatory benefits to the meal. The tomatoes will break down to create a light sauce for the fish, and using the broccoli stalks adds a ton more fibre to support flourishing gut health. If you don't have broccoli, you can use cauliflower, fennel and even aubergine instead.

Preheat the oven to 200°C fan.

Smother the hake fillets in 1 tablespoon of the curry paste, season well and drizzle with 1 tablespoon of oil, then leave to marinate while you continue to cook the rest of the ingredients.

Add the tomatoes, broccoli stalks, the remaining 3 tablespoons of the curry paste and the lentils to a baking tray with 50ml of water and mix thoroughly with your hands.

Drizzle with 1 tablespoon of oil and bake in the oven for 15 minutes until the broccoli stalks are partly cooked, stirring halfway through.

Remove the baking tray and carefully nestle the broccoli florets into the lentils and tomatoes. Place the fish on top of the vegetables and pop back in the oven for 10 minutes until the fish is cooked through.

Serve with coriander leaves, toasted peanuts and a squeeze of lime.

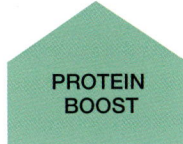

PROTEIN BOOST
Add more fish or peanuts.

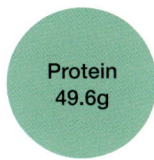

Protein 49.6g
Fibre 13.9g
Plant Points 5

ONE-PAN DINNERS

Monkfish with Capers, Olives and Tomatoes

Prep 10 minutes
Cook 20 minutes

Serves 2

2 tbsp olive oil, plus extra for the radicchio
4 garlic cloves, crushed
200g baby tomatoes, halved
20g capers, drained
10 pitted black olives, halved
2 tsp fresh oregano or 1 tsp dried
Pinch of dried chilli flakes (optional)
20g flat-leaf parsley, stalks and leaves finely chopped
1 x 400g can cannellini beans, drained and rinsed
2 monkfish fillets (about 300g in total)
200g radicchio, leaves torn (Tardivo di Trevisano)

The saltiness of capers with tomatoes and olives is a classic combination that packs this sauce with nutrients, and the tradition may have unique benefits. Research shows that the antioxidant lycopene in tomatoes is better absorbed when tomatoes are cooked with specific ingredients, particularly olive oil, garlic and other vegetables. They contain compounds, such as fat or sulphur compounds, that modify the chemical structure of lycopene, making it easier for our bodies to use. While this recipe transports me to a terrace overlooking an Italian piazza, I'm also reminded of these functional benefits for our health.

Add the olive oil and garlic to a large, lidded sauté pan over a medium heat and cook for 1–2 minutes until the garlic is lightly coloured.

Add the tomatoes, capers, olives, oregano, chilli flakes, if using, and parsley, saving a few leaves to finish, and a splash of water to the pan. Season with salt and pepper, stir, then cover with the lid and cook over a low heat for 5 minutes.

Add the beans, cover with the lid and cook for another 5 minutes until heated through. Add a splash more water if needed. Nestle the monkfish fillets into the tomato and bean sauce, cover, and cook for another 4–5 minutes, turning halfway, until cooked and the fish flakes.

While the fish is cooking, toss the radicchio leaves in olive oil in a serving bowl. Season with a little salt.

Serve the monkfish with the sauce spooned over and the radicchio salad on the side.

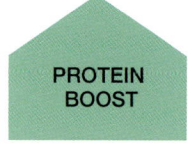

PROTEIN BOOST
Add more fish.

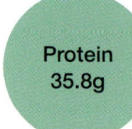

Protein 35.8g | Fibre 16.2g | Plant Points 5.5

ONE-PAN DINNERS

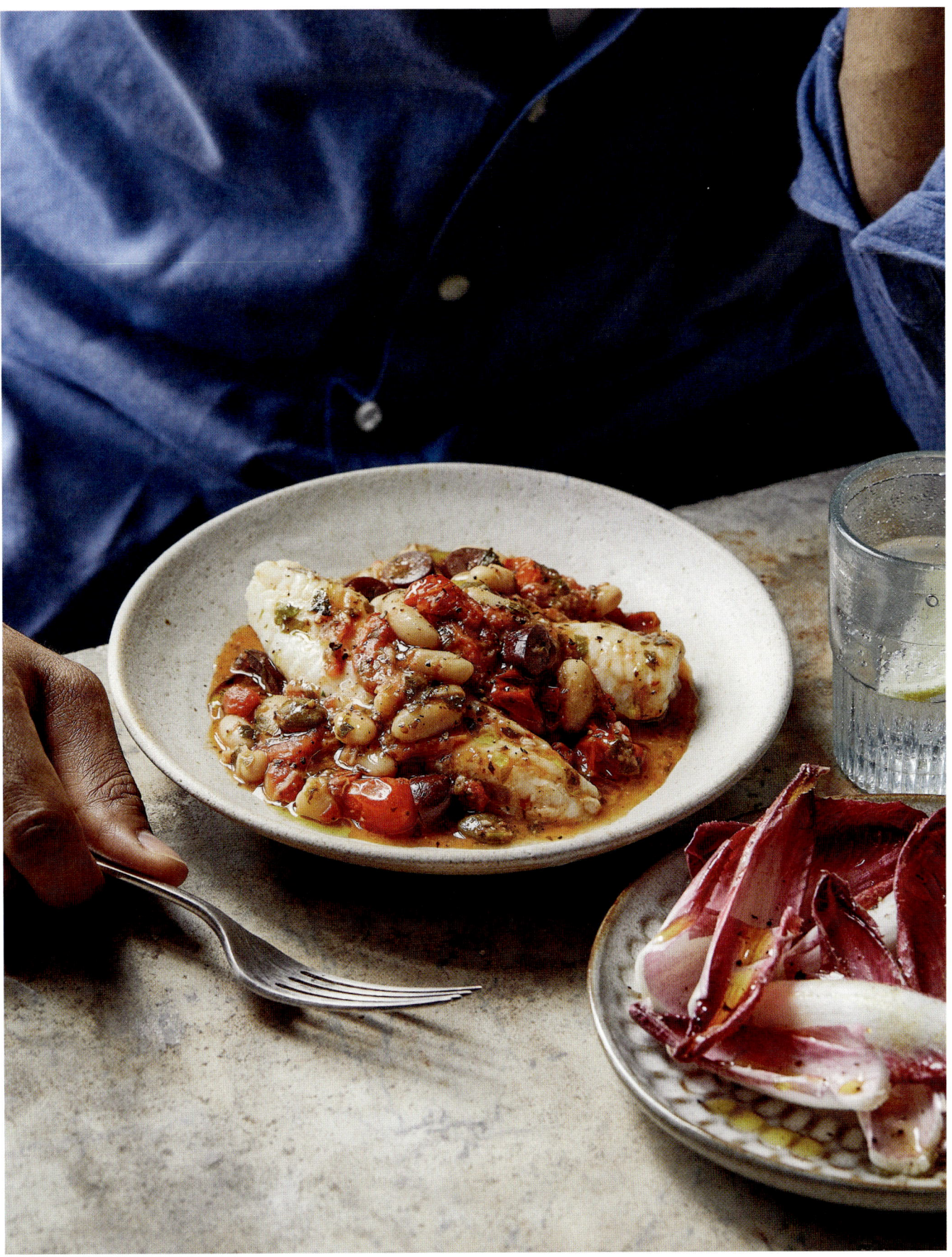

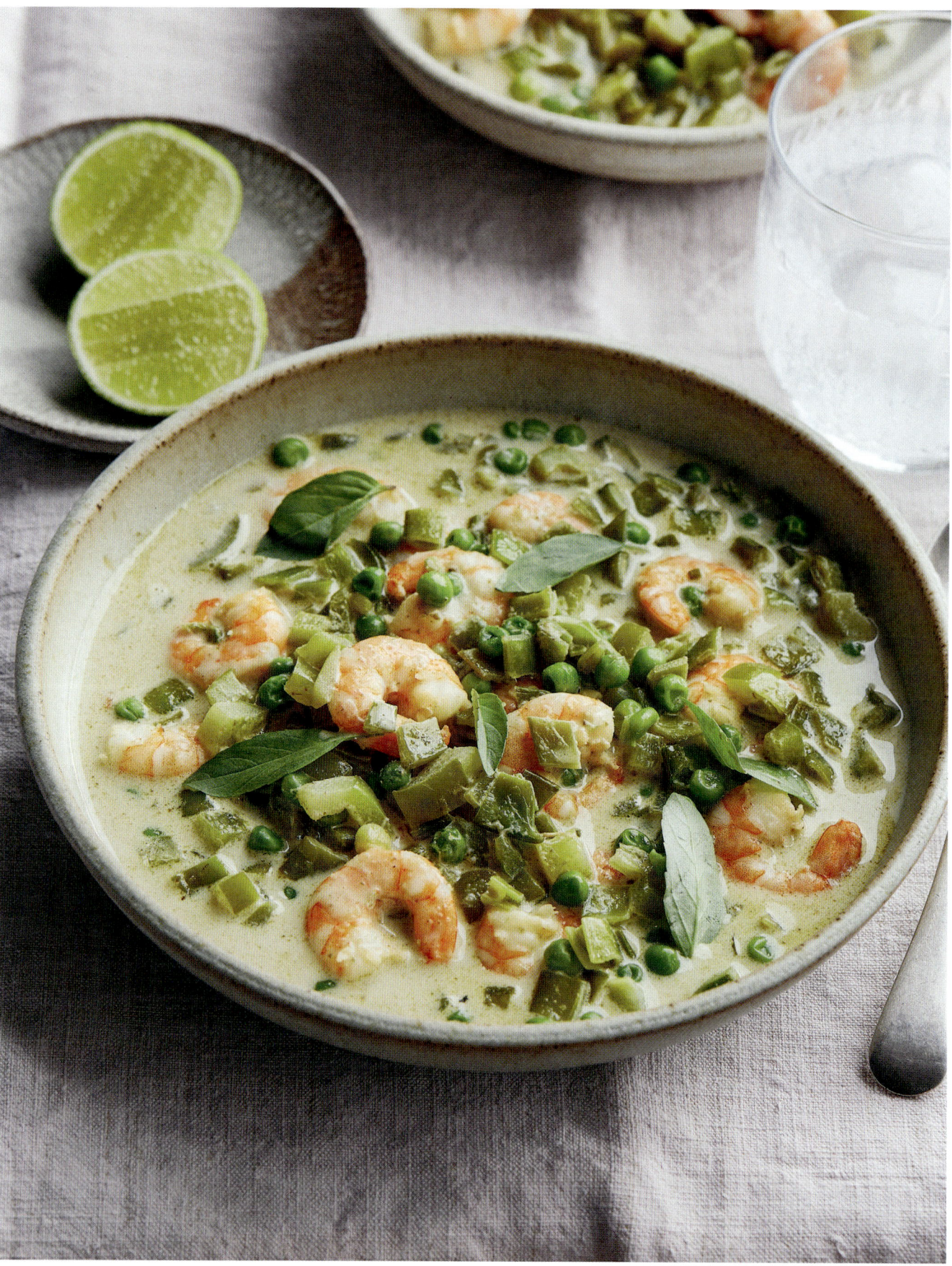

Coconut Prawn Stew with Thai green paste

Prep 10 minutes
Cook 20 minutes

Serves 2

1 tbsp coconut oil
3 tbsp Thai green curry paste
200g green pepper, deseeded and finely diced
150g mangetout or sugar snaps, finely diced
1 x 400ml can light coconut milk
200ml just-boiled water
2 tsp fish sauce
2 tsp soy sauce
200g raw prawns, shelled and deveined
100g peas (fresh or defrosted from frozen)

To serve
15g Thai basil, roughly torn
Juice of 1 lime

I wanted to create a bouillabaisse-like dish but with distinctive Thai flavours. A lot of Thai dishes hail from fishing villages and bouillabaisse is a Provençal fish soup originating in the port city of Marseille. While the green Thai curry flavours are wildly different to bouillabaisse, the method of creating this beautiful protein-packed anti-inflammatory dish shares a similar style. I buy a good-quality Thai green curry paste, with no added sugar or preservatives, to save time, and I use this recipe for a marvellous midweek affair.

Add the coconut oil to a large pan over a medium heat. When it has melted, add the Thai green curry paste and cook, stirring, for 1 minute.

Add the green pepper, mangetout or sugar snaps and cook in the paste for another 3–4 minutes to infuse them with flavour.

Add the light coconut milk, hot water, fish sauce and soy sauce and bring to a very gentle simmer, then cook for 5 minutes, stirring occasionally. Check the seasoning and add more soy or fish sauce as needed.

Carefully add the prawns and peas and cook in the simmering mix for 5 minutes until the prawns are fully cooked. Finish by adding the Thai basil and squeezing over the lime to serve.

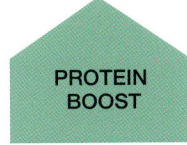

PROTEIN BOOST

Add more prawns or white fish or marinated tempeh.

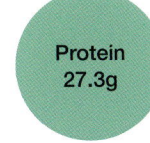

Protein 27.3g
Fibre 8.1g
Plant Points 4.75

ONE-PAN DINNERS

Quick Kale Curry with Lentils

Prep 10 minutes, plus soaking
Cook 30 minutes

Serves 2

1 tbsp olive oil
5cm piece of fresh root ginger, peeled and grated
1 tsp cumin seeds
1 tsp mustard seeds
1 tsp fennel seeds
1 tsp red chilli flakes, plus extra to serve (optional)
1 tsp ground turmeric
100g split red lentils, soaked for 20 minutes, thoroughly rinsed and drained well
200g firm tofu, drained well and finely diced
1 x 400ml can coconut milk
250g cooked beluga lentils
150ml just-boiled water
100g cavolo nero, tough stalks removed and leaves roughly chopped
Juice of 1 lime, cut into wedges

I love combining multiple legumes into a dish. Individually they bring slightly different flavours and textures, plus phytonutrients that add extra diversity to the meal that you'll be presenting to your gut microbes. The beluga and red lentils add a unique richness to this dish, as does the tofu. The spices help with digestion of the pulses, particularly fennel and cumin seeds with their carminative properties.

Heat the olive oil in a large, lidded saucepan over a medium–low heat and add the ginger. Stir for a minute, then add the cumin, mustard and fennel seeds and the chilli flakes. After 30 seconds of cooking, add the turmeric, red lentils and tofu with seasoning and stir to coat them in the spices.

Add the coconut milk, beluga lentils and hot water, then bring to a simmer. Turn the heat to low, cover with the lid and cook for 20 minutes, stirring occasionally, until the red lentils are tender and starting to break down.

Add an extra splash of water, if needed, to loosen the curry. Stir in the cavolo nero and season well. Cover with the lid again and cook for another 3–4 minutes until the greens are cooked through. Serve with the fresh lime and a dash of extra chilli flakes, if you like.

PROTEIN BOOST

Add extra tofu or toasted chopped cashew nuts.

Protein 41.5g

Fibre 14g

Plant Points 7

ONE-PAN DINNERS

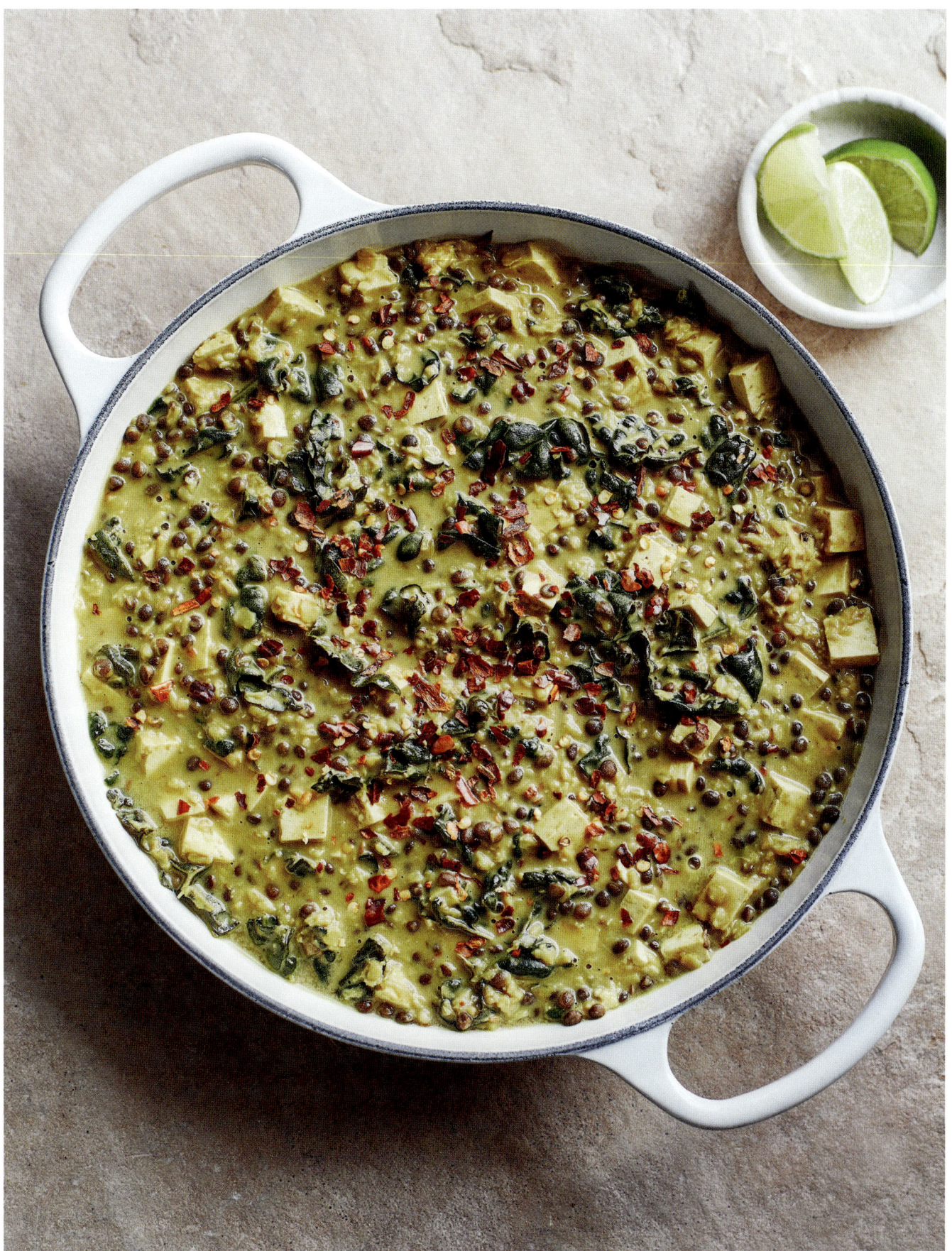

Smoky Masala Red Beans

Prep 10 minutes, plus soaking
Cook 30 minutes

Serves 4

2 tbsp olive oil
100g white onion, finely chopped
4 garlic cloves, grated
5cm piece of fresh root ginger, peeled and grated
100g split red lentils, soaked for 20 minutes, thoroughly rinsed and drained well
1 tsp ground turmeric
2 tsp smoked paprika
1 x 400g can red kidney beans
1 x 400g can whole peeled tomatoes
2 tbsp tomato purée
100ml just-boiled water
100g spinach, chopped
200g smoked firm tofu, cut into 1cm dice
2 tsp garam masala
2 tbsp natural yoghurt

This is my midweek curried bean and lentil recipe. It always gets me out of a pickle when I don't have too many fresh ingredients to hand, or I haven't made it to the shops. Most of the spices I always keep stocked on the spice rack and even if you don't have all of them, the recipe works super well. I try and get a few completely meat-free days in the week and I have come to rely on this high-fibre, gut-boosting, high-protein recipe.

Heat the olive oil in a large, lidded heavy-bottomed pan over a medium heat. Add the onion and cook for 6 minutes until softened, before adding the garlic and ginger with seasoning and stirring for another minute.

Stir in the lentils, then add the turmeric, paprika, kidney beans with their liquid, tomatoes (squeezed into the pan with your hands) and tomato purée with the hot water.

Bring the mixture to a simmer, turn the heat to low, cover with the lid and cook, stirring occasionally, for 10–12 minutes until the lentils are tender. Add more water if needed.

Remove the lid and stir in the spinach, tofu and garam masala. Replace the lid and cook for another few minutes until the spinach has wilted. Using a spoon, marble through the yoghurt and serve.

PROTEIN BOOST

Add extra tofu, cashews or red lentils. Some toasted peanuts or paneer also work well.

Protein 21.2g
Fibre 10g
Plant Points 7.75

ONE-PAN DINNERS

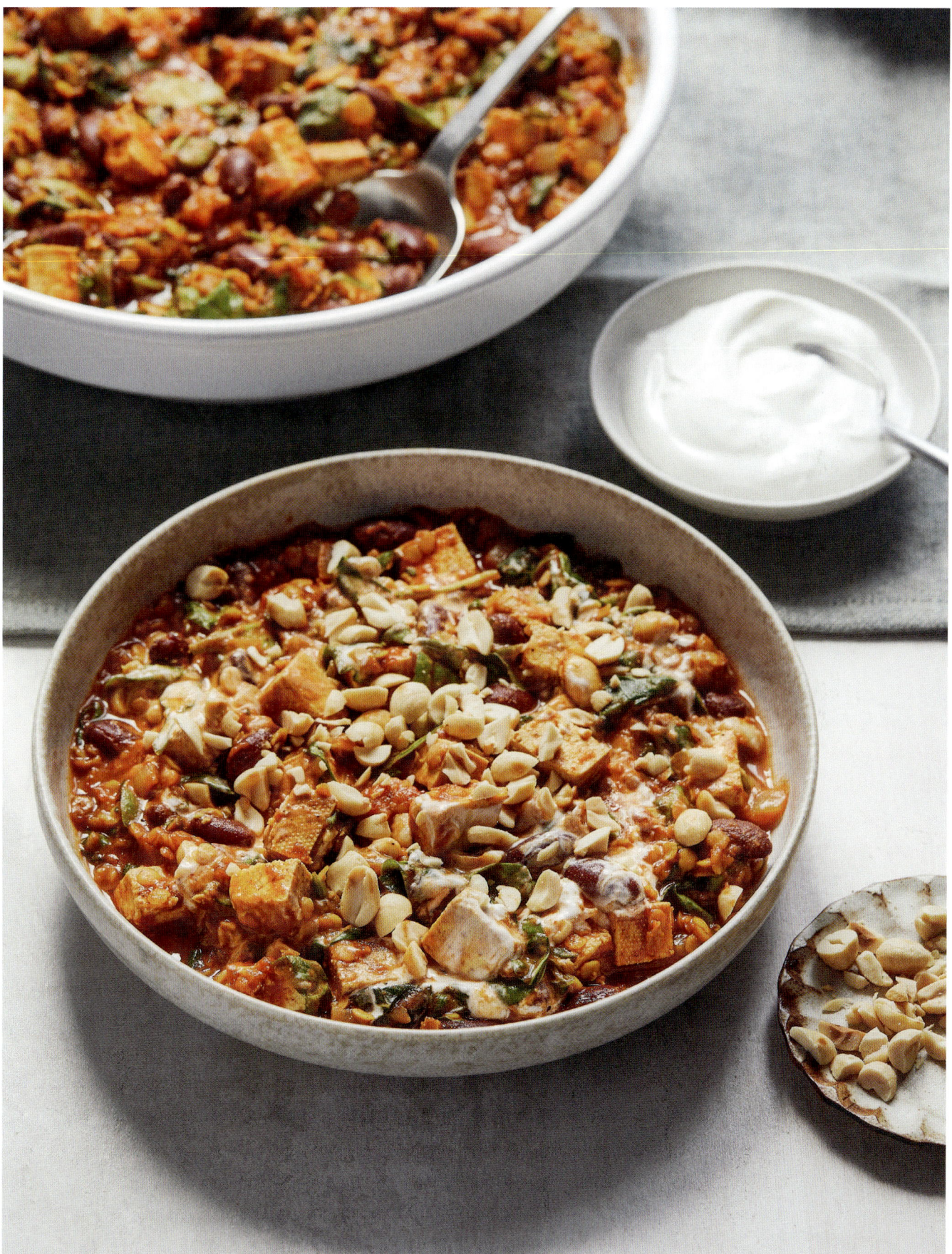

Monkfish with Harissa Chickpeas and Spinach

Prep 5 minutes
Cook 25 minutes

Serves 2

1 x 400g can chickpeas
2 tbsp harissa paste
2 tsp tomato purée
2 garlic cloves, finely grated
200g frozen spinach, defrosted
300g monkfish, cut into 3cm chunks

<u>To serve</u>
Juice of 1 lemon
20g parsley, roughly chopped

Sometimes a jar of quality harissa is all you need to make a delicious, quick meal from minimal ingredients. Chickpeas offer a good dose of prebiotic fibres to help support the function of your microbes to generate metabolites that nourish your gut walls and support the immune system. The light flavour of monkfish takes on the harissa and tomato purée really well. An easy, one-pan crowd-pleaser. Try using different beans like white beans or even green lentils.

Preheat the oven to 180°C fan.

Add the chickpeas with their liquid, the harissa, tomato purée and garlic to a large, ovenproof sauté pan set over a medium heat. Season well with salt and pepper and bring to a simmer. Cook for 6–7 minutes, stirring gently occasionally.

Turn the heat to low–medium, add the spinach and cook, stirring occasionally, for another 5 minutes until heated through.

Remove the pan from the heat, nestle the chunks of monkfish in the sauce and transfer to the oven. Bake for 10 minutes until the monkfish is cooked through.

Add a good squeeze of lemon juice and finish with a scattering of parsley to serve.

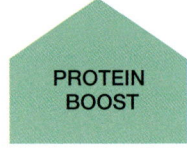
PROTEIN BOOST
Add more fish.

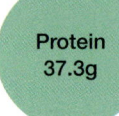
Protein 37.3g | Fibre 12g | Plant Points 3.25

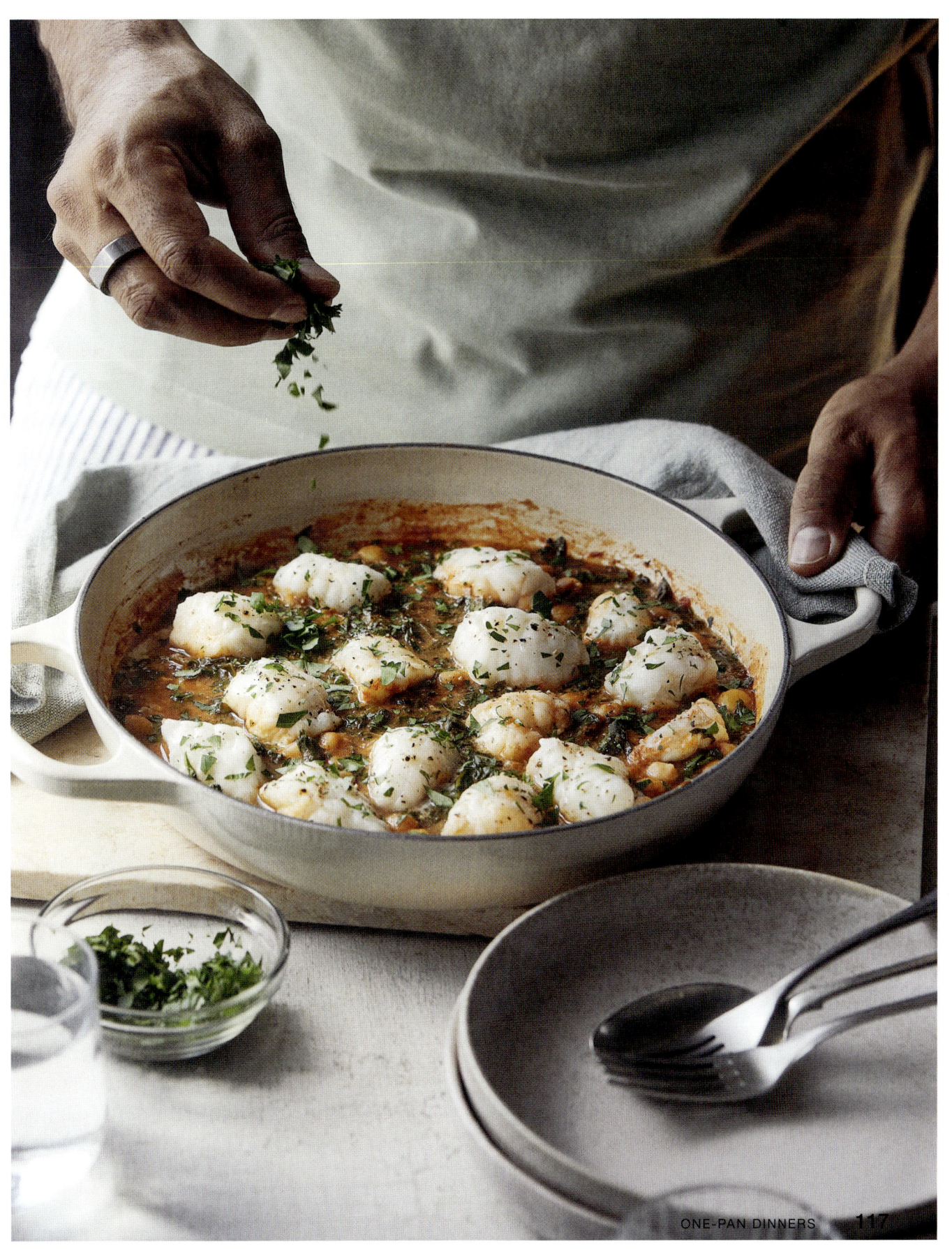

Haricot Bean and Feta Fish Stew

Prep 5 minutes
Cook 25 minutes

Serves 2

200g baby tomatoes, halved
2 tbsp olive oil
2 tbsp harissa paste
50g feta
1 x 400g can haricot beans
200g monkfish, cut into large chunks
100g spinach
30g pistachios, roughly chopped, to serve

When I'm feeling like a 'lazy but healthy' kind of meal, I use this collection of ingredients to create a cosy, delicious one-pan stew packed with wholesome ingredients that comes together so easily. The pistachios contain anti-inflammatory chemicals such as tannins and deliver a beautiful contrasting colour to the rich redness of harissa and tomatoes that have been cooked down to release their gut-friendly polyphenols.

Add the tomatoes and olive oil to a lidded sauté pan over a medium heat with a good pinch of salt.

Add 25ml water and cover with the lid. Cook for 8–10 minutes until the tomatoes have broken down.

Add the harissa paste, crumble in the feta and add the haricot beans with their liquid. Lightly stir the ingredients in the pan together and replace the lid. Cook for another 4–5 minutes until the cheese has melted, creating a creamy spicy sauce.

Add the monkfish, spinach and replace the lid. Cook for another 8 minutes until the fish has fully cooked through.

Finish with the pistachios to serve.

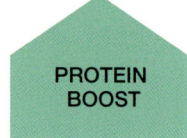

PROTEIN BOOST

Add more fish or pistachios.

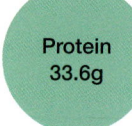

Protein 33.6g | Fibre 13.8g | Plant Points 4.5

ONE-PAN DINNERS

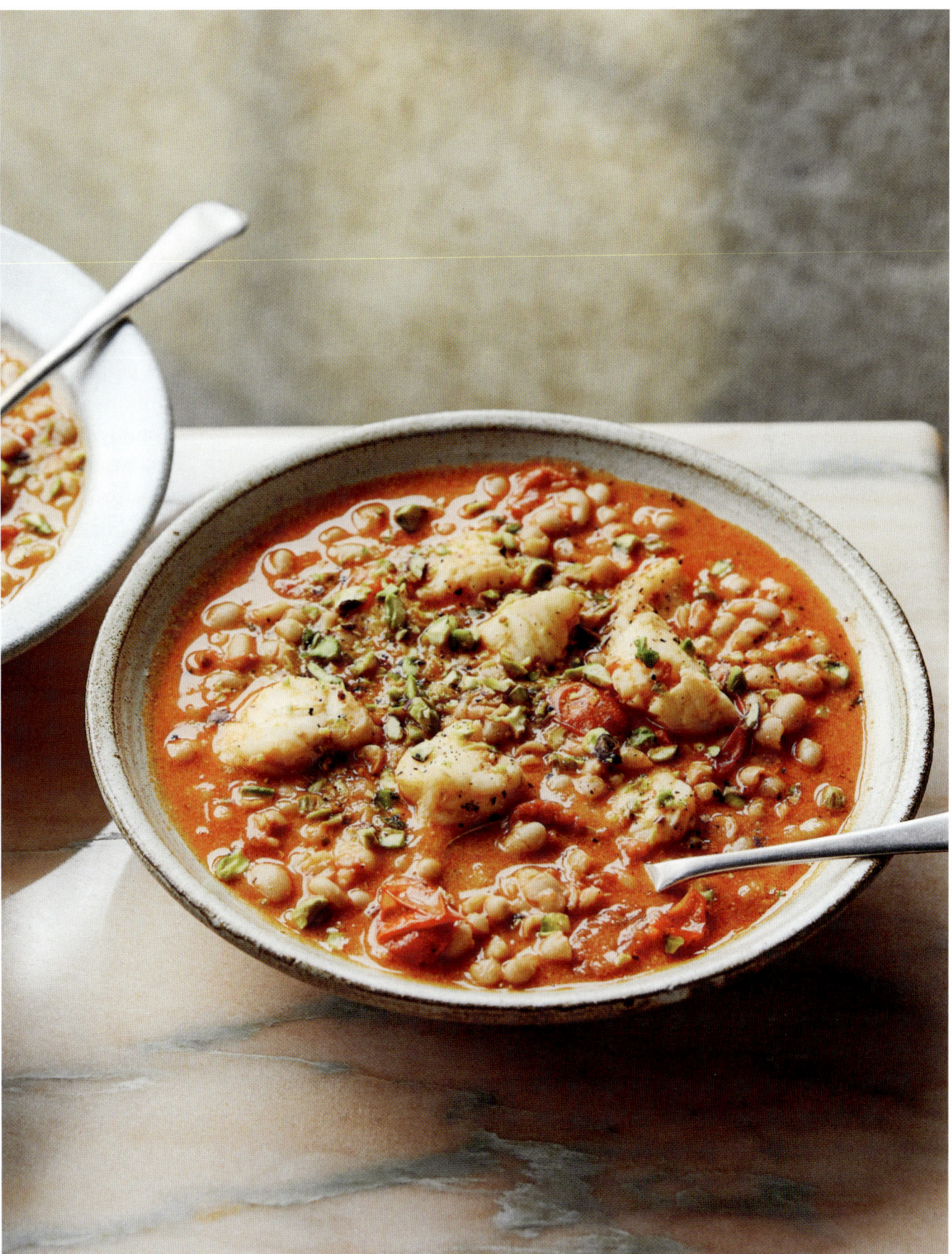

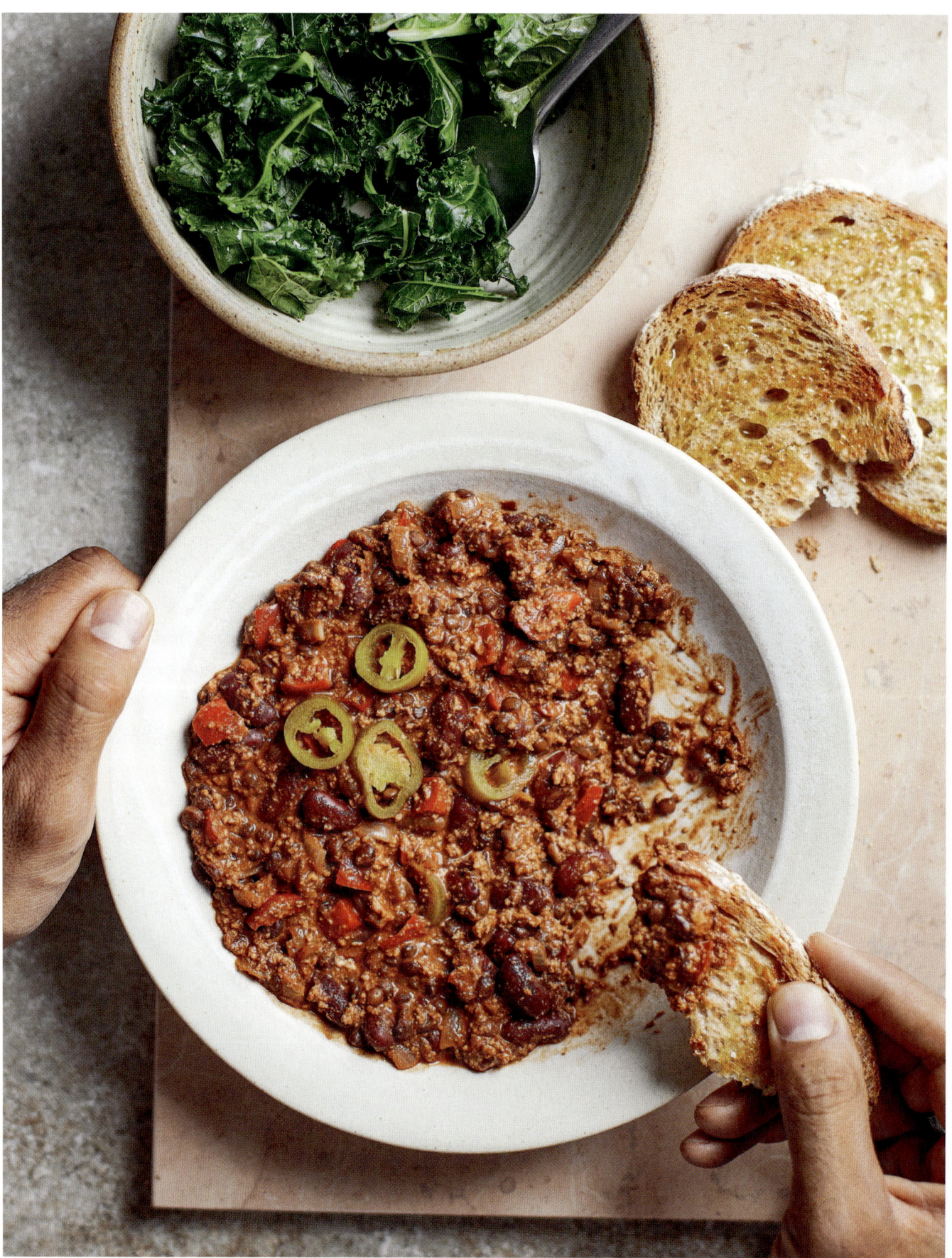

Red Bean Stew with Chocolate and Spices

Prep 15 minutes
Cook 35 minutes

Serves 4

150g onion, finely chopped
2 tbsp olive oil, plus extra to drizzle
100g red pepper, deseeded and finely chopped
2 tsp caraway seeds
1 tsp cumin seeds
400g firm tofu, drained well, finely crumbled
2 tsp smoked paprika
2 tbsp tomato purée
1 tbsp aged balsamic vinegar
200g cooked Puy lentils
1 x 400g can red kidney beans
50g dark chocolate, 75% cocoa solids, finely chopped

To serve
300g kale, stalks removed, and roughly chopped
4 thick slices of rye bread, toasted
40g jalapeños from a jar, sliced

Loosely inspired by the flavours of goulash and mole, this spicy, earthy stew is delicious and wholesome. If you haven't tried it, combining dark chocolate into savoury dishes is magical. The bittersweet polyphenols give a completely new flavour when paired with rich and spicy cumin seeds, paprika and caraway. All these wonderful combinations deliver inflammation and gut-health benefits, plus the tofu packs the protein hit you need. To make the dish even more glorious, try cooking the onions over a low heat for an extra 20 minutes to develop a real savoury-sweet hit. I use firm plain tofu, but smoked tofu would also work really well.

Cook the onion with the olive oil in a heavy-bottomed pan over low–medium heat for 10 minutes until lightly browned, add the red pepper and cook for another 3 minutes, then stir through the caraway and cumin seeds.

Add the tofu, smoked paprika and plenty of seasoning. Stir for 3–4 minutes until the tofu is coated in the spices.

Add the tomato purée, vinegar, lentils and beans with their liquid to the pan. Half-fill the can with water and add to the pan. Stir and simmer very gently over a low heat for 10 minutes to allow all the flavours to infuse.

Add the chopped chocolate and stir until it melts into the sauce.

Meanwhile, steam the kale leaves for 4 minutes in a separate saucepan and drizzle with olive oil.

Serve the stew with the steamed kale, toasted rye bread and jalapeños.

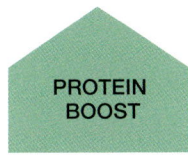

PROTEIN BOOST

You can add extra tofu, pumpkin seeds, peanut butter into the stew. Leftover roast chicken would also work well.

Protein 28.8g
Fibre 15.7g
Plant Points 10.25

ONE-PAN DINNERS

Harissa, Honey and Lentils with Monkfish

Prep 5 minutes
Cook 30 minutes

Serves 4

4 tbsp harissa paste
2 x 400g cans beluga or Puy lentils
2 tbsp honey
3 tbsp tomato purée
600g monkfish, on the bone
200g peas (fresh or defrosted from frozen)
200g frozen spinach, defrosted
2 tbsp olive oil

To serve
20g coriander, leaves finely chopped
30g walnuts, finely chopped

A simple one-pan dish packed with a variety of gut-health-boosting ingredients including lentils and peas. The harissa does the heavy lifting of injecting flavour into this recipe, and pairing it with a good dose of honey mellows the heat. The pulses and fish give this Mediterranean-style dish more than ample healthy protein and the lavish use of greens keeps it anti-inflammatory.

Preheat the oven to 200°C fan.

Add the harissa paste, lentils with their liquid, honey and tomato purée to an ovenproof lidded pan over a medium heat and stir.

Cook for 4–5 minutes until the contents start bubbling, then lay the monkfish into the lentil mixture and cook for 5 minutes with the lid off. Add a bit of hot water if the mixture is looking a little dry and add your peas and spinach, then stir for a minute to combine.

Drizzle with the olive oil, add a good pinch of salt and place in the oven for 15 minutes until the fish is cooked through and golden on top. Depending on the thickness of your monkfish, you may need to cook it in the oven for longer.

Garnish with the coriander and walnuts to serve.

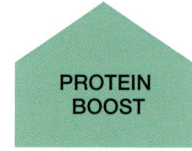

PROTEIN BOOST

Add more monkfish or lentils.

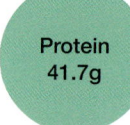

Protein 41.7g

Fibre 12.1g

Plant Points 5

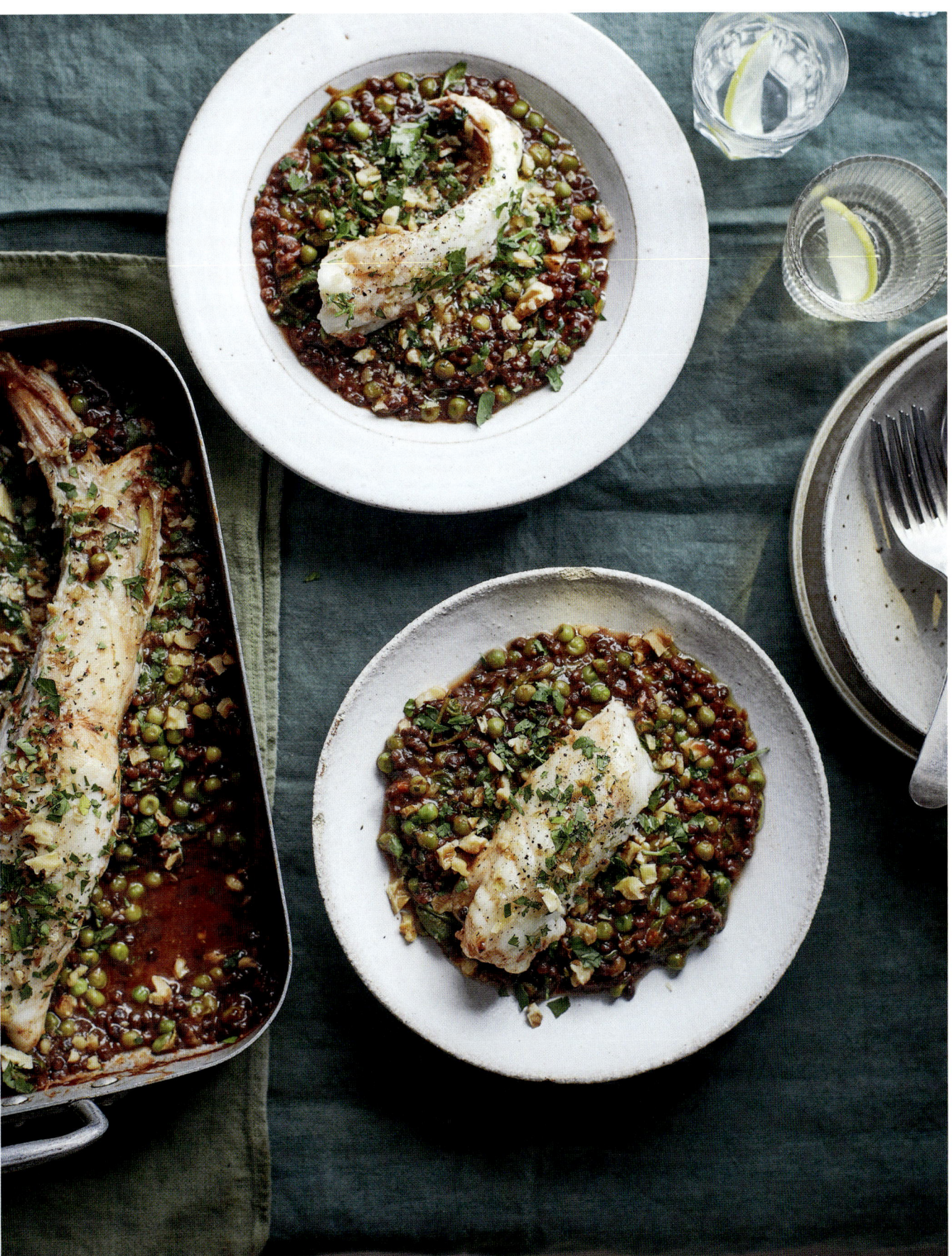

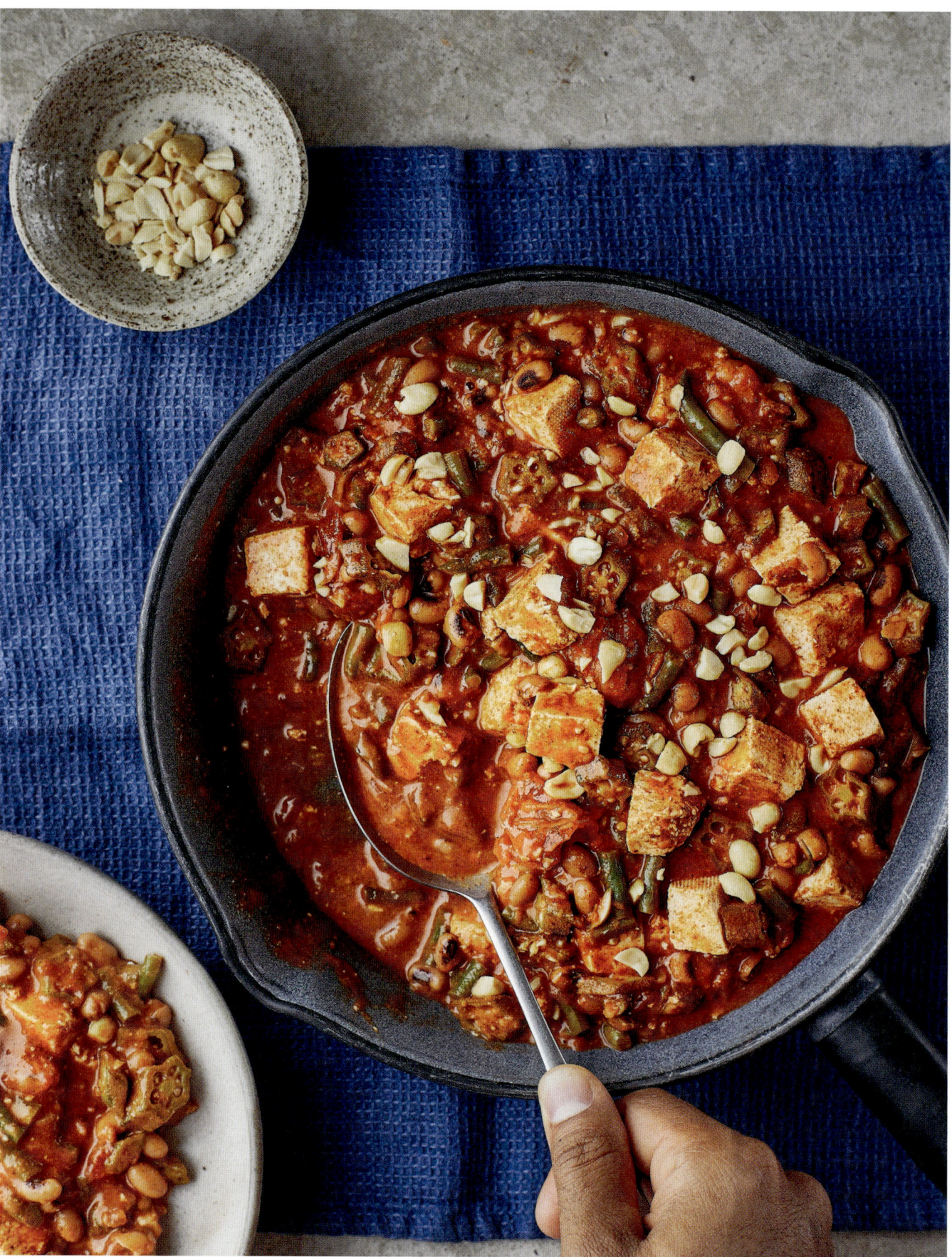

Paprika, Peanut and Okra Stew with Cinnamon

Prep 5 minutes
Cook 25 minutes

Serves 2

- 2 tbsp olive oil
- 4 garlic cloves, grated
- 200g okra, cut into 1cm thick slices
- 200g smoked extra-firm tofu, drained and cut into 1cm cubes
- 200g fine green beans, sliced into 1cm pieces
- 1 tsp ground cinnamon
- 2 tsp smoked paprika
- 1 x 400g can black-eyed peas
- 1 x 400g can peeled plum tomatoes
- 2 tbsp crunchy peanut butter
- 30g roasted peanuts, roughly chopped, to serve

A Zimbabwean chef first showed me how to add peanut butter to curries, and I love this approach. It adds a wealth of flavour as well as a healthy dose of protein and fats to a curry that is difficult to mimic with other ingredients. The okra gives a delicious body and it also contains soluble fibres that help your microbes maintain a healthy gut barrier and reduce inflammation. This smoky dish with the paprika and flavoured tofu is a delicious one-pan mid-week affair which I turn to time and time again.

Heat the olive oil in a large lidded sauté pan over a medium heat. Add the garlic and cook, stirring, for 1 minute before adding the okra, tofu and beans.

Cook for 3–4 minutes until starting to soften, then add the spices and seasoning and stir for another minute to infuse their flavours.

Add the black-eyed peas with their liquid, then crush the whole tomatoes into the pan with your hands. Pour in 100ml water and bring to a simmer, then stir in the peanut butter. Turn the heat to low, cover with the lid and cook for 12–15 minutes until cooked through, adding a splash more water if the sauce looks dry.

Serve the stew topped with the chopped peanuts.

PROTEIN BOOST

Add more tofu, peanut butter. You could also use leftover roast chicken in this dish.

Protein 40.5g
Fibre 21.6g
Plant Points 8

ONE-PAN DINNERS

3 WAYS WITH NUT AND SEED BUTTERS

1. Give some body and a nutritional boost to curries

When making a curry, particularly an Indian or African-style curry with tomatoes, add a tablespoon of smooth peanut butter. It'll give a lot more body to the curry as well as extra protein and healthy, inflammation-lowering fats.

2. Stir-fry

Try adding sesame paste or almond butter to the base of a stir-fry for extra protein and healthy fats. It'll add an extra flavour and a bit of a thicker sauce, especially when mixed with fish sauce or soy sauce.

3. Try it in a sauce

Blending seed and nut butters into sauces is a great way of adding a little extra protein that will go a long way to providing your daily needs. You can also simply use nut butters on their own to provide those nutrients, such as pistachio butter on Greek yoghurt with berries. Try it as a dip for pears and apple with a dash of ground cinnamon, or on top of frozen yoghurt for a boost of flavour.

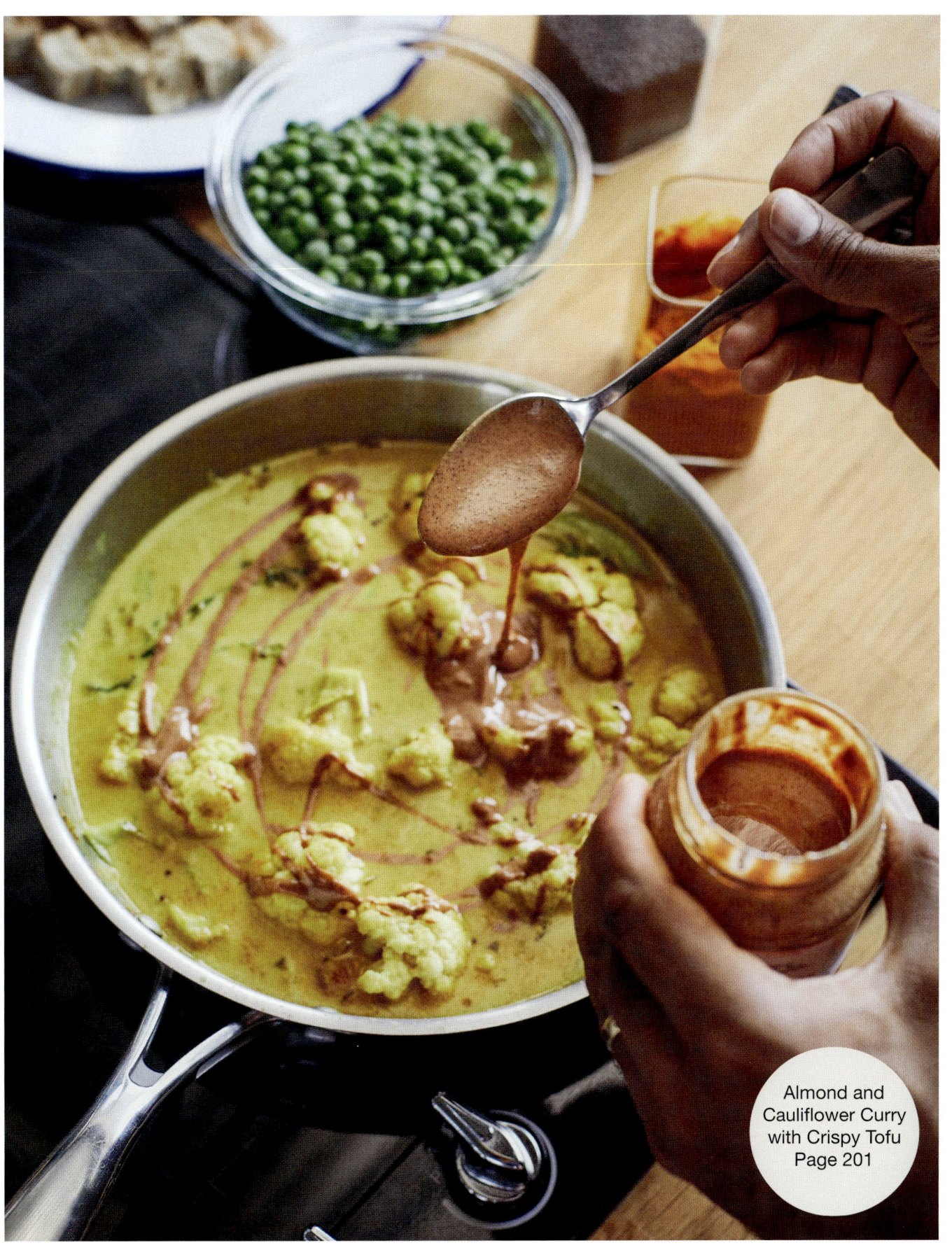

Almond and Cauliflower Curry with Crispy Tofu
Page 201

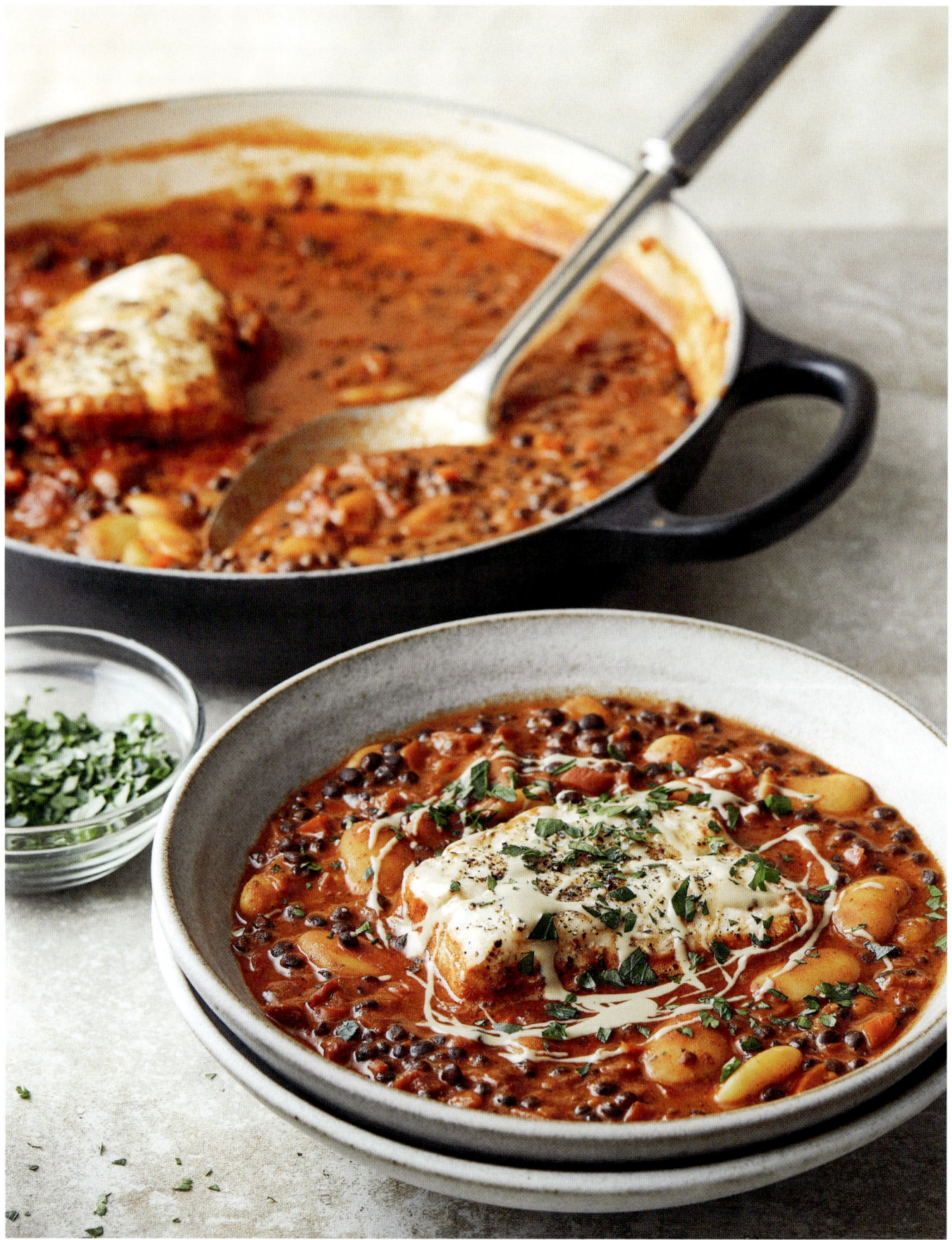

Sundried Tomato and Red Pepper Beans with Hake

Prep 5 minutes
Cook 40 minutes

Serves 2

- 2 tbsp olive oil
- 150g red pepper, deseeded and finely diced
- 30g sundried tomatoes, chopped
- 2 tsp smoked paprika
- 1 tbsp aged balsamic vinegar
- 25g nutritional yeast
- 200ml passata
- 250g cooked beluga lentils
- 1 x 400g can butter beans
- 200g skinless hake fillets
- 3 tbsp tahini
- 10g parsley, finely chopped

Sundried tomatoes are a go-to flavour booster of mine. They're rich in concentrated, tomato, umami goodness, and pack a lot of polyphenols with strong antioxidant activity. In fact, they may reduce the risk of certain cancers as well as age-related eye disease. Combined with smoked paprika, aged balsamic vinegar and nutritional yeast, you have a real rich flavour that works wonderfully with the gut-supporting beluga lentils, butter beans and delicate white fish.

Add the olive oil and red pepper to a large lidded casserole dish over a medium heat and sauté for 10–12 minutes until nicely caramelised.

Add the sundried tomatoes, smoked paprika, vinegar and nutritional yeast, salt and pepper, and stir into the red pepper for a minute.

Add the passata, lentils, beans and 100ml of water and bring to a simmer for 15 minutes, stirring occasionally

Lightly season the hake, then place the fillets into the simmering mixture, cover with the lid and cook for another 5–6 minutes until the fish is cooked through.

Drizzle over the tahini and scatter with the parsley to serve.

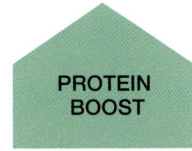

PROTEIN BOOST

Add more hake, tahini, lentils.

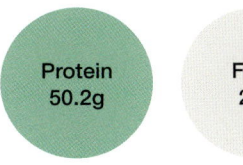

Protein 50.2g · Fibre 23g

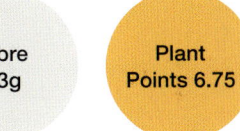

Plant Points 6.75

ONE-PAN DINNERS

Sticky Sweet Chilli Salmon with Roasted Cauliflower

Prep 10 minutes, plus marinating
Cook 55 minutes

Serves 4

For the sweet chilli salmon
3 tbsp dark soy sauce
1 tbsp rice wine vinegar
1 tbsp brown or coconut sugar
1 tsp chilli powder
½ tsp ground cinnamon
500g salmon fillet, skin-on, cut into 4cm square chunks

For the roasted cauliflower
400g cauliflower, broken into florets
200g red onion, cut into thick wedges
200g green pepper, deseeded and cut into large pieces
2 tbsp rice wine vinegar
1 tbsp olive oil
1 x 400g can beluga lentils, drained and rinsed

To serve
20g sesame seeds
30g coriander leaves, finely chopped

The sugar in the rice vinegar caramelises along with the other ingredients to give a delicious, sweet sharp flavour that marries with the buttery soft salmon beautifully. The brassica vegetable, cauliflower, matched with the omega-3 fats of the fish and the fibre content of the lentils, makes for a phenomenally healthy dish that you'll thoroughly enjoy, especially if you love Asian cuisine combinations. A one-tray dish that is perfect for some midweek indulgence with minimal clean-up.

Mix together the soy sauce, rice wine vinegar, sugar and spices in a large bowl. Add the salmon pieces and turn in the marinade until coated. Cover and leave to marinate in the fridge for at least 20 minutes or an hour for maximum flavour.

When you are ready to cook, preheat the oven to 200°C fan.

Spread out the cauliflower, onion and green pepper on a large baking tray. Pour over the rice wine vinegar and olive oil, then toss with your hands until combined. Roast the vegetables for 30 minutes, turning halfway through. Remove the tray from the oven and pour the marinade from the salmon over the vegetables, leaving the salmon pieces in the bowl. Return the baking tray to the oven for another 10 minutes.

Remove the tray from the oven, stir the lentils into the vegetables and place the salmon pieces on top. Return to the oven to cook for a final 8 minutes. The salmon should be cooked through and caramelised and the juices in the tray dark and sticky.

Finish the dish with a sprinkling of sesame seeds and coriander.

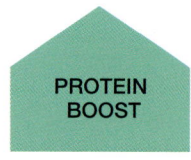

PROTEIN BOOST

Add more fish.

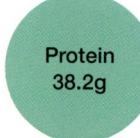

Protein 38.2g | Fibre 8.3g | Plant Points 5

130 ONE-PAN DINNERS

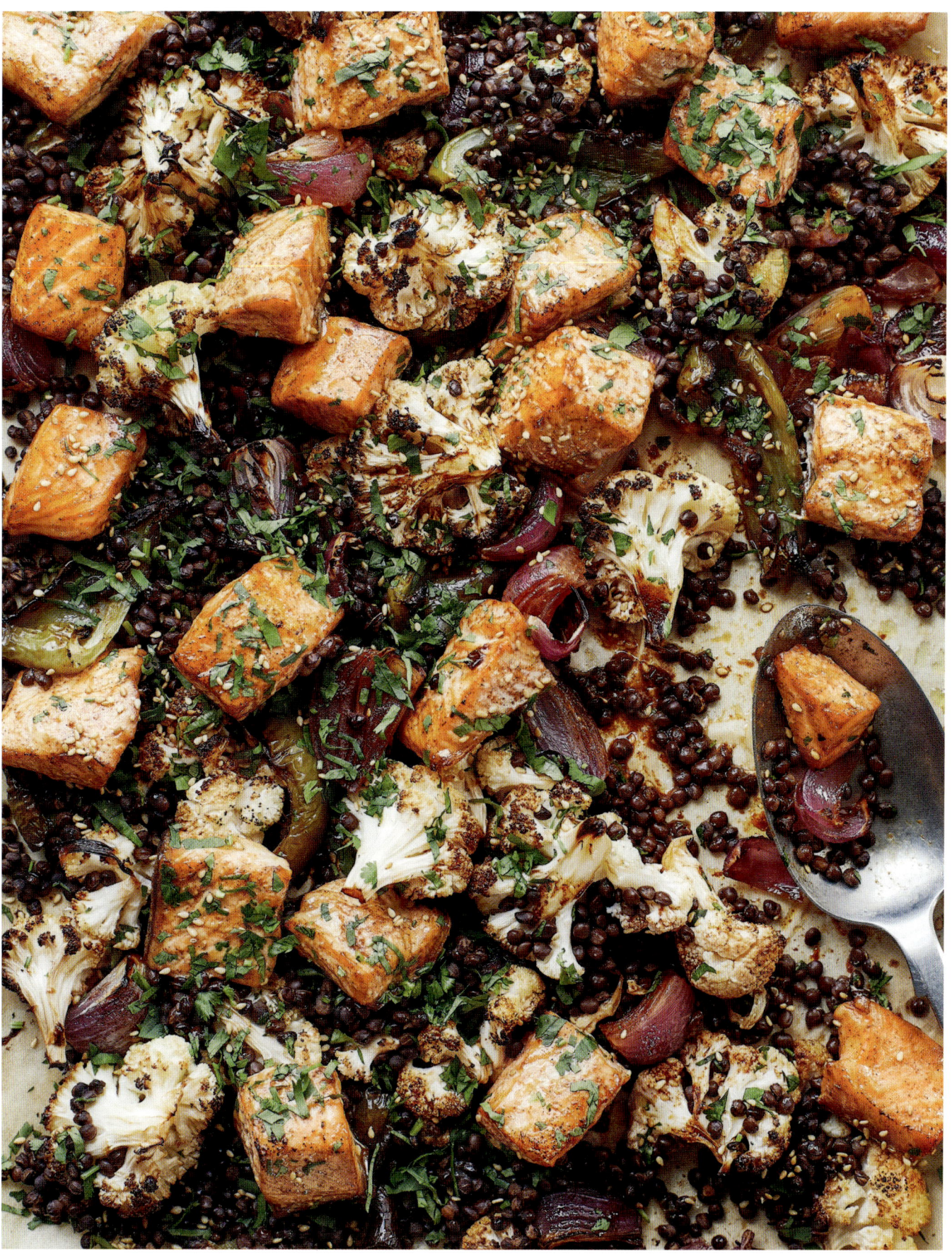

Lazy Coconut Fish Curry

Prep 5 minutes
Cook 25 minutes

Serves 2

- 1 tbsp olive oil
- 15g fresh root ginger, peeled and grated
- 2 tsp mustard seeds
- 10–12 curry leaves
- 1 ground tsp turmeric
- 1 tsp Kashmiri chilli powder or sweet paprika
- 200g peas (fresh or defrosted from frozen)
- 1 x 400g can green lentils, drained and rinsed
- 100g frozen spinach, defrosted
- 1 x 400ml can full-fat coconut milk
- 150ml just-boiled water
- 350g skinless haddock fillet, cut into 5cm chunks
- Juice and finely grated zest of 1 lime
- 2 tsp dried fenugreek leaves or fresh coriander leaves (optional)

I rely on this dish when I want to impress my wife with minimal effort. And it surprises me every time just how impactful these glorious, nutrient-rich spices are at transforming coconut milk into a gorgeous, flavourful sauce for the fish. It's so simple and uses largely store-cupboard ingredients. If I see a good piece of white fish at the fishmongers and I feel like something lazy but healthy, I make this easy dish. You can use coriander leaves instead of the fenugreek at the end to garnish, but if you can get these dried leaves, they make a world of difference to the flavour.

Add the olive oil to a large sauté pan over a medium heat. Stir in the ginger, mustard seeds and curry leaves, then cook for about 1 minute until the mustard seeds start to pop.

Stir in the turmeric and chilli powder or paprika before adding the peas and lentils. Stir until combined, then add the spinach and coconut milk with the hot water and bring to a simmer. Turn the heat to low and cook for 10 minutes, stirring occasionally, to infuse the flavours. Season with salt and pepper.

Rub the fish in half of the lime juice and add it to the simmering coconut curry. Cook for 6–8 minutes until the fish is opaque white and starting to flake. Finish with a sprinkling of fenugreek or coriander leaves, if you like, as well as the remaining lime juice and the zest.

PROTEIN BOOST

Add more haddock, use extra lentils.

- Protein 51.2g
- Fibre 12g
- Plant Points 6

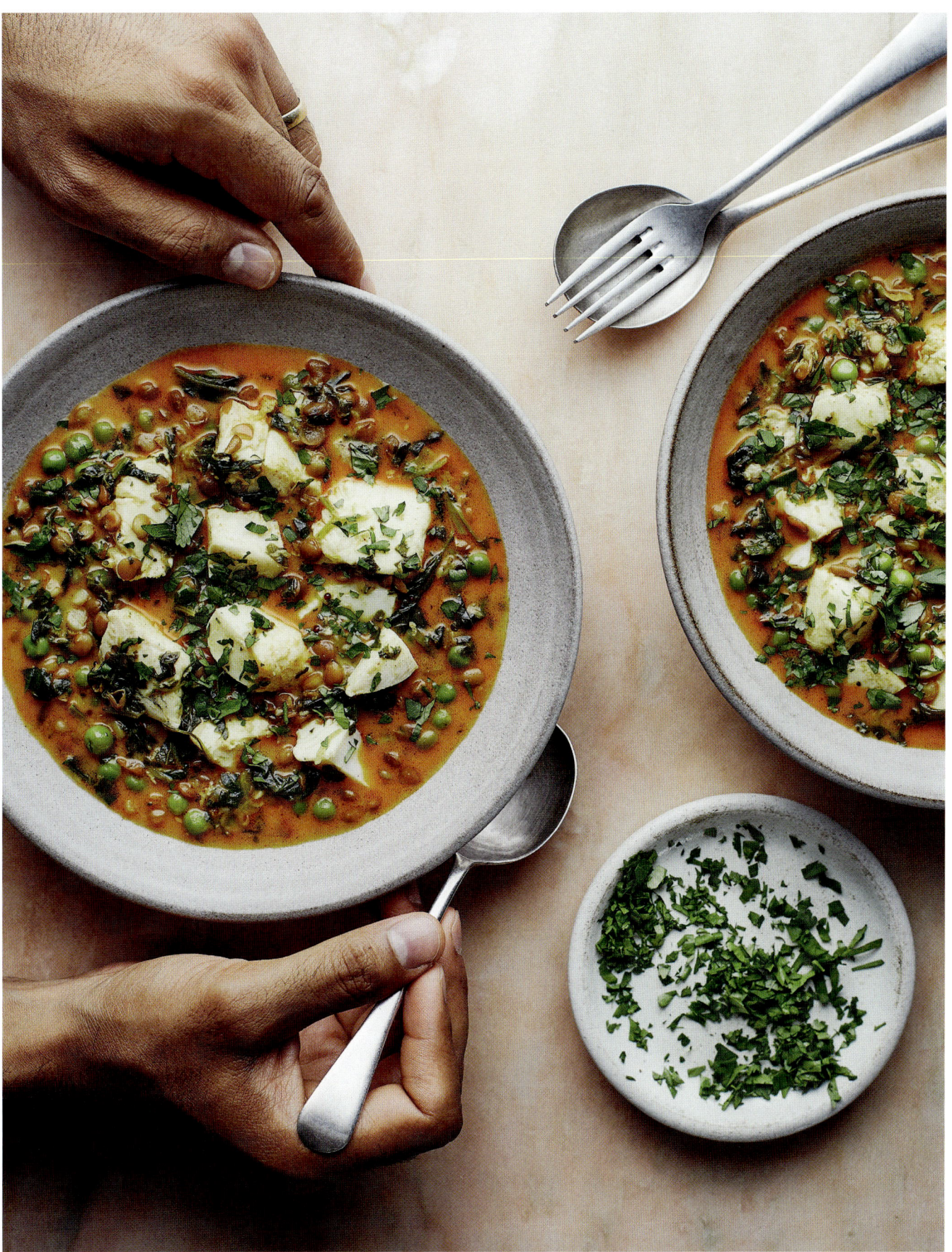

Rich and Silky Beans with Nachos

Prep 10 minutes
Cook 35 minutes

Serves 2

2 tbsp olive oil
200g red onion, finely diced
200g red pepper, deseeded and finely diced
5 garlic cloves, thinly sliced
2 tsp smoked paprika
1 tsp cumin seeds
1 tsp ground cinnamon
2 tbsp raw cacao
1 x 400g can black beans
250g cooked beluga lentils
2 tsp raw honey
200ml just-boiled water

To serve
150g corn tortilla baked chips
Zest and juice of 1 lime
50g queso fresco or light feta, crumbled
1 avocado, halved, stoned removed and sliced thinly
50g baby tomatoes, halved

This dish is a nod to a mole stew, the traditional dish of Oaxaca, in Mexico, which I visited during my medical elective. I'd never experienced the flavours of raw cacao and smoky chilli in a dish before. I was instantly hooked. The cacao in this bean and lentil stew gives a rich and complex sour flavour which needs a touch of honey to round it out. The benefits of cacao are vast, ranging from promoting heart health to brain-boosting properties, so I love combining it into dishes as much as possible. The extra collection of spices further adds to the anti-inflammatory properties and this makes a perfect casual meal with good-quality 100% corn tortilla baked chips. The black beans also have the highest protein content of any bean. This is a generous dish which will probably leave you with some leftovers that are perfect for a snack the next day.

Put a large saucepan over low–medium heat and add the olive oil. Sauté the red onion, red pepper and garlic in the oil, season with salt and pepper and cook for 15–20 minutes, stirring occasionally, until jammy and caramelised.

Add the spices and cacao and cook for another minute before adding the beans with their liquid, lentils, honey and the hot water. Simmer for another 15 minutes to intensify the flavours.

Scatter the tortilla chips over a platter, top with the beans, sprinkle over the lime zest and juice and cheese and serve with the avocado and tomatoes with a sprinkle of paprika.

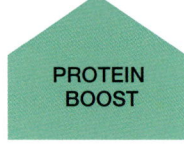

PROTEIN BOOST

Add more cheese, lentils.

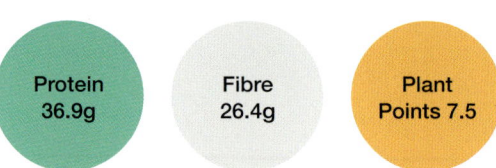

Protein 36.9g
Fibre 26.4g
Plant Points 7.5

134 ONE-PAN DINNERS

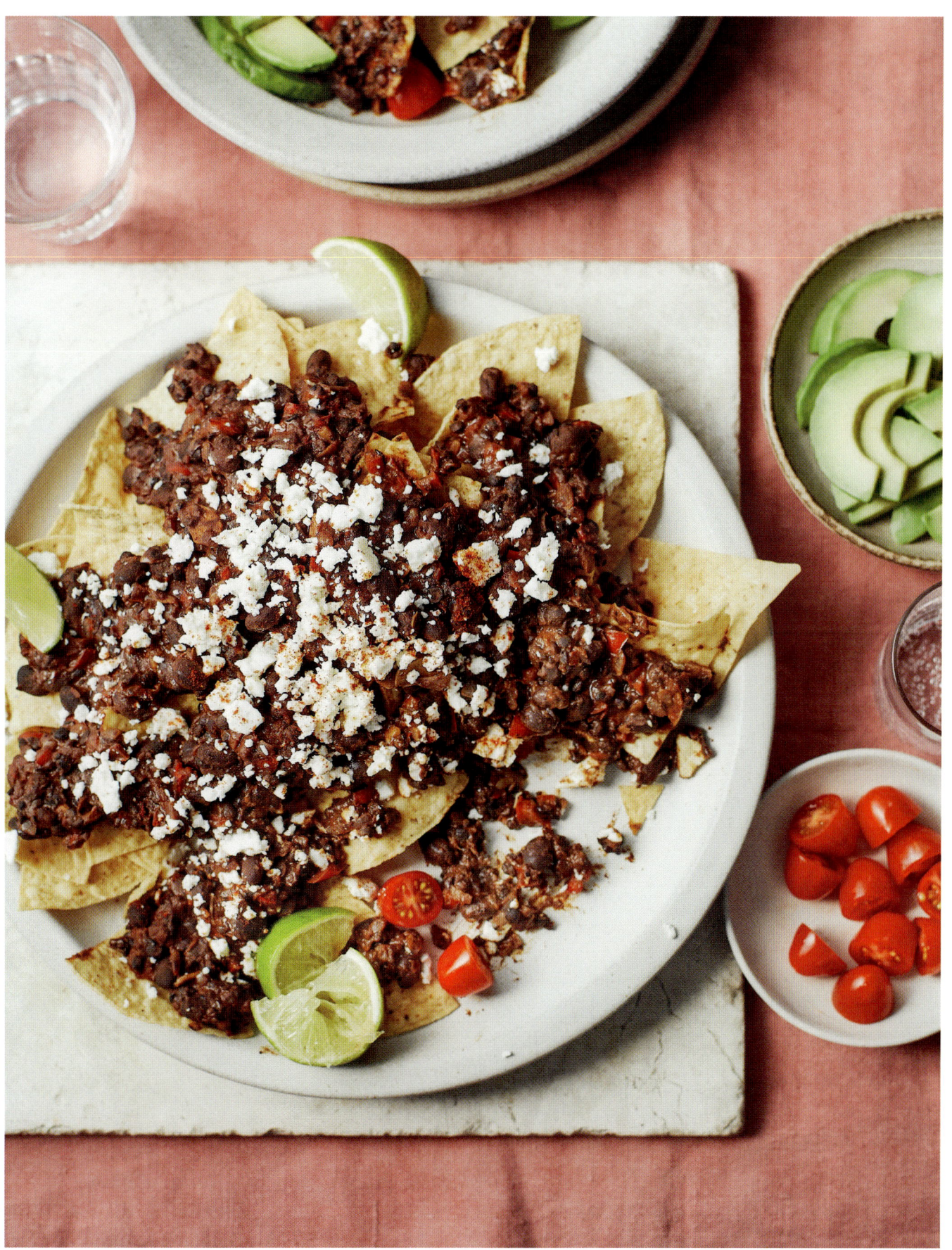

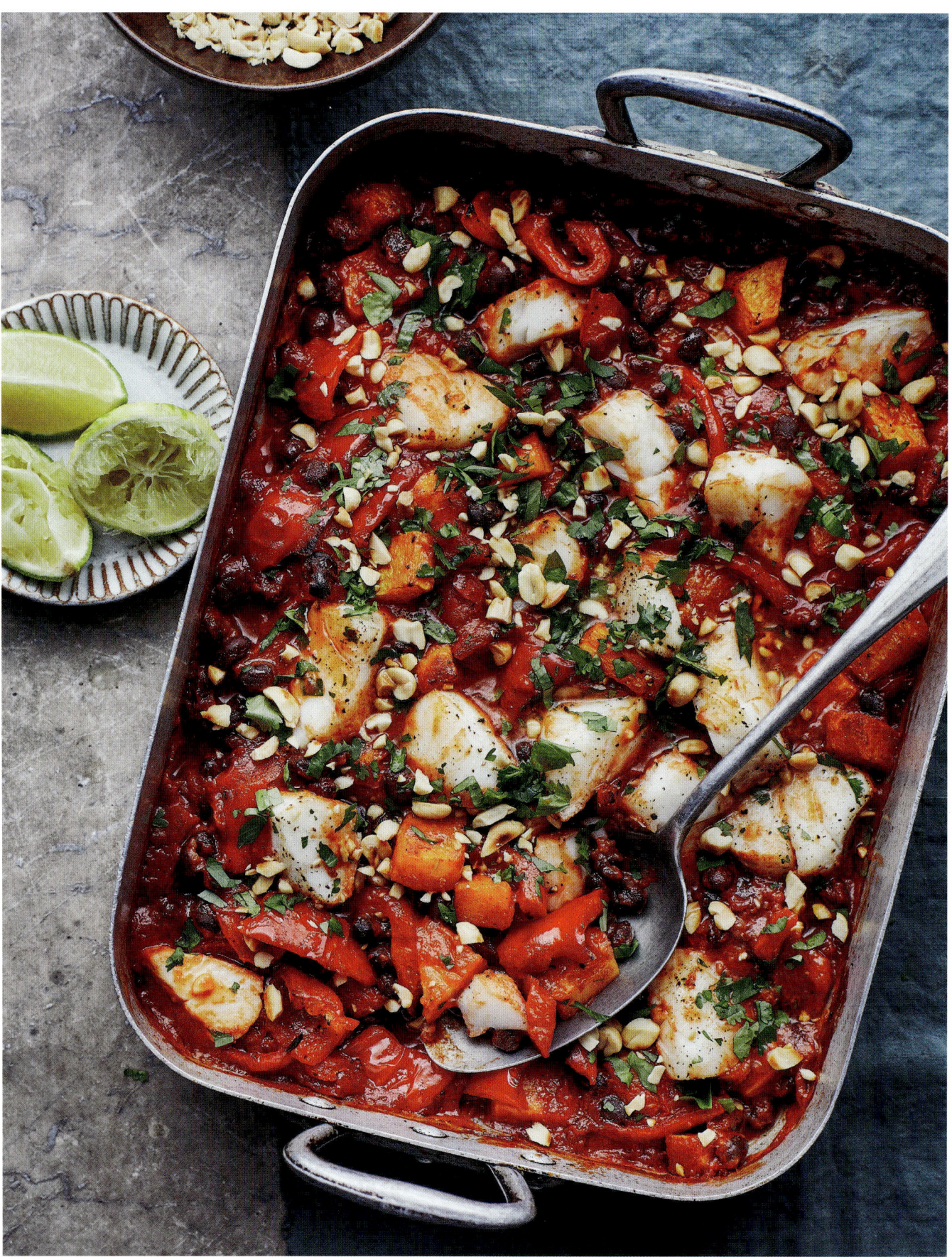

Spicy Gochujang Bake with Cod and Toasted Peanuts

Prep 10 minutes
Cook 45 minutes

Serves 2

250g butternut squash, cut into 3cm cubes
200g red pepper, deseeded and cut into 3cm chunks
2 tbsp olive oil
300ml passata
2 tbsp gochujang
1 x 400g can black beans, drained and rinsed
300g cod fillet, cut into 3cm chunks

To serve
Juice of 1 lime
10g coriander leaves, chopped (optional)
40g peanuts, lightly toasted and crushed

A super-lazy meal that packs flavour with the simple addition of gochujang. By roasting the squash we add further natural sweetness to our meals, plus black beans and peanuts are delivering extra protein and fibre to our white fish. A simple collection of ingredients all brought together effortlessly into one tray. A perfect, no-fuss midweek meal for two.

Preheat the oven to 200°C fan.

Add the squash and pepper to a deep baking tray, season well with salt and pepper and drizzle over 1 tablespoon of oil. Toss with your hands to coat the vegetables in the oil, then roast in the oven for 25 minutes, turning halfway through.

Mix together the passata and gochujang in a mixing bowl, then add the black beans and stir to combine. Remove the baking tray, add the black bean mixture, stir through the squash and peppers and return to the oven for 8 minutes.

Remove the tray again, nestle in the chunks of fish, drizzle with the remaining olive oil, season the fish and cook for a further 8 minutes until the ingredients are bubbling and slightly charred in areas, and the fish is cooked through.

Add a good squeeze of lime juice, scatter over coriander leaves, if using, and top with the toasted peanuts to serve.

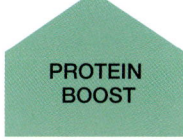

PROTEIN BOOST
Add more fish or peanuts.

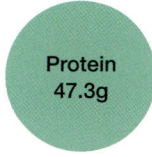

Protein 47.3g | Fibre 12.5g | Plant Points 6

ONE-PAN DINNERS

Sweet Spring Harissa Beans with Pecorino

Prep 10 minutes
Cook 15 minutes

Serves 2

2 tbsp olive oil
100g white onion, finely chopped
4 garlic cloves, thinly sliced
200g courgette, cut into small chunks
150g asparagus, stalks thinly sliced and tips left whole
100g kale, tough stalks removed and leaves roughly chopped
1 x 400g can white beans
1 tbsp harissa paste
50g pecorino, coarsely grated
10g dill, finely chopped
2 tsp honey, to serve

The typical combinations with in-season asparagus are to allow the subtle flavours of this vegetable to sing as loudly as possible. But I think a touch of heat with harissa and a hit of saltiness with pecorino make good partners. You might shudder at the thought of all these ingredients in the pan, but they work well. I've packed this with three types of greens to ensure the gut health and inflammation benefits are met too.

Add the oil to a large sauté pan over a medium heat. Add the onion and cook for 5 minutes until softened, then add the garlic and cook for another minute until lightly browned.

Add the courgette and asparagus stalks and cook, stirring occasionally, for 3–4 minutes until softened, before adding the kale and asparagus tips.

Tip in the white beans with their liquid, the harissa paste and a splash of water to loosen. Stir to combine and bring to a gentle simmer over a low–medium heat. Cook for 4–5 minutes until the vegetables are just tender. Season with salt and pepper.

Stir in the pecorino and dill and finish with a drizzle of honey to serve.

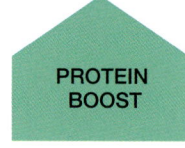

PROTEIN BOOST
Add more white beans.

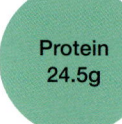

Protein 24.5g
Fibre 17.3g
Plant Points 6

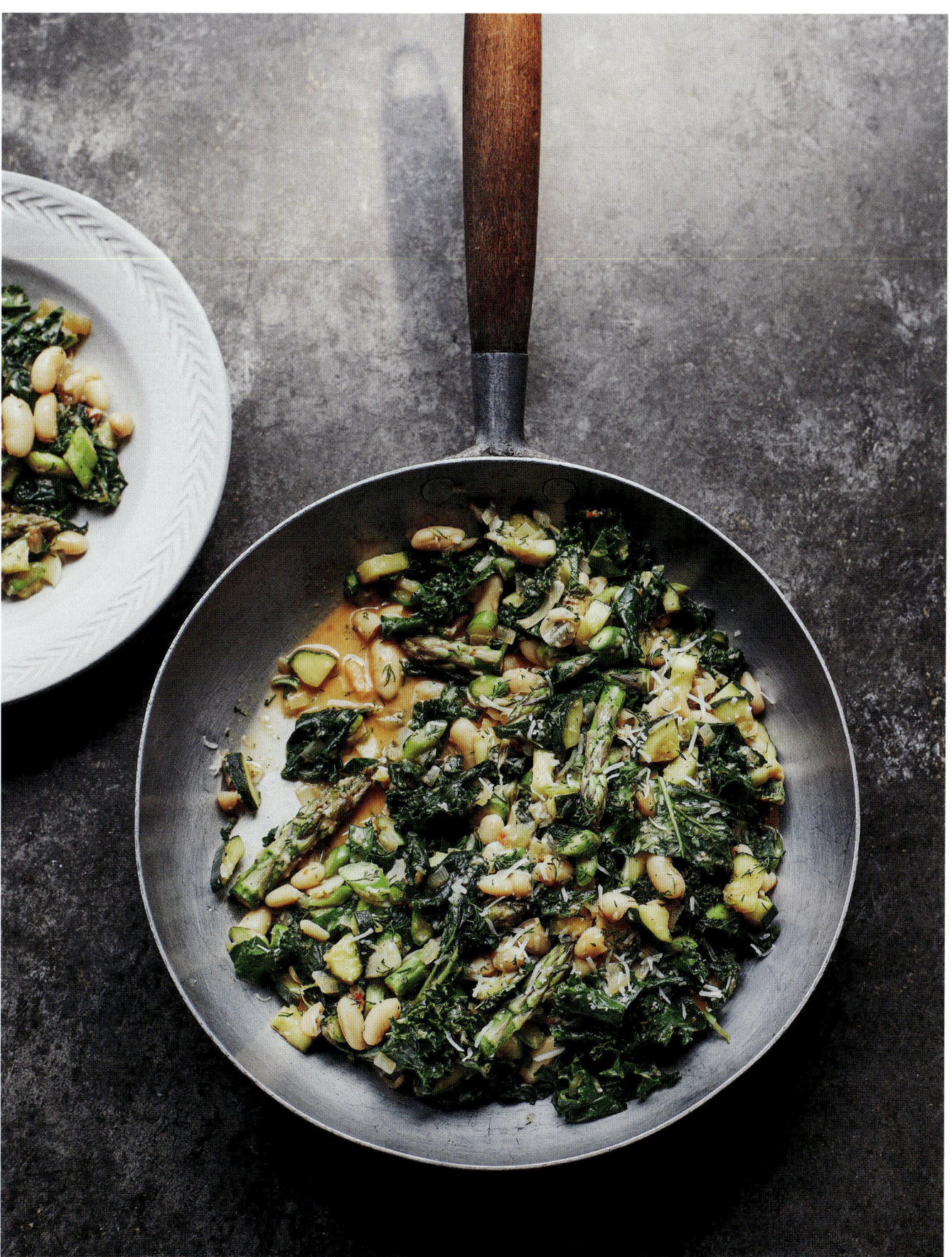

Smoky Paprika Lentils with Hake and Dill

Prep 15 minutes, plus soaking
Cook 35 minutes

Serves 2

- 2 tbsp olive oil
- 150g celery, finely diced
- 150g fennel, finely diced
- 100g baby tomatoes, roughly chopped
- 1 tsp fennel seeds
- 1 tsp smoked paprika
- 1 tsp English mustard powder
- ½ tsp dried chilli flakes
- 100g split red lentils, soaked for 20 minutes, thoroughly rinsed and drained well
- 300ml vegetable stock
- 100g frozen spinach, defrosted
- 200g thick skinless hake fillet, cut into thick 3cm chunks
- 20g dill, finely chopped, to serve

Smoky paprika with fish and soft herbs transport me to the Mediterranean in an instant. The vibrant red colours and delicate white fish are a beautiful combination that works so well. I like to mix up the aromatics used at the start of the dish every now and then. Celery, fennel and baby tomatoes have delicious flavours when lightly sautéed together, and you'll appreciate these as much as onion and garlic. The variety of vegetables used in this dish will keep your microbes happy and deliver on those anti-inflammatory benefits that you want.

Heat the olive oil in a large, lidded sauté pan over a low–medium heat. Add the celery, fennel and tomatoes and cook, covered with the lid, for 10 minutes until the vegetables are tender and starting to colour.

Add the fennel seeds, spices and lentils and stir for a minute, before adding the vegetable stock, then bring to a simmer. Turn the heat to low, cover with the lid and cook gently for 15 minutes until the stock has almost been absorbed and the lentils have cooked through.

Stir in the spinach and heat through, season with salt and pepper, then sit the chunks of hake into the lentils. Turn up the heat to medium and cook, covered, for 5 minutes until the fish is cooked through. Spoon into shallow serving bowls and garnish with dill to serve.

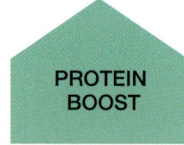

PROTEIN BOOST

Add more fish, red lentils.

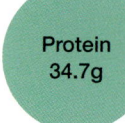

Protein 34.7g | Fibre 10g | Plant Points 6.5

140 ONE-PAN DINNERS

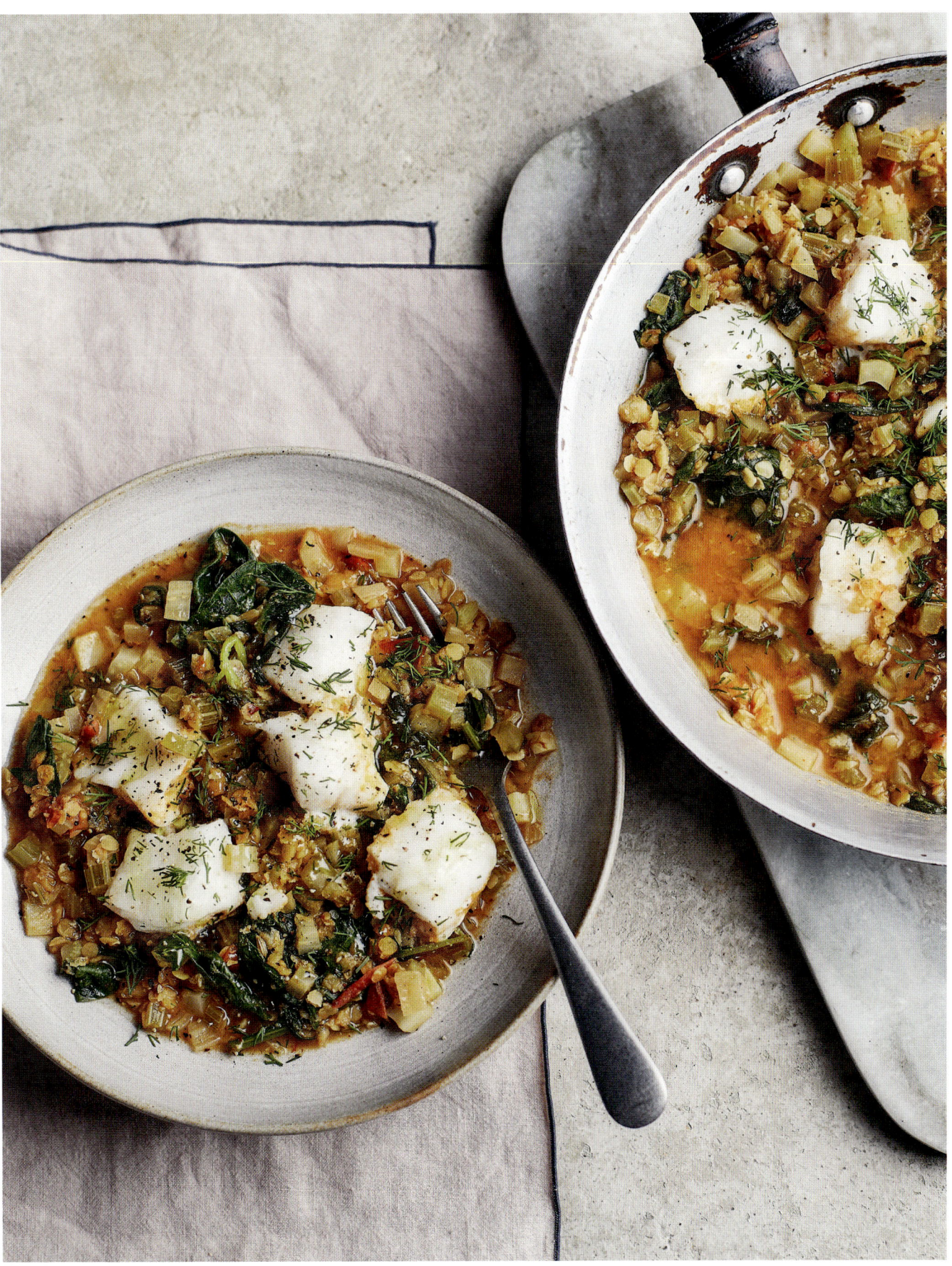

HIGH-
PROTEIN

DIVER-
SITY
BOWLS

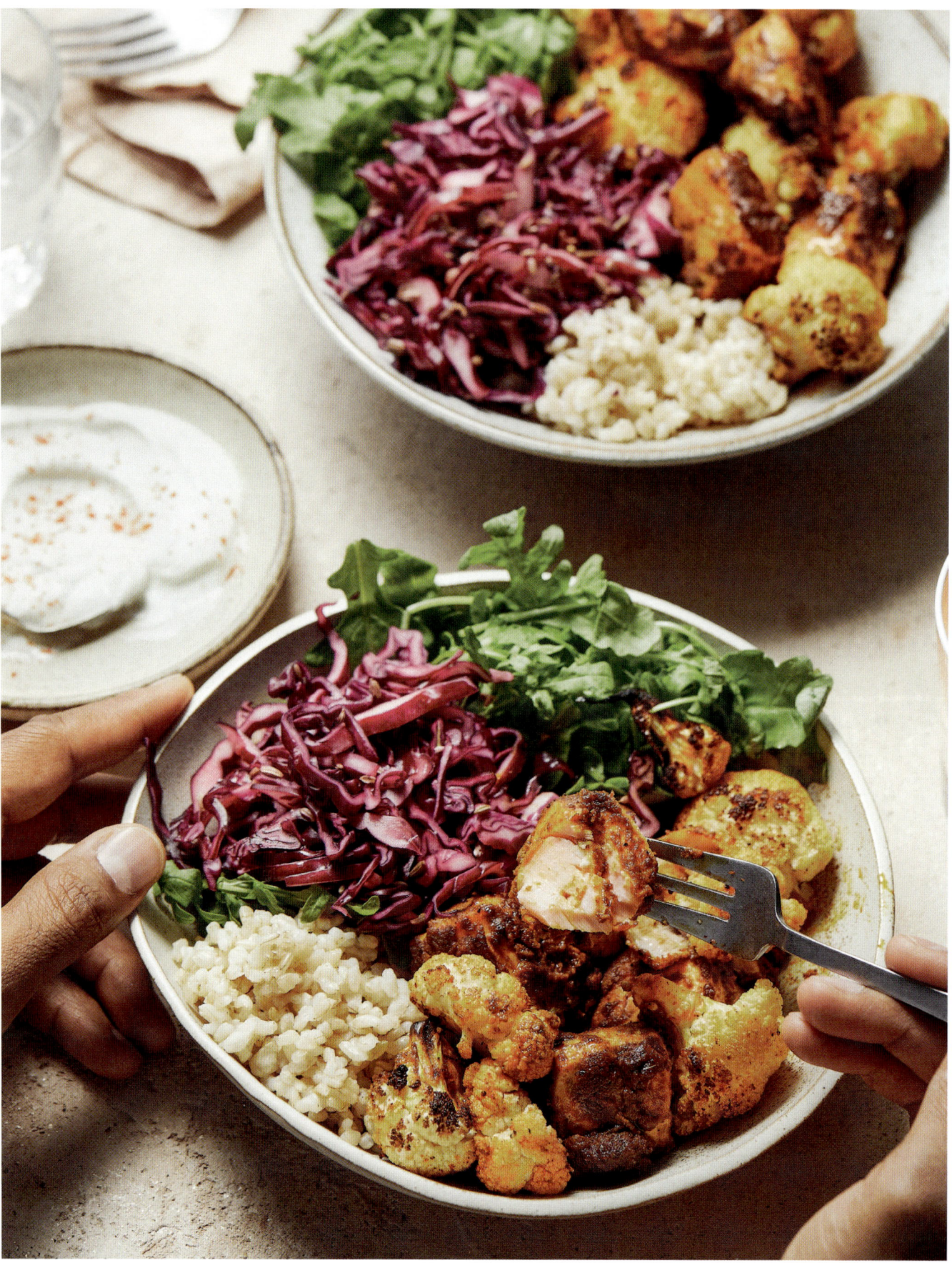

Salmon Tikka Bowls with a Quick Fennel and Cabbage Pickle

Prep 10 minutes, plus marinating
Cook 30 minutes

Serves 2

300g salmon, skin on, cut into thick 4cm chunks
2 tbsp tikka masala paste or mild curry paste
300g cauliflower, broken into 2cm florets
1 tsp mustard seeds
½ tsp ground turmeric
½ tsp Kashmiri chilli or sweet paprika
1 tbsp olive oil, plus extra to drizzle

For the fennel and cabbage pickle
100g red cabbage, finely shredded with a mandolin
2 tsp fennel seeds
4 tsp red wine vinegar
4 tsp apple juice or 1 tsp sugar
½ tsp salt

To serve
150g cooked short-grain brown rice, warmed
2 tbsp Greek yoghurt
100g rocket leaves

Every Tuesday in the Doctor's Kitchen household, it's salmon bowl night. We use a single tray to make the most delicious and easy bowls, packed with vegetables, grains and high-protein oily fish. It's something I always look forward to. You can easily use an air fryer to cook the salmon instead in half the time, and if you want a recipe for a curry paste that's low in sugar, use the one on page 249.

Preheat the oven to 200°C fan.

Smother the salmon in the curry paste and cover with foil in a bowl. Leave to marinate in the fridge for 20 minutes (it's even better overnight).

Add the cauliflower to a baking tray, sprinkle over the spices and drizzle over the olive oil and mix well. Then season well and bake for 15 minutes.

Meanwhile, add the cabbage, fennel seeds, vinegar, apple juice or sugar and salt to a mixing bowl and scrunch everything together with your hands for 30 seconds. Set aside.

Remove the tray from the oven, toss the cauliflower florets and turn up the heat to 220°C fan. Nestle the salmon, skin-side up, between the cauliflower florets and bake for another 10–12 minutes until the salmon is cooked through and golden coloured with some charring.

Build your bowls with the warmed rice, fennel and cabbage pickle, dollops of yoghurt, salmon and cauliflower, and rocket leaves with a drizzle of oil.

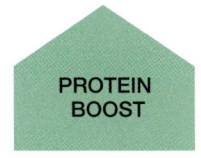

PROTEIN BOOST
Add more salmon.

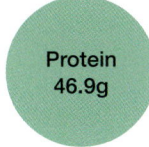
Protein 46.9g

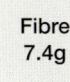
Fibre 7.4g

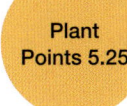
Plant Points 5.25

HIGH-PROTEIN DIVERSITY BOWLS

Air-fried Cajun Chicken with Fennel Slaw and Watermelon

Prep 10 minutes
Cook 25 minutes

Serves 2

200g boneless, skinless chicken thighs, cut into 3cm chunks
2 tsp Cajun or Creole spice mix
1 tbsp soy sauce
2 tsp cornflour or rice flour
1 tbsp olive oil

For the fennel slaw
150g fennel, finely shredded with a mandolin
4 tsp white wine vinegar
2 tsp orange juice or 1 tsp sugar
1 tsp coriander seeds
½ tsp salt

To serve
150g mixed salad leaves, torn
100g cooked short-grain brown rice, warmed
150g watermelon, cut into 2cm chunks
1 avocado, sliced
1 tbsp chipotle or chilli sauce

Fried chicken has always been my kryptonite. And when I started playing around with air fryers a couple of years ago, I became determined to mimic that crunch and crispy texture of breaded and fried chicken in a slightly healthier way. While I don't think this is quite the same, it does satisfy the urge for an unhealthy takeaway. The salty, spicy, herby Cajun spice mix pairs beautifully with the sharp slaw and sweetness of the watermelon. Plus, with the collection of ingredients in these amounts, it's designed to be gut friendly too!

Preheat your air fryer to 205°C and rub the chicken in the spices, seasoning and soy sauce. Leave to marinate while you make your slaw.

Add the shredded fennel to a mixing bowl with the vinegar, juice or sugar, coriander seeds and salt. Mix thoroughly together scrunching with your hands to break down the fennel shreds and then set aside.

Toss the chicken through the cornflour or rice flour to coat, then drizzle with the olive oil and add to the air fryer. Cook for 12 minutes until crispy and cooked through.

Build your bowls with the slaw, salad leaves, warmed rice, watermelon, avocado and chicken. Lightly dress the chipotle or chilli sauce on top of the bowls (using a sauce bottle with a fine nozzle if you have one).

Note
You can also use the oven, preheated to 220°C fan, to cook the chicken. Bake the chicken for 15 minutes until cooked through.

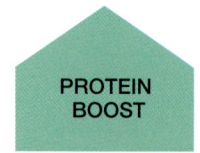

PROTEIN BOOST

Add more chicken. Air-fried white beans (page 156) would also work well.

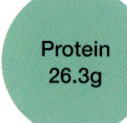

Protein 26.3g

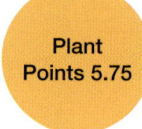

Fibre 7.4g

Plant Points 5.75

HIGH-PROTEIN DIVERSITY BOWLS

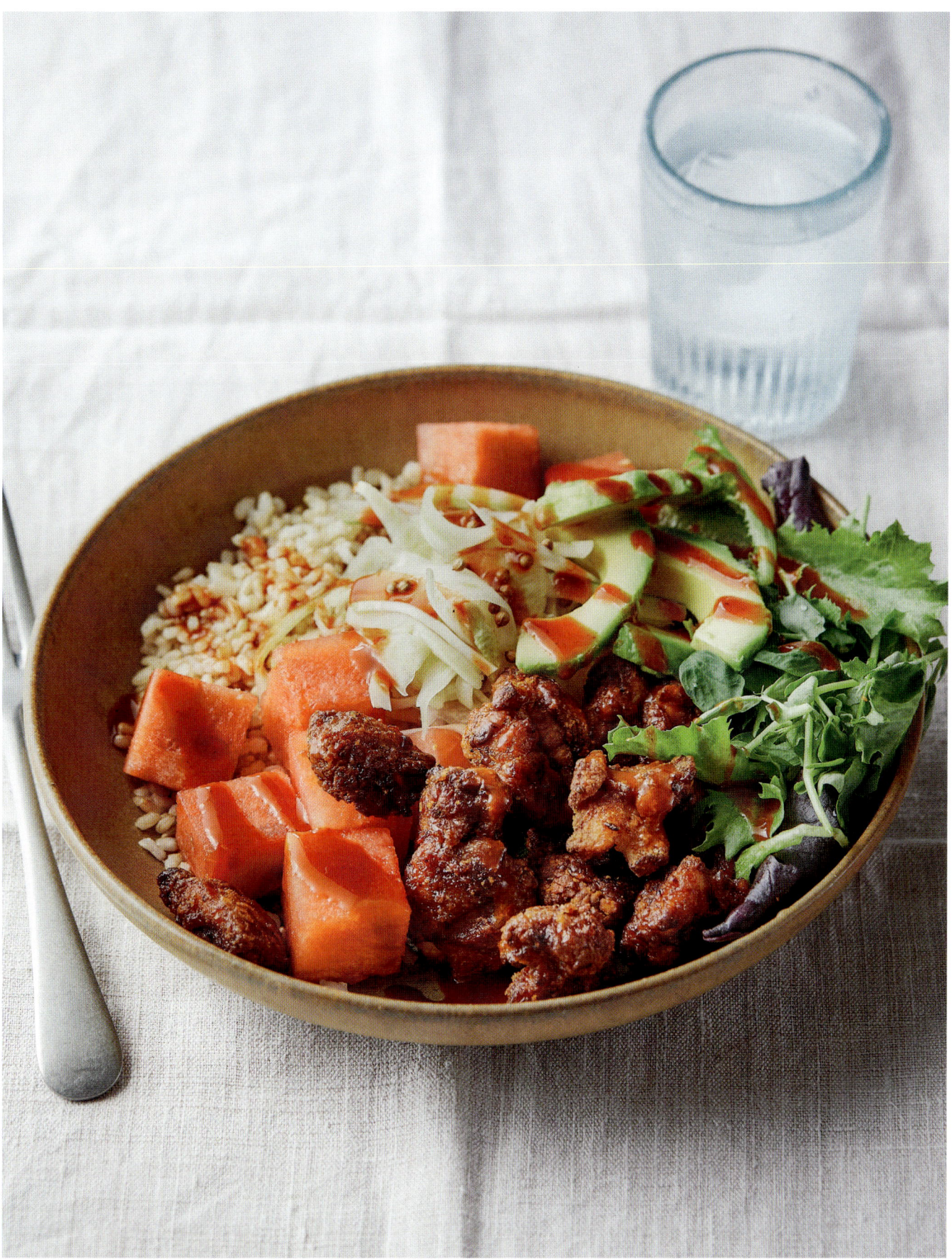

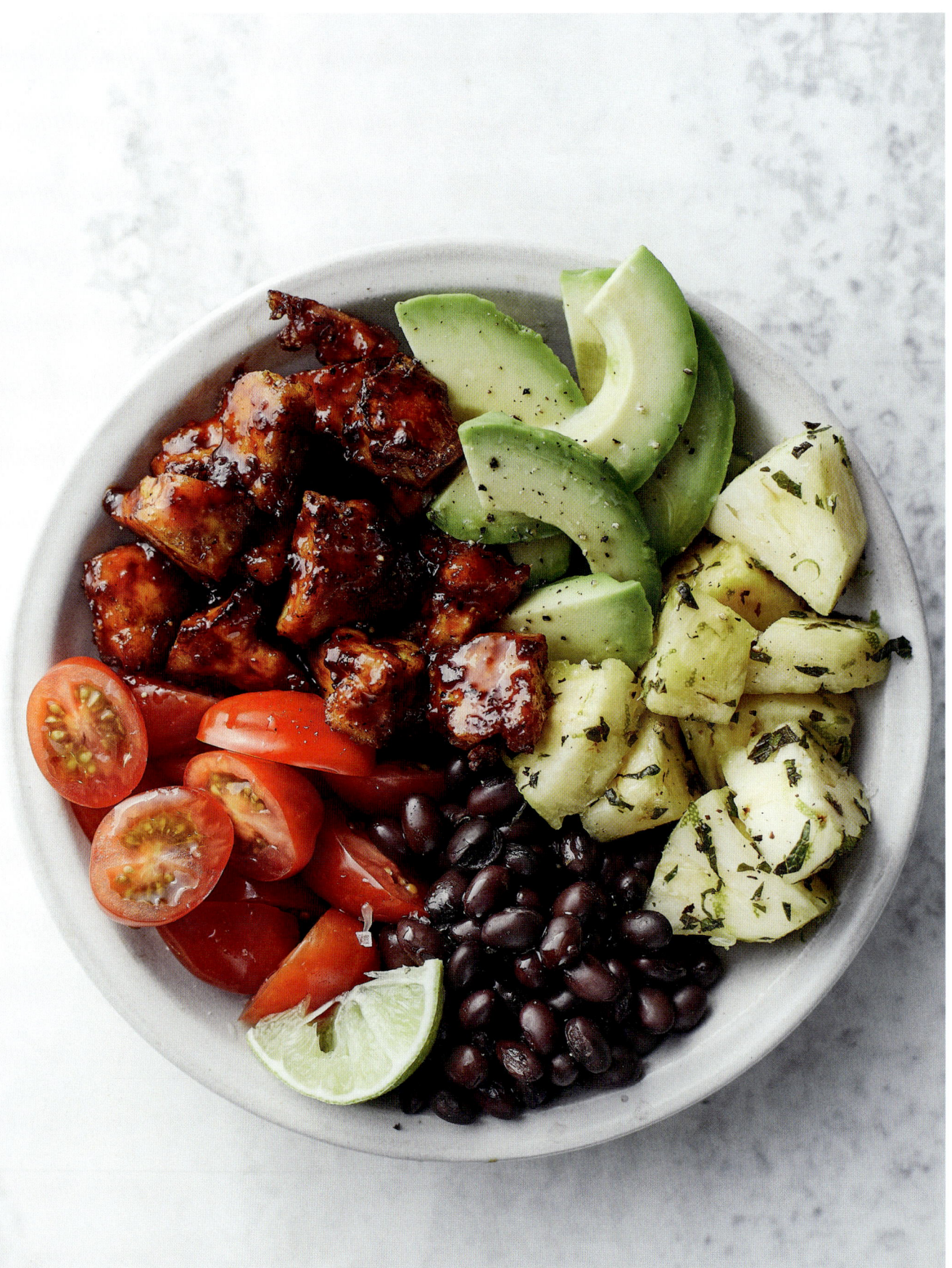

Chipotle and Honey Air-fried Tofu Bowls with Black Beans and Pineapple

Prep 5 minutes
Cook 30 minutes

Serves 2

300g firm tofu, broken into 2cm chunks
2 tbsp soy sauce
1 tbsp cornflour
1 tbsp olive oil

For the sauce
½ tbsp chipotle paste
1 tbsp honey

To serve
Zest and juice of 1 lime
1 avocado, sliced
1 x 400g can black beans, drained and rinsed
150g pineapple, cut into 2cm cubes
10g mint, finely chopped
150g baby tomatoes, halved
1 tbsp olive oil

This technique of making tofu crispy is such a versatile method that I use in many different dishes. It's ignited my excitement for what is otherwise a fairly bland ingredient. But with a crispier texture and combined with these spicy, sweet ingredients it can taste glorious. Check your chipotle sauce before you use it, they can be very hot! Use less accordingly, to taste, and remember, this will also work well with harissa paste. The meal provides anti-inflammatory flavones from the tofu, plus extra protein and fibre from the black beans. Pineapple is also anti-inflammatory and balances the heat in this dish with its tropical sweetness.

Mix the firm tofu with the soy sauce and season well, then toss through the cornflour and drizzle with the oil. Preheat your air fryer to 200°C and air fry for 15 minutes until crispy at the edges, turning halfway through. Alternatively, to crisp the tofu in the oven, spread it over a baking sheet and cook at 220°C fan for 20–25 minutes, or longer if it needs more crisping.

Meanwhile, prepare the sauce by adding the chipotle paste, honey and 2 tablespoons of water to a sauté pan. Gently warm through over a low–medium heat, stirring the ingredients together.

Once the crispy tofu has been cooked, add to the sauce, mix thoroughly and take off the heat.

Squeeze some of the lime juice over the avocado. Then add the avocado and black beans to your bowls. Toss the pineapple chunks in the mint and lime zest and add to the bowls with the tofu and tomatoes. Squeeze over the remaining lime juice and drizzle with the olive oil to finish.

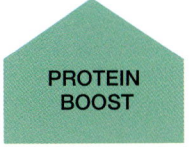

PROTEIN BOOST
Add more tofu, black beans.

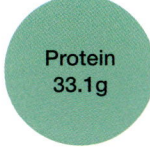

Protein 33.1g · Fibre 11.5g · Plant Points 5.75

HIGH-PROTEIN DIVERSITY BOWLS

5 Spice Mince Bowls with Kimchi Mayo

Prep 10 minutes, plus soaking
Cook 30 minutes

Serves 2

150g sunflower seeds, soaked in boiling water for 20 minutes
200g extra-firm tofu, coarsely grated
2 tbsp olive oil, plus extra to drizzle
2 tbsp Chinese 5 spice seasoning
1 tbsp soy sauce
2 tbsp tomato purée
200g pak choi, halved

<u>To serve</u>
80g kimchi and the liquid
2 tbsp mayonnaise
1 avocado, sliced
100g cooked brown short-grain rice, warmed
1 red chilli, thinly sliced

People always roll their eyes when I call this prepared tofu 'mince', but you have to try it to believe it. It has real umami, there's a slight chew that resembles beef and, with the tang of kimchi against the beautiful 5 spice aromatics, it's a gorgeous, healthful, delicious bowl. The clove and cinnamon in the 5 spice deliver so much anti-inflammatory punch, plus the sunflower seeds give body and a textural component to the tofu that makes it even more nutritious and enjoyable to eat. Always warm your rice, it's much nicer to have it reheated thoroughly. Serve with a dash of the kimchi liquid or a splash of rice wine vinegar if you have some.

Preheat the oven to 220°C fan.

Pulse the soaked sunflower seeds in a bullet blender or food processor to break them up slightly and add to a mixing bowl with the tofu, olive oil and 5 spice seasoning and mix thoroughly.

Combine the soy sauce and tomato purée in a small mixing bowl before adding to the seed and tofu mixture and mixing well.

Spread out the mixture onto a baking tray and bake for 25 minutes until the mixture has dried and become charred in places.

Meanwhile, sauté the pak choi cut-side down in a pan over a medium heat with a drizzle of oil for 5 minutes until slightly charred. Flip and cook for another 2 minutes before setting aside.

Squeeze out the salty liquid from the kimchi into a mixing bowl and add the mayonnaise. Whisk thoroughly to create a kimchi mayo.

Build your bowls with the 'mince', sautéed greens, kimchi, avocado, warmed brown rice and chilli and finish with the kimchi mayo.

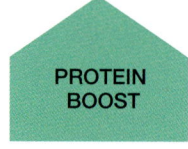

PROTEIN BOOST

Add more tofu or try adding cooked edamame or black beans.

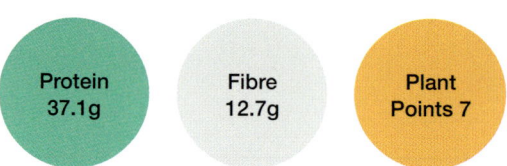

Protein 37.1g
Fibre 12.7g
Plant Points 7

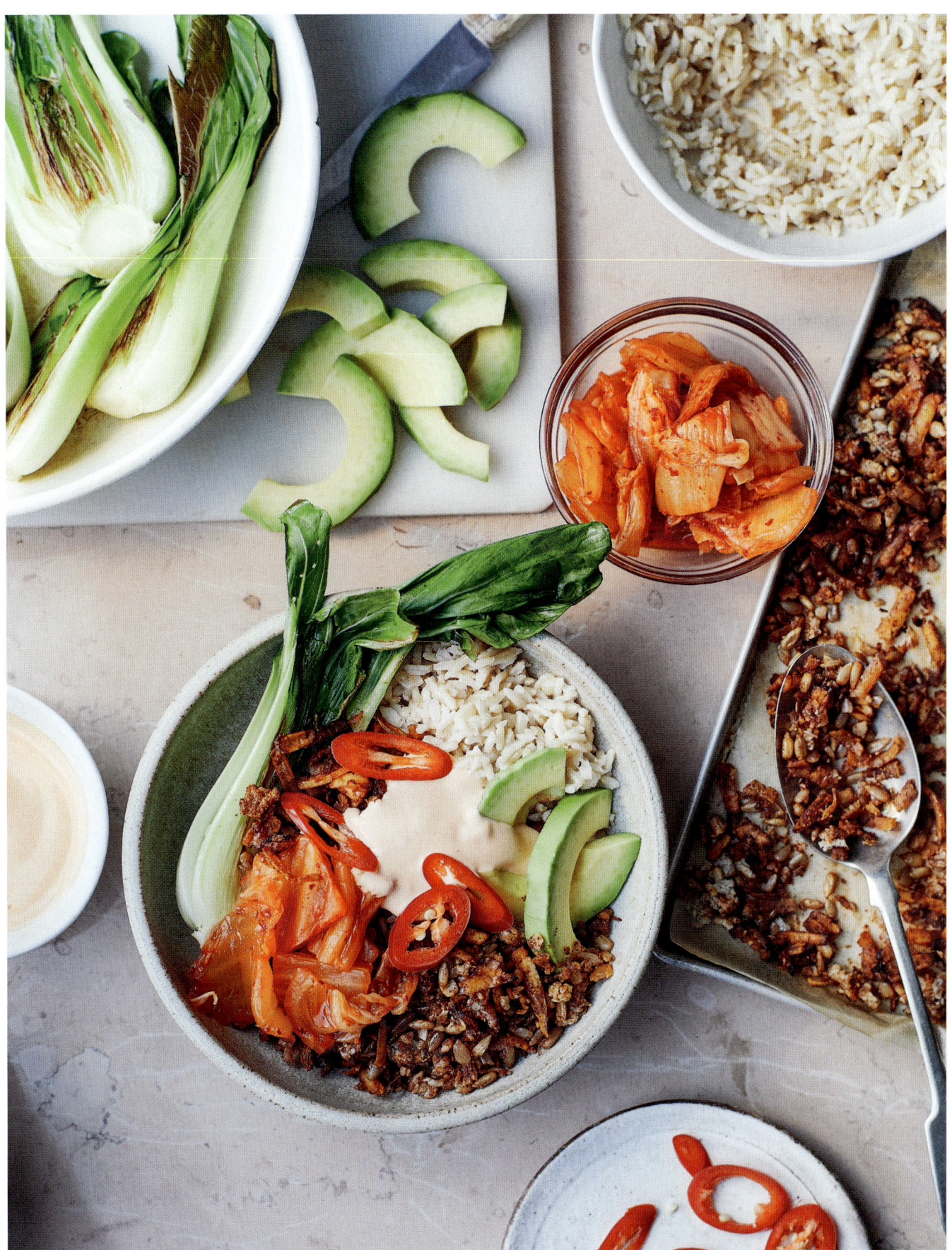

Pinto Bean Bowl with Spicy Prawns, Sweet Potato and Corn

Prep 10 minutes
Cook 30 minutes

Serves 2

200g sweet potato, cut into 2cm cubes
2 tbsp olive oil, plus extra to serve
250g extra-large prawns, shelled and deveined (450–500g when whole)
1 tbsp fajita or taco seasoning
200g sweetcorn (fresh or defrosted from frozen)

For the spicy mayonnaise
2 tbsp mayonnaise
1 tsp sweet paprika

To serve
1 x 400g can pinto beans, drained and rinsed
100g roasted red peppers, from a jar, roughly chopped, plus 1 tbsp of the juice, for the spicy mayonnaise (see above)
10g dill, stalks removed, finely chopped

A simple and delicious collection of ingredients that I always reach for when I want a nourishing, spicy bowl of goodness. The natural sweetness in the potato, corn and peppers is a great match for the taco seasoning and paprika and I love using dill to bring it together. Each element contributes its own unique blend of fibre and anti-inflammatory phytonutrients, plus the prawns are packed with protein. Have fun with variations of this dish such as using black beans, lentils and white fish.

Preheat the oven to 200°C fan.

Scatter the sweet potato on a baking sheet, drizzle with the olive oil and season well. Bake for 20–25 minutes until cooked through.

Meanwhile, rub the prawns in the fajita or taco seasoning and a pinch of salt, then sauté in a lidded dry pan over a medium heat. This will create a nice charring effect that makes the prawns delicious and golden; do remember to keep the extractor fan on high. Cook for a couple of minutes on each side until cooked through and set aside.

Add the corn to the pan and cover with the lid to cook through for a couple of minutes and absorb some of the flavours from the seasoning.

Whisk the mayonnaise with the paprika, 1 tbsp of the liquid from the jar of red peppers and a pinch of salt to make a spicy mayonnaise.

Build your bowls with the sweet potato, corn, pinto beans, peppers and charred prawns. Garnish with the spicy mayonnaise, a drizzle of oil and finely chopped dill.

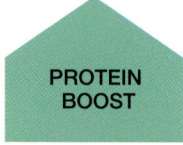

PROTEIN BOOST
Add more prawns, pinto beans or use black beans.

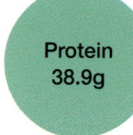

Protein 38.9g | Fibre 6.5g | Plant Points 5

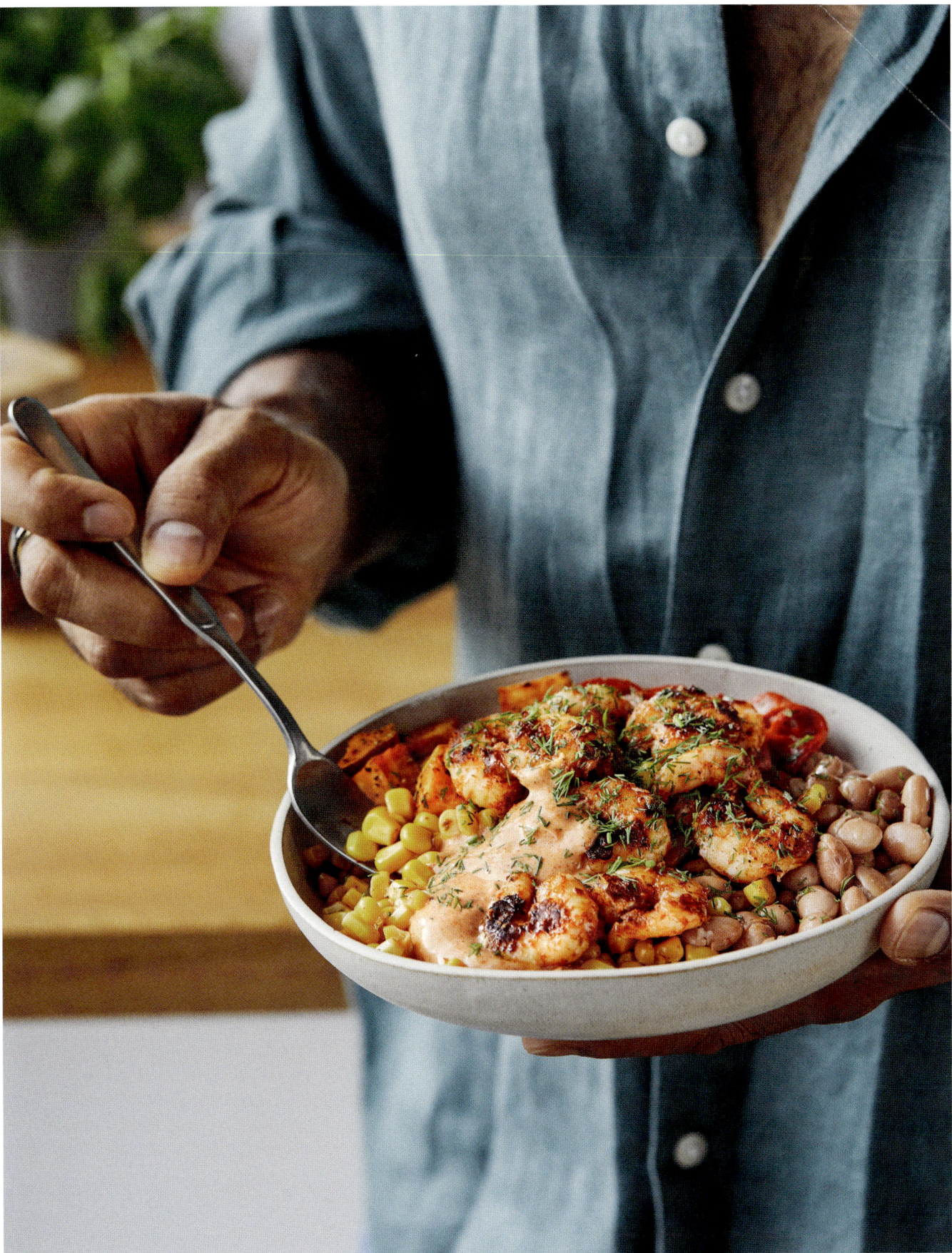

Spicy Gochujang Bowls with Green Apple Slaw and Brown Rice

Prep 10 minutes
Cook 15 minutes

Serves 2

1 tbsp olive oil
200g turkey mince
2 tsp gochujang

For the green apple slaw
1 green apple, finely diced
200g green or white cabbage, finely shredded
50g spring onion, thinly sliced
20g jalapeños from a jar, chopped
1 tbsp apple cider vinegar
25g coriander, chopped
100g Greek yoghurt
Juice of 1 lime

To serve
200g cooked short-grain brown rice, warmed
1 avocado, halved, stone removed and thinly sliced
100g tomatoes, diced
50g peanuts, toasted and chopped

The flavour of turkey with the spicy sweetness of gochujang works incredibly in this bowl with apple, jalapeños and green cabbage slaw to cut through the rich flavour. This is the sort of bowl that makes you feel healthy instantly by just looking at it. You can try cooking other protein-rich foods in the same way as the turkey, such as chicken mince or even tempeh.

Mix the ingredients for the slaw together thoroughly in a large mixing bowl. Set aside until ready to serve.

To cook the mince, heat the oil in a large frying pan over a medium–high heat. Add the mince and cook for 5 minutes, breaking it up with a spatula, until starting to turn golden. Stir in the gochujang to coat the mince and cook for another 1–2 minutes until the mince crisps up slightly. Season with salt and pepper.

Prepare the bowls by adding the warm cooked rice, avocado and tomatoes. Scoop the mince into the bowls and serve with a large spoonful of the green apple slaw and toasted peanuts.

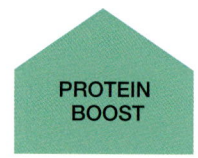

PROTEIN BOOST

Add more mince; you can also try chicken or tempeh cut into chunks.

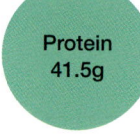

Protein 41.5g | Fibre 12.1g | Plant Points 8

154　HIGH-PROTEIN DIVERSITY BOWLS

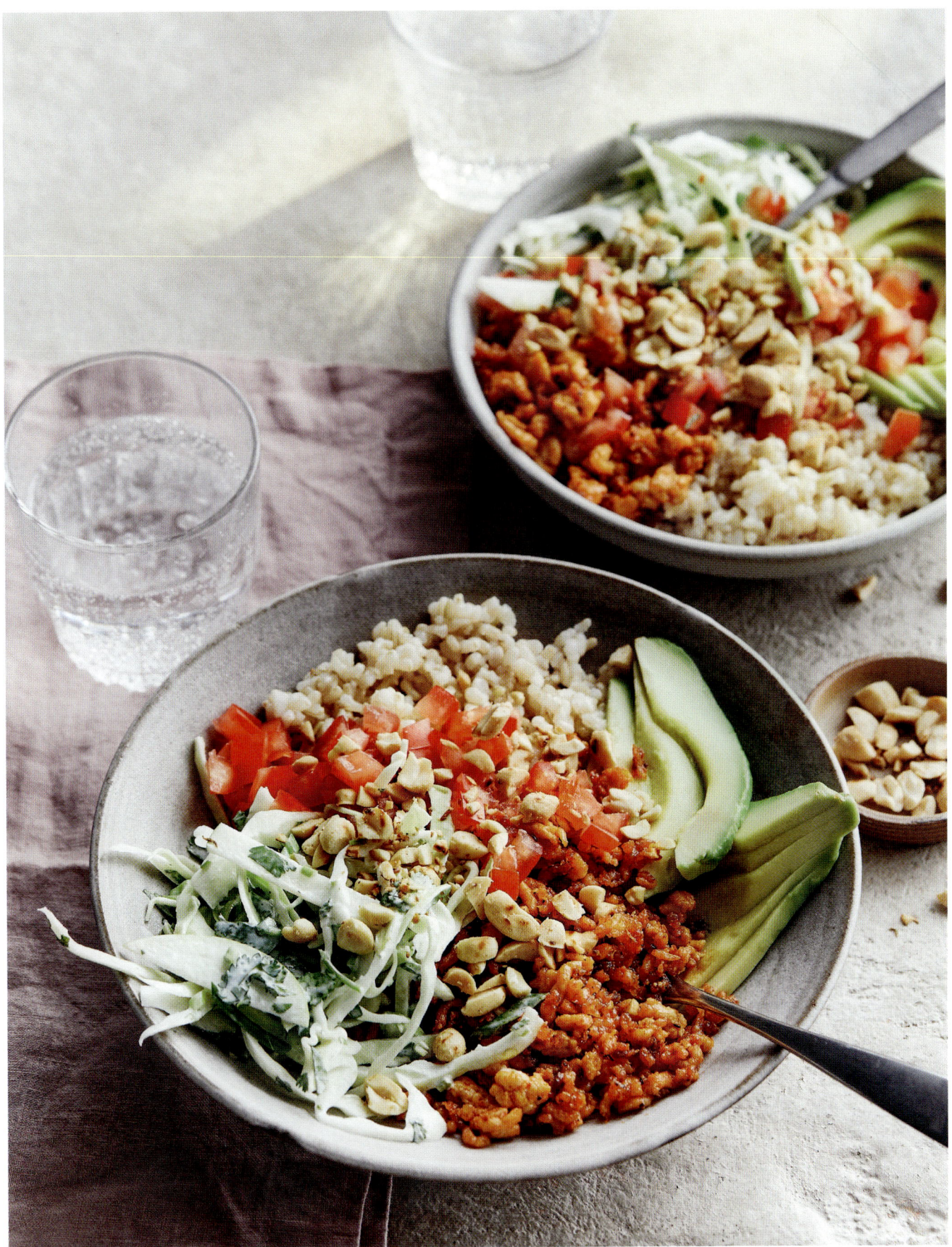

3 WAYS WITH BEANS

1. Simply add to a stew

Need some extra fibre in your family casserole recipe? Just add beans from a jar or can, and you've instantly added extra protein and fibre per serving, effortlessly.

2. Beans = dips

You can pretty much make any bean into a dip. Try this with cannellini, butter beans, chickpeas, red kidney beans, pinto or black beans. Or green lentils also work well.

Drain a **400g can of beans** and thoroughly rinse (or use 240g weight of cooked beans) and add to a food processor with **100ml hot water, 1 tbsp olive oil** and **plenty of seasoning**. Blend into a dip and enjoy with baked vegetable chips, rice cakes, rye bread or simply with crudités for a gut-boosting snack that also contains some protein.

3. Crispy toppers

Instead of shallow-fried onions or nuts, you can try adding crispy beans, which is one of my favourite ways to add texture to a bean soup or green salad. You can again do this with any cooked bean, but my favourite to use are large white butter beans.

Rinse and drain a **400g can or jar of butter beans**, and dry them thoroughly with kitchen paper. Smother them in **1 tbsp olive oil**. Season them well and dust in **1 tsp sweet paprika**. Air fry at 200°C for 10 minutes (or oven bake at 200°C fan for 22 minutes) until golden and crispy. Make sure to shake them halfway through cooking. Enjoy as a snack or as a meal topper.

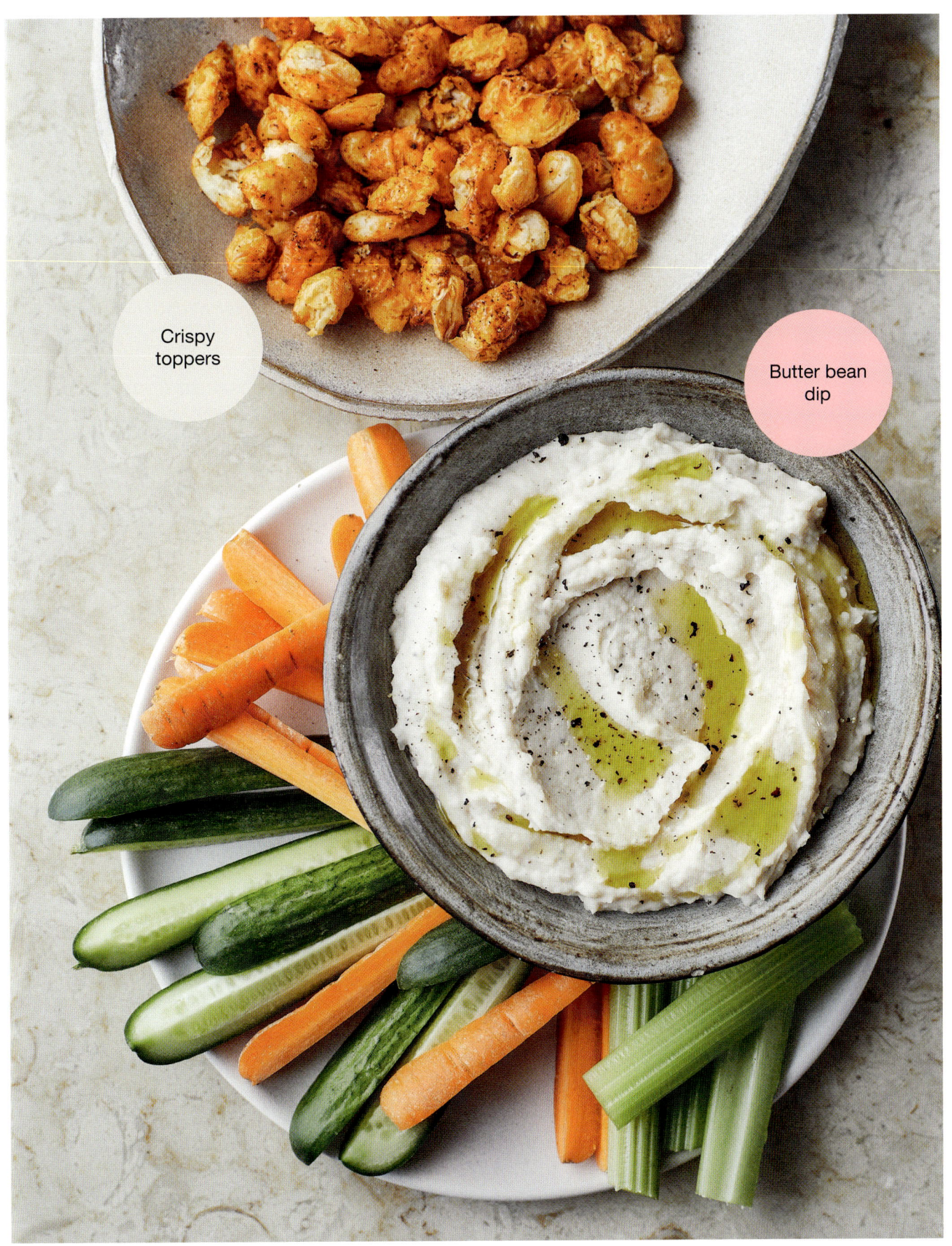

Paccheri with red mullet and pistachio

Prep 10 minutes
Cook 30 minutes

Serves 2

2 tbsp olive oil, plus extra to serve
50g shallot, finely chopped
6 garlic cloves, crushed
200g baby tomatoes, quartered
¼ tsp ground cinnamon
½ tsp dried chilli flakes
Pinch of saffron
100ml fish stock
150g dried paccheri pasta
100g spinach, roughly chopped
300g red mullet fillet (you can also use sea bass, snapper, amberjack or grouper), cut into 3cm pieces

To serve
20g parsley, finely chopped
50g pistachio nuts, gently toasted and finely chopped
Juice of 1 lemon

I had the best paccheri of my life in Ischia, a small fishing island close to Naples. Paccheri is a type of pasta shape, and the tomato sauce it was bathed in was light, yet rich with flavour. The catch of the day was beautifully fresh and vibrant and the pasta perfectly al dente. I've been trying to recreate it ever since and this is the closest I've come. If you have the time to make the fish stock from scratch, with fresh bones, do it. It adds so much more flavour and voluptuousness to the dish, it's incredible.

Heat the olive oil in a lidded pan over a medium heat. Add the shallot and cook for 4–5 minutes until lightly coloured, then add the garlic and cook for another minute.

Add the baby tomatoes and stir through for 2 minutes, allowing them to start to break down. Stir in the cinnamon, chilli flakes and saffron, then pour in the fish stock.

Reduce the heat to low and simmer the sauce, part-covered with the lid, for 10 minutes until the tomatoes break down and the sauce is reduced slightly.

Meanwhile, cook the pasta in plenty of boiling salted water according to the packet instructions.

Stir the spinach into the sauce and simmer for another 2 minutes until wilted. Turn the heat to medium, then add the fish pieces to the simmering sauce and cook for 4–5 minutes, carefully turning them once until cooked. Add a ladleful of the pasta cooking water to loosen the sauce if needed and check for seasoning, adding salt and pepper if needed.

Transfer the pasta to the sauce with a slotted spoon. Toss through the sauce and finish with the parsley. Serve with the toasted pistachios, a squeeze of lemon and an extra drizzle of olive oil.

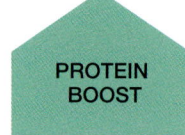

PROTEIN BOOST
Add more fish or pistachios.

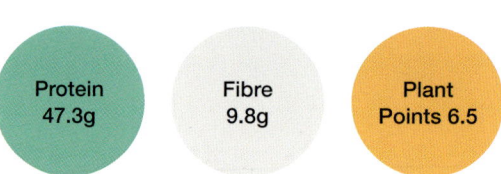

Protein 47.3g
Fibre 9.8g
Plant Points 6.5

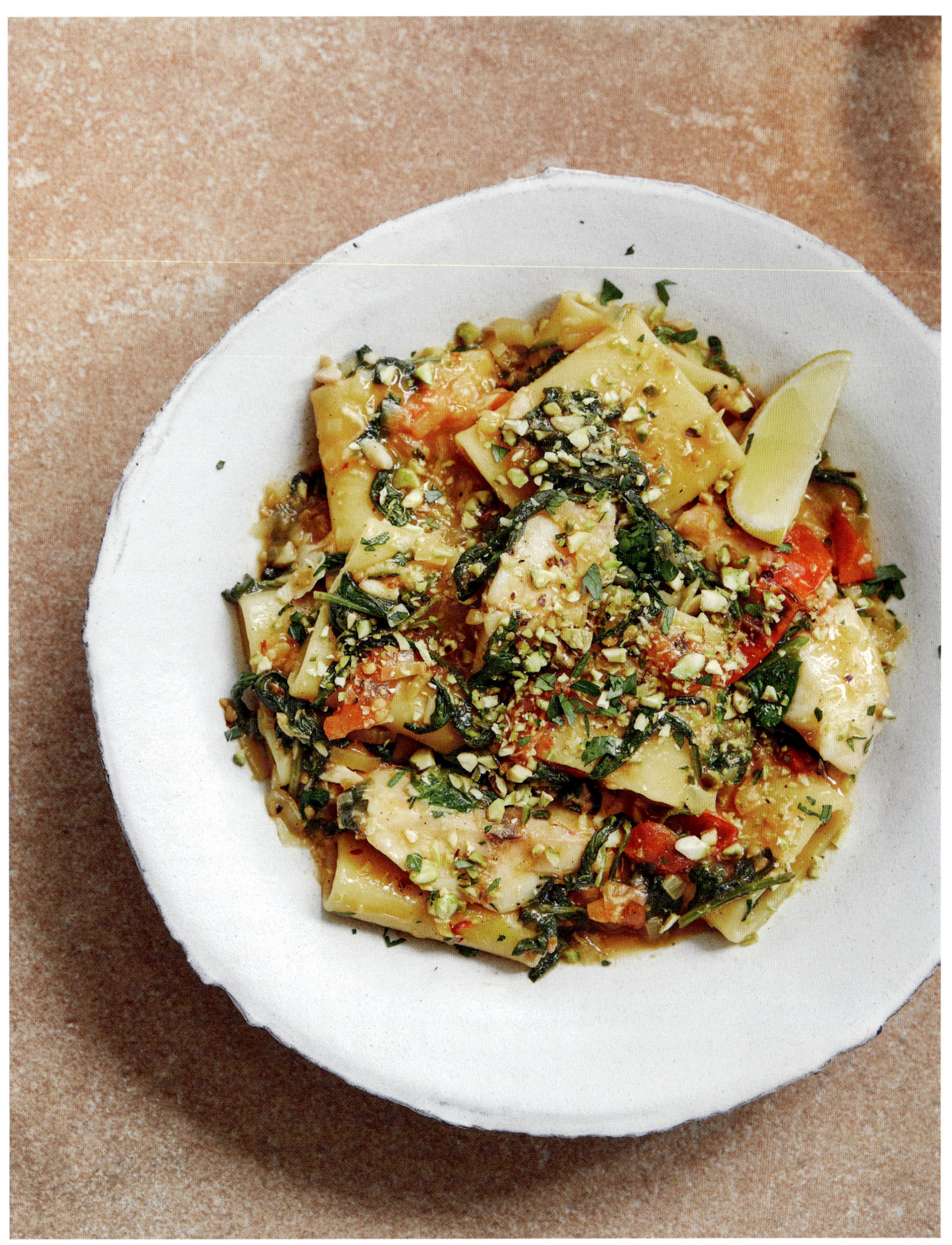

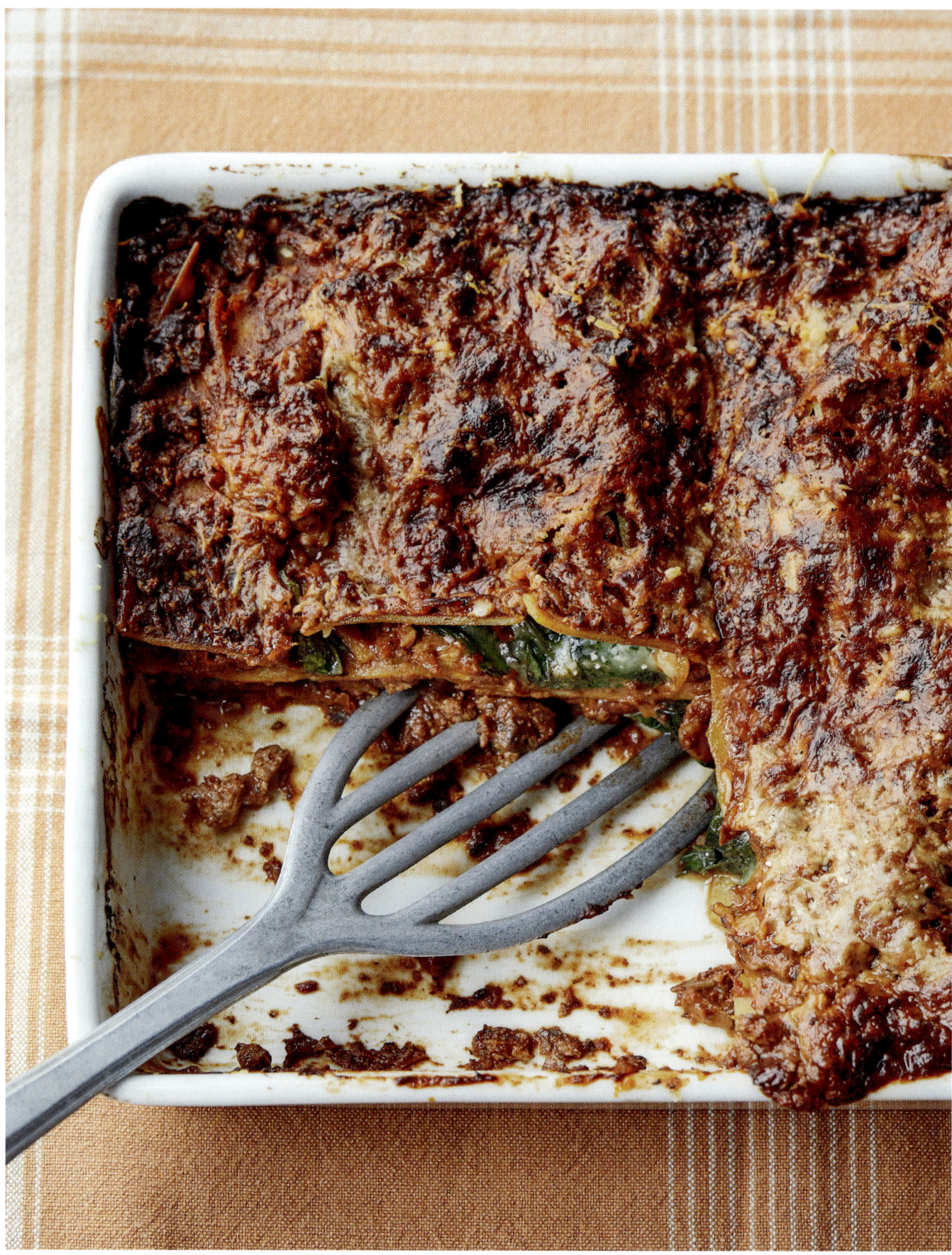

Plant-powered Lasagne with Mushroom and Tofu

Prep 10 minutes, plus soaking
Cook 55 minutes

Serves 4

200g baby spinach
30g dried mushrooms
2 tbsp olive oil, plus extra to drizzle
6 large garlic cloves, finely diced
80g walnuts, coarsely blitzed or finely chopped
3 tbsp oregano
1–2 tsp red chilli flakes
400g firm tofu, drained, pressed well and patted dry with kitchen paper
3 tbsp aged balsamic vinegar
3 tbsp tomato purée
40g nutritional yeast
2 x 400g cans whole peeled tomatoes
1 vegetable stock cube
150g–200g dried lentil or regular lasagne sheets (about 9–12 sheets)
100g Parmesan, coarsely grated

I've prepared all the ingredients for this crowd-pleasing dish in less than 30 minutes, ready for either freezing or delivering to a friend's house for them to easily put in the oven. It's so simple once you've got the hang of doing it and it's one of those dishes to cook and keep in the freezer for times when you want a healthy comfort meal. The dried mushrooms deliver a gorgeous deep, earthy flavour and the tofu, walnuts and nutritional yeast pack this with a decent amount of protein. Feel free to use regular lasagne sheets, but the lentil-based version adds even more fibre and protein to your meal. Trust me, you won't feel heavy after this pasta!

Put the spinach in a sieve over a bowl and pour boiling water over the leaves to wilt them. Save the water and press the spinach with the back of a spoon to extract as much water as possible, then place on a plate lined with kitchen paper.

Measure 200ml of the reserved water and pour it over the dried mushrooms in a bowl to cover, then leave them to rehydrate for 15 minutes. Drain the mushrooms in a sieve, then roughly chop them, saving the soaking liquid.

Heat the olive oil in a large saucepan over a medium heat, add the garlic and cook for 1 minute until softened. Add the rehydrated mushrooms, walnuts, oregano and chilli flakes and stir for a minute, then crumble in the drained tofu. Stir to coat it in the flavourings and cook over a low–medium heat for another 5–6 minutes until thoroughly combined and the tofu is fully broken down.

Add the balsamic vinegar, tomato purée, nutritional yeast and mushroom soaking liquid, stir to combine and cook gently for 2–3 minutes to intensify the flavour.

Add the tomatoes, squeezing them into the saucepan or using a fork to mash them into the sauce, and crumble in the vegetable stock cube. Bring the mixture to a simmer and cook without a lid for 15 minutes. Check the seasoning and season with salt and pepper if needed.

Meanwhile, preheat the oven to 200°C fan.

Select a deep lasagne dish, about 28 x 20cm, spoon a thin layer of the sauce over the base, add a layer of lasagne sheets, about 3–4, snapping them to fit in an even layer. Top with a third of the sauce, then layer over the spinach and half the Parmesan. Repeat with another layer of the lasagne sheets and another third of the sauce. Top with a final layer of lasagne sheets and the rest of the sauce, then scatter with the remaining Parmesan.

Drizzle over extra olive oil and bake for 20–25 minutes until the lasagne sheets are cooked through and the top is brown and crispy.

If you're using regular wheat lasagne sheets you'll need this extra step. Reduce the heat to 180°C fan, cover the dish with foil to stop the top burning and cook for another 20–25 minutes until the lasagne sheets are cooked through.

Leave to rest out of the oven for 5 minutes and serve.

PROTEIN BOOST

Add more tofu; use beef mince if you prefer. Add ricotta or a béchamel sauce for a more traditional take.

Protein 43.7g

Fibre 12.9g

Plant Points 7

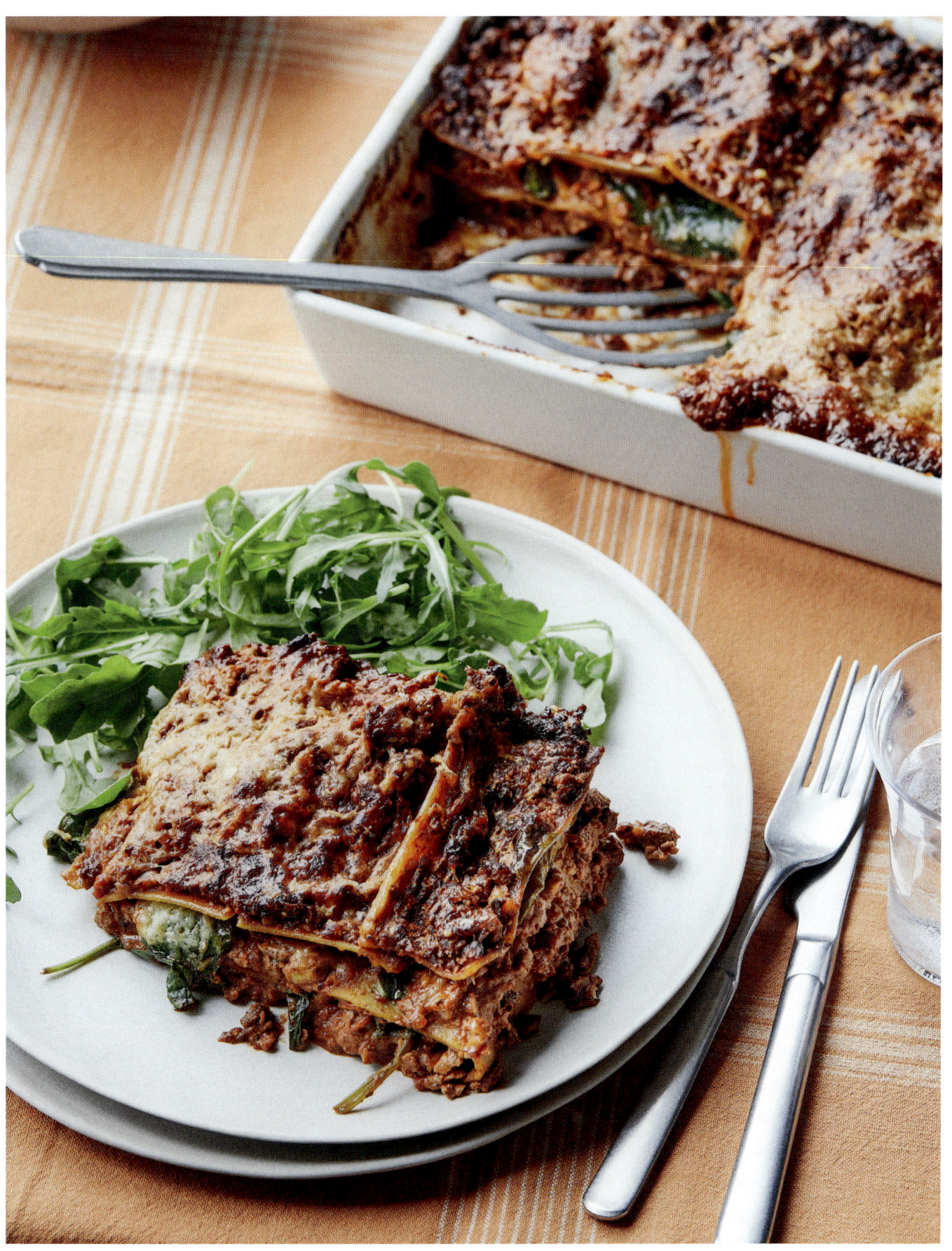

Rupy's High-protein Rigatoni

Prep 10 minutes
Cook 40 minutes

Serves 2

2 tbsp olive oil, plus extra to serve
100g onion, finely chopped
4 garlic cloves, finely chopped
3 tsp dried mixed herbs
2 tbsp tomato purée
100ml red wine
100g walnuts, roughly chopped or pulsed into a coarse crumb
200g tempeh, roughly chopped or pulsed into a coarse crumb
200ml vegetable stock
200ml passata
1 tbsp aged balsamic vinegar
200g cooked Puy lentils
100g cavolo nero, stalks removed, and leaves massaged and roughly chopped
150g dried rigatoni pasta
20g Parmesan, finely grated, to serve

The walnut, tempeh, Puy lentil blend in this recipe delivers on the protein and fibre needs for your gut wellbeing, and the texture and flavour of this combination are phenomenal. With red wine and mixed herbs plus a bit of time you get a gorgeous bowl of food that is nourishing and delicious. Try it with different pasta varieties if you wish and, for more protein, use a lentil- or bean-based pasta.

Heat the olive oil in a large lidded casserole pan over a medium heat, add the onion and cook, stirring occasionally, for 10 minutes until softened and starting to turn golden. Add the garlic and plenty of seasoning and cook for another minute before adding the mixed herbs and tomato purée. You want to cook the purée for 3–4 minutes to intensify the flavour.

Pour the red wine into the pan and cook for another 3 minutes until there is no smell of alcohol and the mixture becomes thick and sticky.

Add the walnuts and tempeh and stir to coat them in the sticky mixture. Cook for 2 minutes, stirring, then pour in the stock, passata and vinegar and add the lentils. Reduce the heat to low–medium, stir until combined and simmer, part-covered with the lid, for 15 minutes. Toss in the massaged cavolo nero for the last 2 minutes of cooking.

Meanwhile, cook the pasta in plenty of boiling salted water according to the packet instructions. Drain, reserving a mugful of the cooking water. Add the pasta to the sauce with enough of the pasta cooking water to loosen. Serve in bowls, drizzled with olive oil and with the Parmesan scattered over.

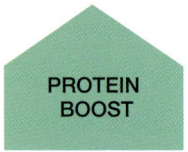

PROTEIN BOOST

Add more tempeh and walnuts. You can also use lean beef mince instead of tempeh, just add 150g mince to the onions, garlic, tomato purée and herbs, and cook for 5 minutes before adding the red wine.

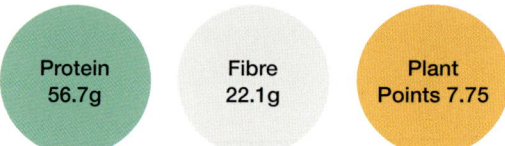

Protein 56.7g · Fibre 22.1g · Plant Points 7.75

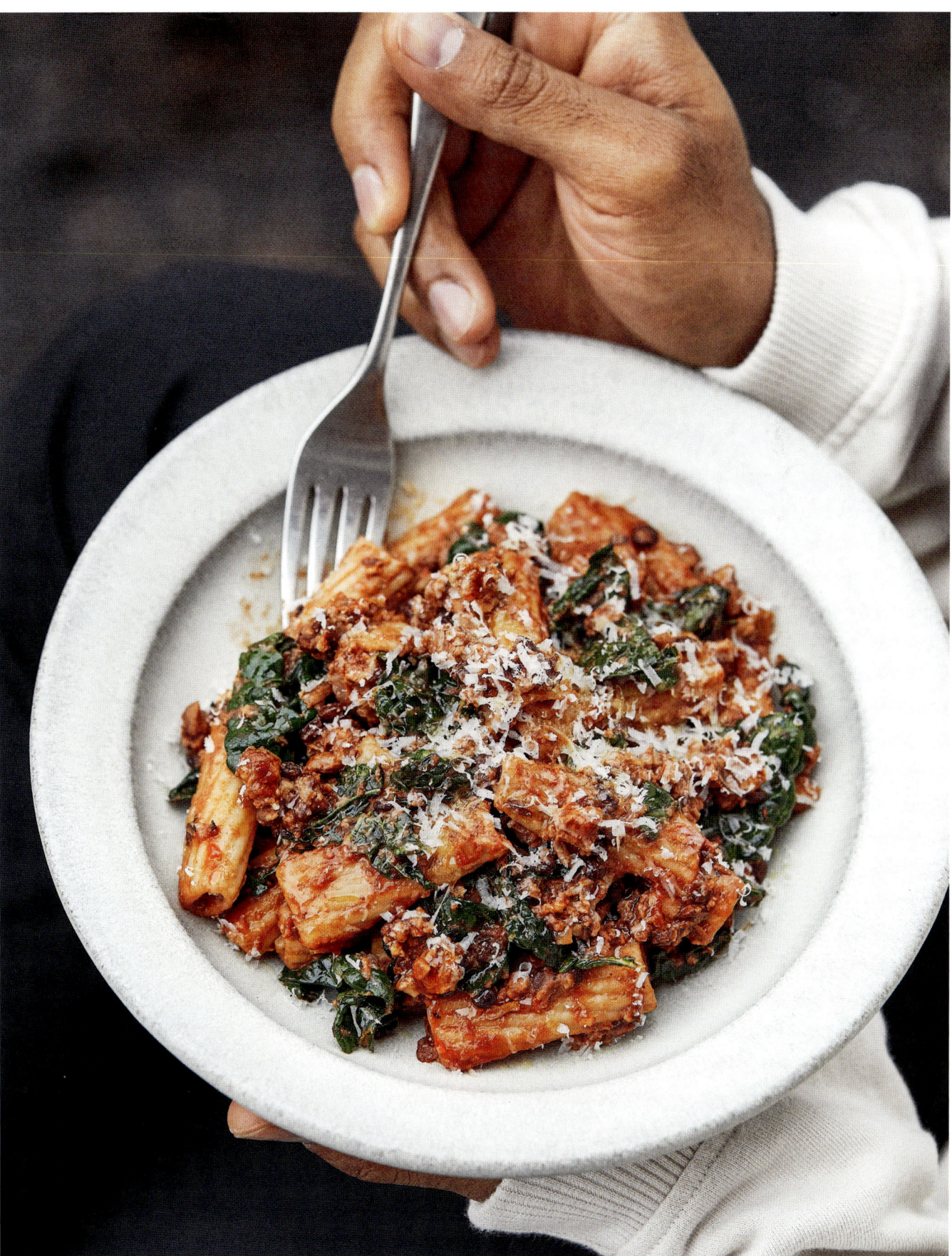

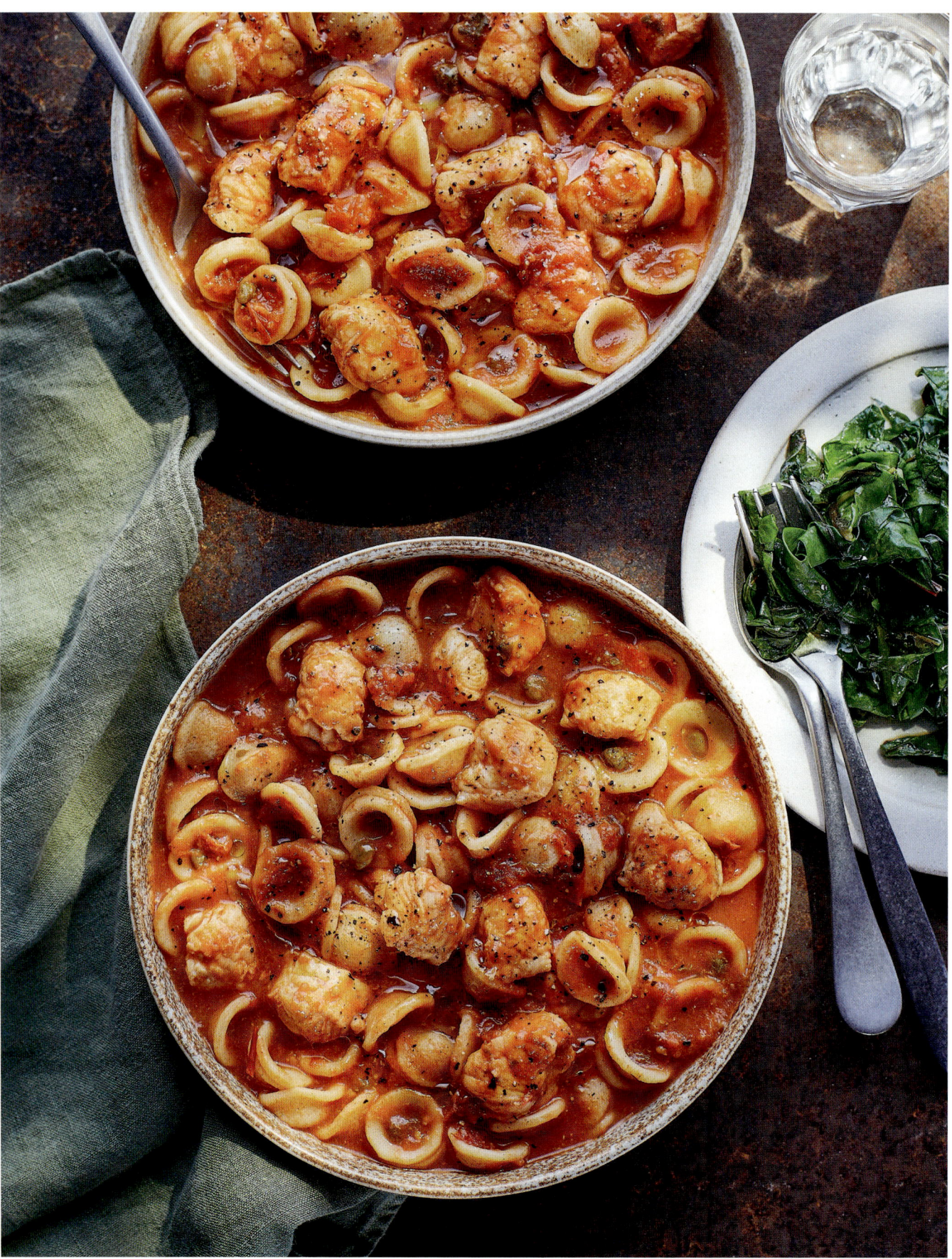

Tomato, Caper and Fish Stew with Orecchiette

Prep 5 minutes
Cook 45 minutes

Serves 4

- 2 tbsp olive oil, plus extra to drizzle
- 6 garlic cloves, finely diced
- 2 tsp fish sauce
- 3 tbsp tomato purée
- 2 tbsp capers, drained
- 2 tbsp aged balsamic vinegar
- 400g tomatoes, roughly chopped
- 150ml fish stock
- 300ml passata
- 600g monkfish, cut into 2.5cm chunks
- 300g dried orecchiette pasta
- 400g puntarelle, Swiss chard or spring greens, tough stalks removed, leaves roughly chopped

This delicious ragù-style sauce with fish sounds unconventional but it honestly works super well. The rich flavours of fish sauce, salty capers and aged balsamic transform the sauce into a deep, rich, umami occasion that the monkfish takes to really well. Puntarelle is a bitter green vegetable, typical of Italian cuisine, that packs an incredible amount of anti-inflammatory chemicals, but use spring greens or watercress – which are equally bitter and potent – if you can't source it. You can also use plant-protein pastas, such as lentil fusilli and penne, if you can't find orecchiette.

Heat the oil in heavy-based saucepan or casserole dish over a medium heat. Add the garlic and sauté for a few minutes, then add the fish sauce, tomato purée and capers and cook, stirring, for another 2 minutes until dark red in colour.

Add the balsamic vinegar, fresh tomatoes, fish stock and passata and bring to a gentle simmer. Cook over a low heat, without a lid, stirring every so often, for 20–25 minutes until the sauce has reduced and thickened. Season with salt and pepper.

Add the fish and cook for another 8–10 minutes until cooked through.

Meanwhile, cook the pasta in plenty of boiling salted water according to the packet instructions. Drain and gently stir into the fish stew to combine with the sauce.

To cook the greens, put them in a lidded sauté pan with a splash of water, a drizzle of oil and a pinch of salt. Cover with the lid and cook over a low–medium heat for 3–4 minutes until the greens wilt and the water evaporates.

Serve the fish stew in large bowls with the greens on the side and a good drizzle of olive oil.

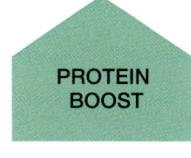

PROTEIN BOOST

Add more fish

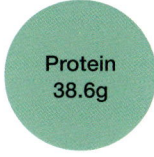

Protein 38.6g | Fibre 11g | Plant Points 4.75

HIGH-PROTEIN DIVERSITY BOWLS

FRESH

& LIGHT
PLATES

Thai-style Pomelo Salad with Crispy Tofu

Prep 15 minutes
Cook 30 minutes

Serves 2

300g extra-firm tofu, ripped into 3cm chunks
2 tbsp soy sauce
1 tbsp cornflour
1 tbsp olive oil

For the dressing
2 tsp fish sauce
2 tbsp soy sauce
Juice and zest of 1 lime
1 tsp coconut sugar
2 tbsp sesame oil
1 red chilli, thinly sliced

For the salad
250g pomelo, cut into segments
100g bean sprouts
150g mangetout, thinly sliced on an angle
50g spring onions, thinly sliced on an angle
50g peanuts, toasted and roughly chopped, plus extra to serve
20g Thai basil, torn
20g coriander, chopped

This sweet, sharp and salty combo is delicious. The rich use of herbs is brilliant for your gut microbes and the tofu and peanuts are bringing the protein punch as well as crispy, crunchy texture. There are plenty of greens and spices in here to keep inflammation low, it's a fantastic all-rounder salad. You can also use orange segments instead. Other citrus like blood orange or grapefruit would be wonderful too.

Preheat the oven to 220°C fan and line a baking sheet with baking paper.

Mix the tofu chunks with the soy sauce and then dust over the cornflour and mix again until all the chunks are covered.

Spread the pieces out on the baking sheet, drizzle with the oil and bake for 20–25 minutes or air fry the tofu on the highest heat for 15 minutes.

Meanwhile, mix the dressing ingredients and set aside.

Add the pomelo, bean sprouts, mangetout, spring onion and peanuts to a large mixing bowl, along with half the green herbs, then toss gently together with your hands.

When the tofu is ready add it the bowl then pour over half the dressing and toss to coat evenly.

To serve, drizzle over the remaining dressing, sprinkle with the remaining green herbs and extra peanuts.

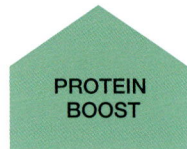

PROTEIN BOOST

Add more tofu or peanuts. You can also add cooked prawns.

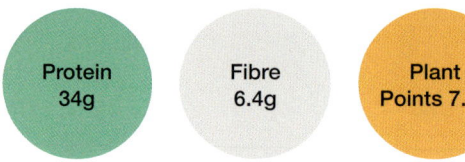

Protein 34g
Fibre 6.4g
Plant Points 7.25

170 FRESH & LIGHT PLATES

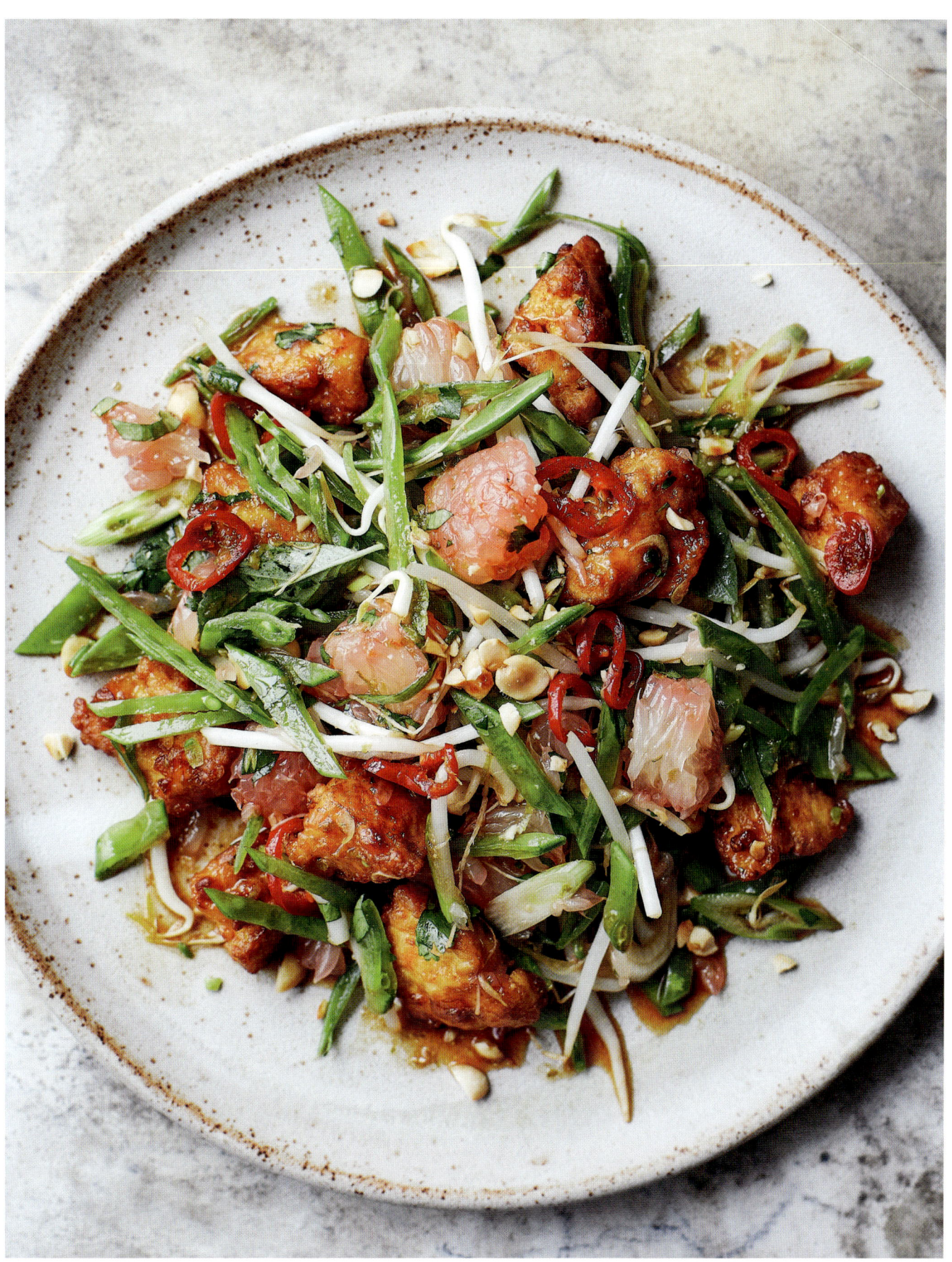

Silken Soup with Crispy Masala Chickpeas and Soft Herbs

Prep 10 minutes
Cook 25 minutes

Serves 2

For the crispy masala chickpeas
1 x 400g can chickpeas, drained and rinsed
1 tbsp olive oil, plus extra to drizzle
2 tsp garam masala

For the soup
300g silken tofu
20g nutritional yeast
50g pecans, crushed
10g dill, chopped
10g mint, chopped
100g cucumber, finely diced
Ice cubes
1 tsp sumac

Inspired by a traditional Persian yoghurt soup dish, I've given this a high-protein twist with tofu, nuts and chickpeas. This is perfect for a hot summer's day when you want something cooling, nourishing and easy to prepare without much effort. The nutritional yeast gives a delightful rich flavour and umami depth that is mellowed with the mint and dill. The warm and cold contrasts work so well in this dish. You can also cook the chickpeas in an air fryer at 200°C for half the time of the oven.

Preheat the oven to 200°C.

Thoroughly dry the chickpeas on kitchen paper, then tip them onto a baking tray and rub in the olive oil and garam masala. Sprinkle with salt and roast for 20 minutes, turning once, until crispy.

Meanwhile, make the soup. In a blender, blitz together the silken tofu, 300ml of water, seasoning and the nutritional yeast. The mixture should come together like very thin yoghurt. Check the seasoning and adjust as needed.

Pour the tofu mixture into 2 serving bowls and stir in a handful of ice cubes, three-quarters of the pecans and herbs, all the cucumber and a couple of ice cubes.

To serve, scatter over the rest of the pecans, crispy chickpeas, the remaining herbs and sumac. Finish with an extra drizzle of olive oil.

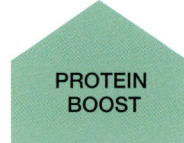

PROTEIN BOOST
Add more pecans. You can also use walnuts.

Protein 30.2g | Fibre 11.1g | Plant Points 5.25

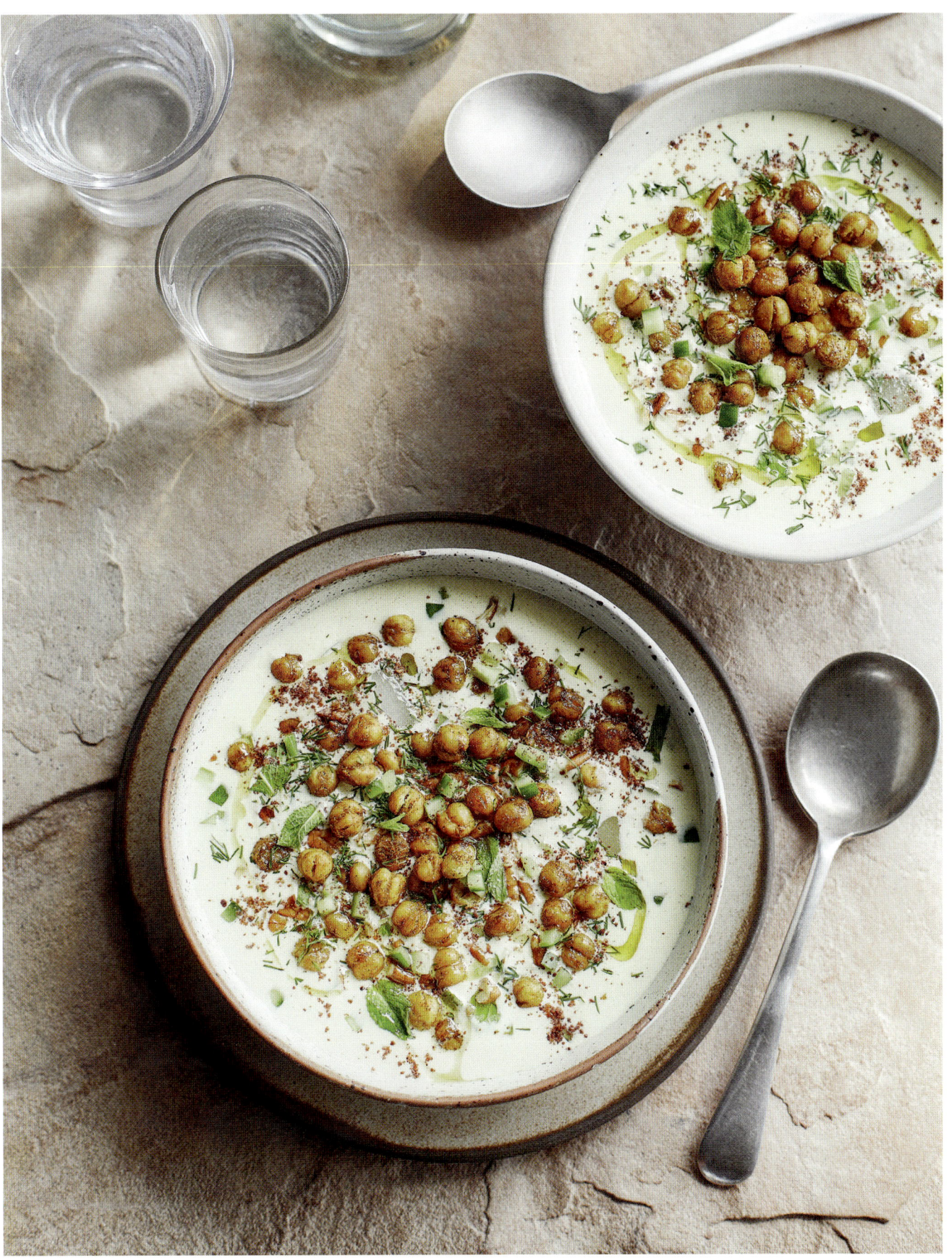

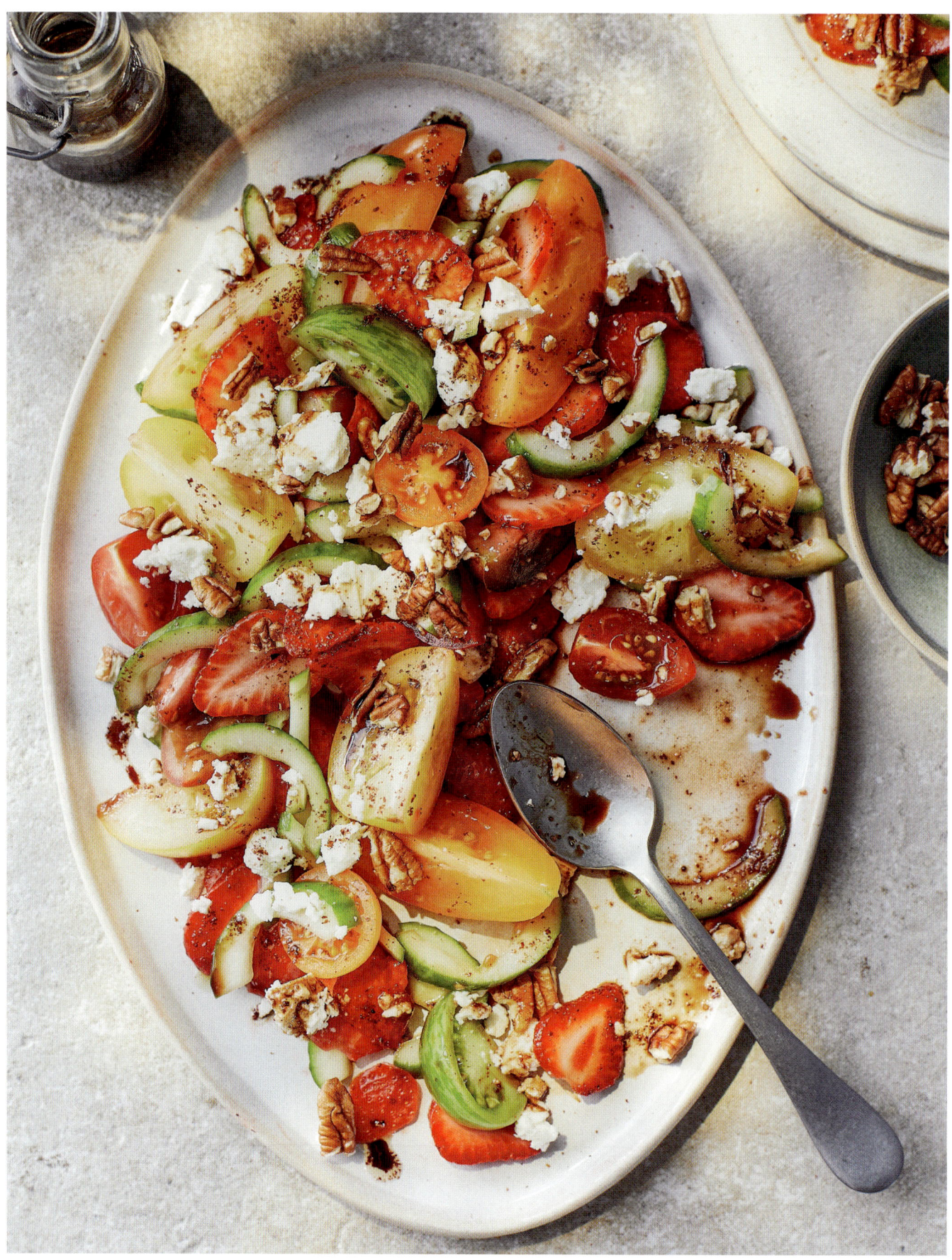

Heritage Tomatoes, Strawberries and Feta

Prep 10 minutes, plus marinating

Serves 2

250g heritage tomatoes, halved or quartered if large
100g strawberries, very thinly sliced
120g cucumber, halved lengthways, seeds scooped out, sliced on an angle or chopped into small chunks
75g feta
30g pecans, toasted and chopped

For the dressing
2 tbsp olive oil
1 tsp sumac
2 tsp aged balsamic vinegar

The combination of sweet strawberries with feta and tomatoes sounds slightly odd but, trust me, this combination works phenomenally well. The seasonal ingredients blend beautifully together and the sharp sweetness of aged balsamic is a welcome flavour. The polyphenols in strawberries deliver an anti-inflammatory dose and the feta is a good source of protein. This would make a brilliant side to simply cooked fish to boost up the protein.

Add the tomatoes, strawberries and cucumber to a mixing bowl, season with salt and gently mix together (the salt will help to release some of the juices in the salad ingredients). Set aside for 10 minutes.

With your hands, transfer the salad ingredients to a shallow serving bowl and to the remaining liquid in the mixing bowl, add the dressing ingredients and whisk together. It should taste slightly sweet from the juices, with sharpness from the olive oil and sumac. Add seasoning, if needed, and drizzle the dressing over the salad.

Crumble the feta over the salad in small chunks, drizzle over some more balsamic vinegar and finish with the pecans.

PROTEIN BOOST

Try adding air-fried white beans (see page 156). You could also serve this with boquerones (pickled anchovies) for a salty protein hit.

Protein 9.1g | Fibre 4.5g | Plant Points 4.5

FRESH & LIGHT PLATES

Salmon, Squash and Grilled Peach Salad with Tahini Herb Dressing

Prep 10 minutes
Cook 35 minutes

Serves 2

300g butternut squash, skin on, cut into 2cm chunks
2 tbsp olive oil, plus extra to drizzle
250g salmon fillet, skinless
2 tsp sumac
2 peaches, halved, stone removed and each half cut into wedges
100g watercress, roughly torn
50g walnuts, toasted and roughly chopped

For the tahini herb dressing
50g tahini
75ml boiled water
Juice of 1 lemon
20g dill, tough stalks removed
20g basil, tough stalks removed

A bright, summery dish with a gorgeous, simple dressing. The soft herbs and tahini are a favourite combination of mine and it pairs beautifully with the oily salmon, rubbed in red, tangy sumac. The beautiful orange squash and peaches contain carotenoids that support inflammation balance and add a diversity of fibres to support your gut, along with the high protein salmon.

Preheat the oven to 200°C fan.

Add the squash to a baking sheet, drizzle with 1 tbsp of olive oil, massage with salt and roast for 20 minutes.

Rub the salmon with the sumac and a drizzle of olive oil.

Remove the tray from the oven, turn up the heat to 220°C fan and nestle the salmon in the tray and bake for another 10 minutes until the salmon is nicely coloured and is cooked through.

Meanwhile, heat a ridged griddle pan over a medium–high heat. Rub the peaches in the remaining olive oil add them to the pan and cook for a few minutes on each side until lightly charred.

Meanwhile, blitz the dressing ingredients in a bullet blender into a smooth green dressing. Season with salt and pepper.

Put the watercress and walnuts into a large serving bowl and toss in the peaches and squash. Flake over the salmon in large chunks and drizzle with the tahini dressing.

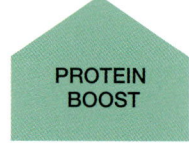

PROTEIN BOOST
Add more salmon, walnuts or tahini.

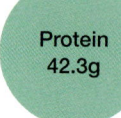

Protein 42.3g
Fibre 9.8g
Plant Points 6.25

176 FRESH & LIGHT PLATES

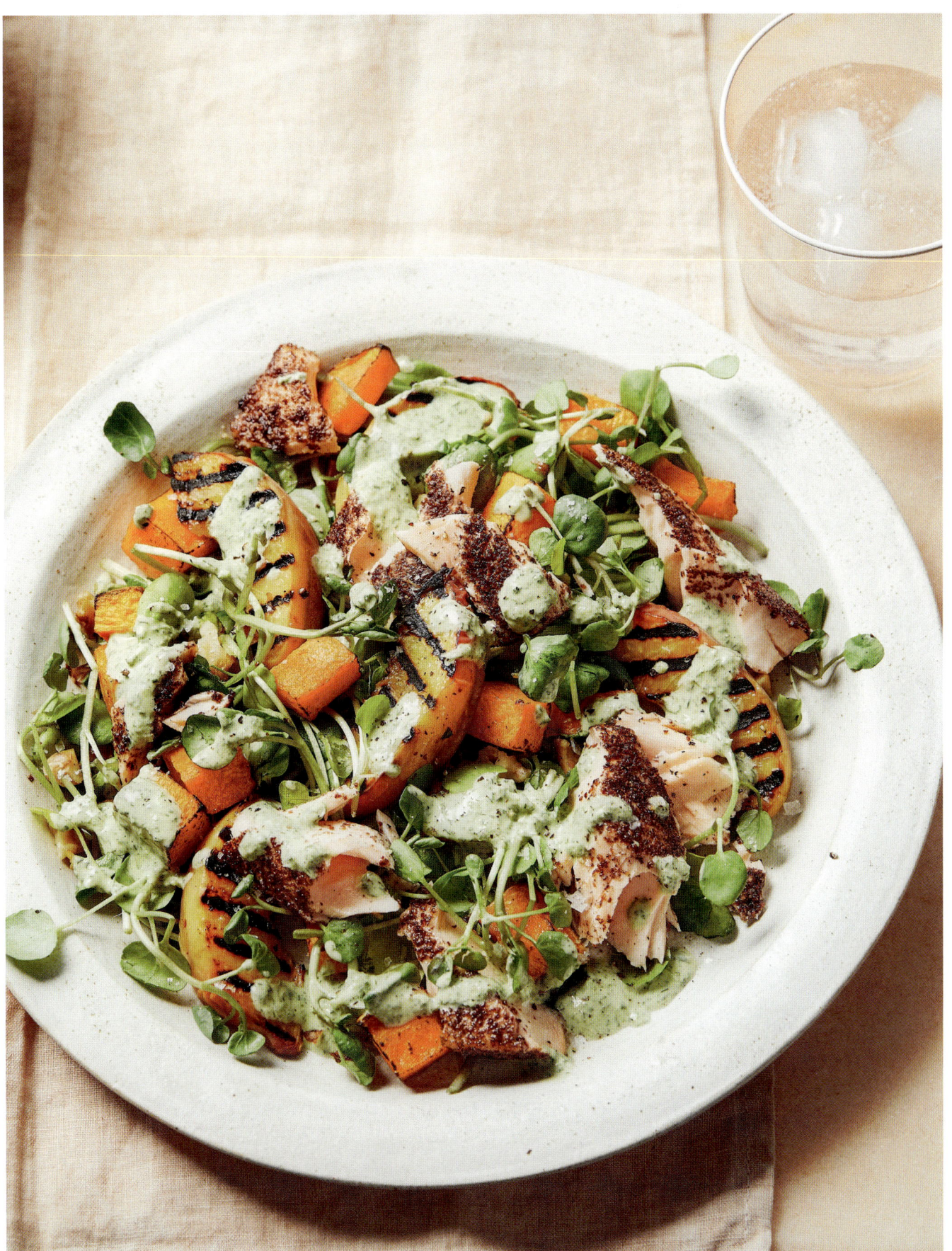

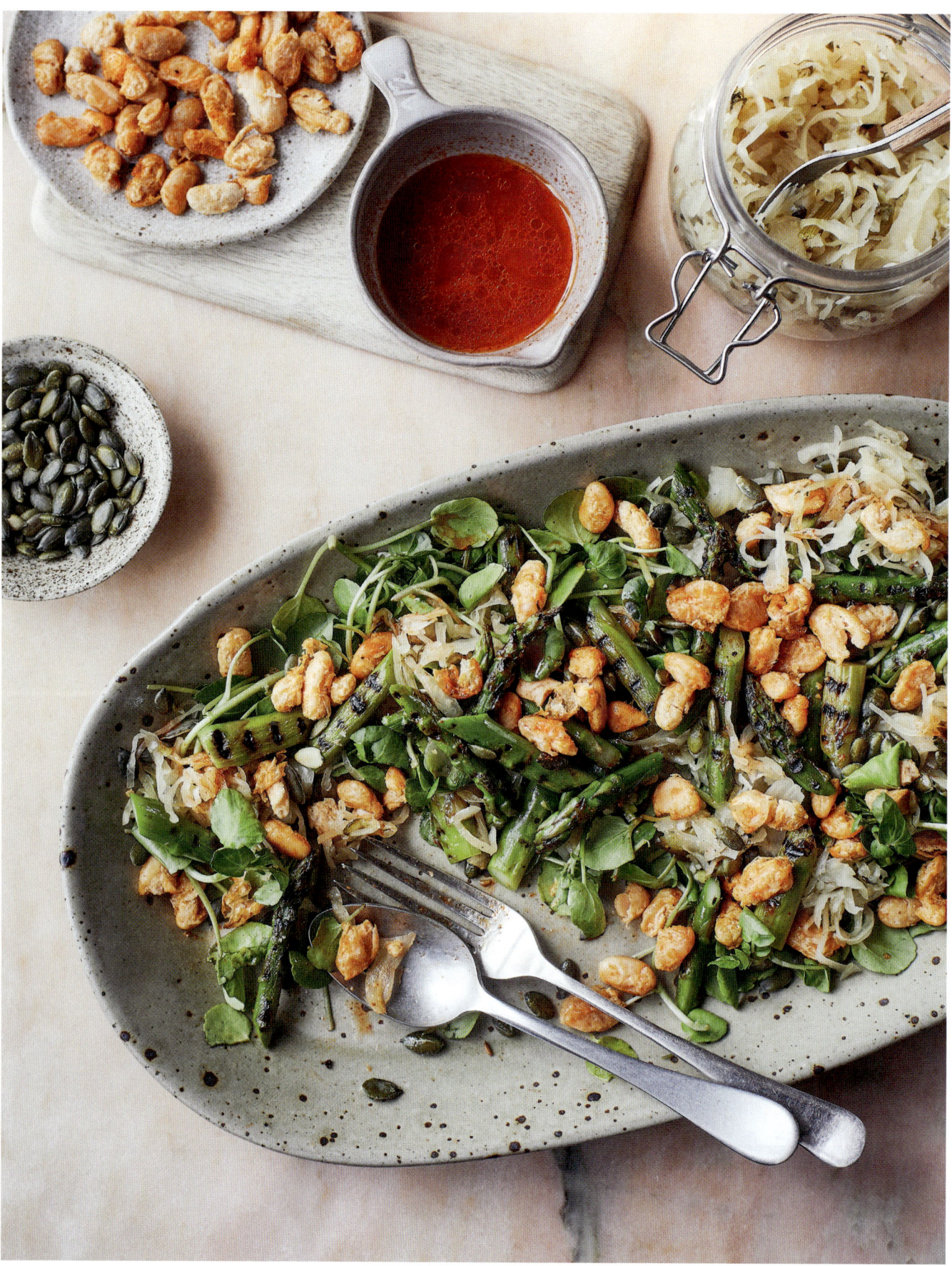

Crispy Bean and Kraut Salad with Pumpkin Seeds

Prep 5 minutes
Cook 30 minutes

Serves 2

- 1 x 400g can large white beans, drained and rinsed
- 2 tbsp olive oil, plus extra for frying
- 1 tsp sweet paprika
- 150g asparagus
- 75g sauerkraut, with the juice
- 100g watercress
- 50g pumpkin seeds, lightly toasted

One of my favourite uses of the air fryer is to make these crispy beans. The crunchy outer shells with soft warm centres are like mini roast potatoes, perfectly cooked and beautifully seasoned. As a salad topper these provide a good dose of fibre and, coupled with the pumpkin seeds to add more texture, you're getting some good-quality fats. You can also use Tenderstem broccoli or mini leeks instead of asparagus.

To make the crispy beans, thoroughly dry the white beans on kitchen paper, then add to a bowl and drizzle with a little of the oil and half of the paprika. Season with salt and mix gently with your hands until combined.

Air fry at 200°C for 10 minutes (or oven bake at 200°C fan for 20–22 minutes) until golden and crispy. Make sure you shake them halfway through cooking.

Meanwhile, brush the asparagus with a little oil. Heat a sauté pan or griddle pan over a medium heat, add the asparagus and cook for 5 minutes, turning occasionally, until just tender with a slight bite. Set aside to cool, then slice the stalks diagonally, leaving the tips whole.

Squeeze the juice from the sauerkraut into a small mixing bowl, then whisk in 2 tablespoons of the olive oil and the remaining paprika. Season with salt and pepper and set aside.

To build your salad, start with the watercress leaves on the base and top with the pumpkin seeds, asparagus and sauerkraut, then drizzle over the simple sauerkraut-infused paprika dressing. Scatter over the crispy beans to finish.

PROTEIN BOOST

Try serving this with cooked tempeh chunks or leftover chicken.

Protein 18.9g

Fibre 13.8g

Plant Points 5.5

FRESH & LIGHT PLATES

Orange and Olive Freekeh with Grilled Trout

Prep 10 minutes
Cook 15 minutes

Serves 2

a bunch of spring onions, thinly sliced
50g pitted black olives, halved
50g flat-leaf parsley, finely chopped
100g cooked freekeh
200g cooked Puy lentils
1 large orange, cut into segments
300g trout fillets, skin on

For the dressing
2 tbsp extra-virgin olive oil, plus extra for rubbing
1 tbsp sour cherry or pomegranate molasses
1 tsp Aleppo pepper

The oily fish is anti-inflammatory, we have a beautiful diversity of ingredients and polyphenols from the oranges and olives plus a good amount of fibre and protein which will keep you satiated and strong. Simply use short-grain brown rice if you can't find freekeh or need a gluten-free swap, but I do enjoy the nutty flavour and harder texture of freekeh. This will also work well with salmon, mackerel, sardines or by adding chickpeas instead of Puy lentils.

First make the dressing. Whisk together the ingredients, season with salt and pepper and set aside.

Add the spring onions, olives, parsley, freekeh, lentils and orange segments to a large serving bowl and gently toss together.

Rub the trout fillets with a little olive oil and season. Heat a sauté pan or griddle pan over a medium heat, place the fillets, skin-side down, and cook for 3–4 minutes, then turn over and cook for another 2–3 minutes, depending on their thickness.

Pour the dressing over the salad, toss to combine and check for seasoning. Transfer the salad to plates or shallow serving bowls and top each one with a trout fillet.

PROTEIN BOOST
Add more trout or lentils.

Protein 42.5g | Fibre 9.9g | Plant Points 5.75

FRESH & LIGHT PLATES

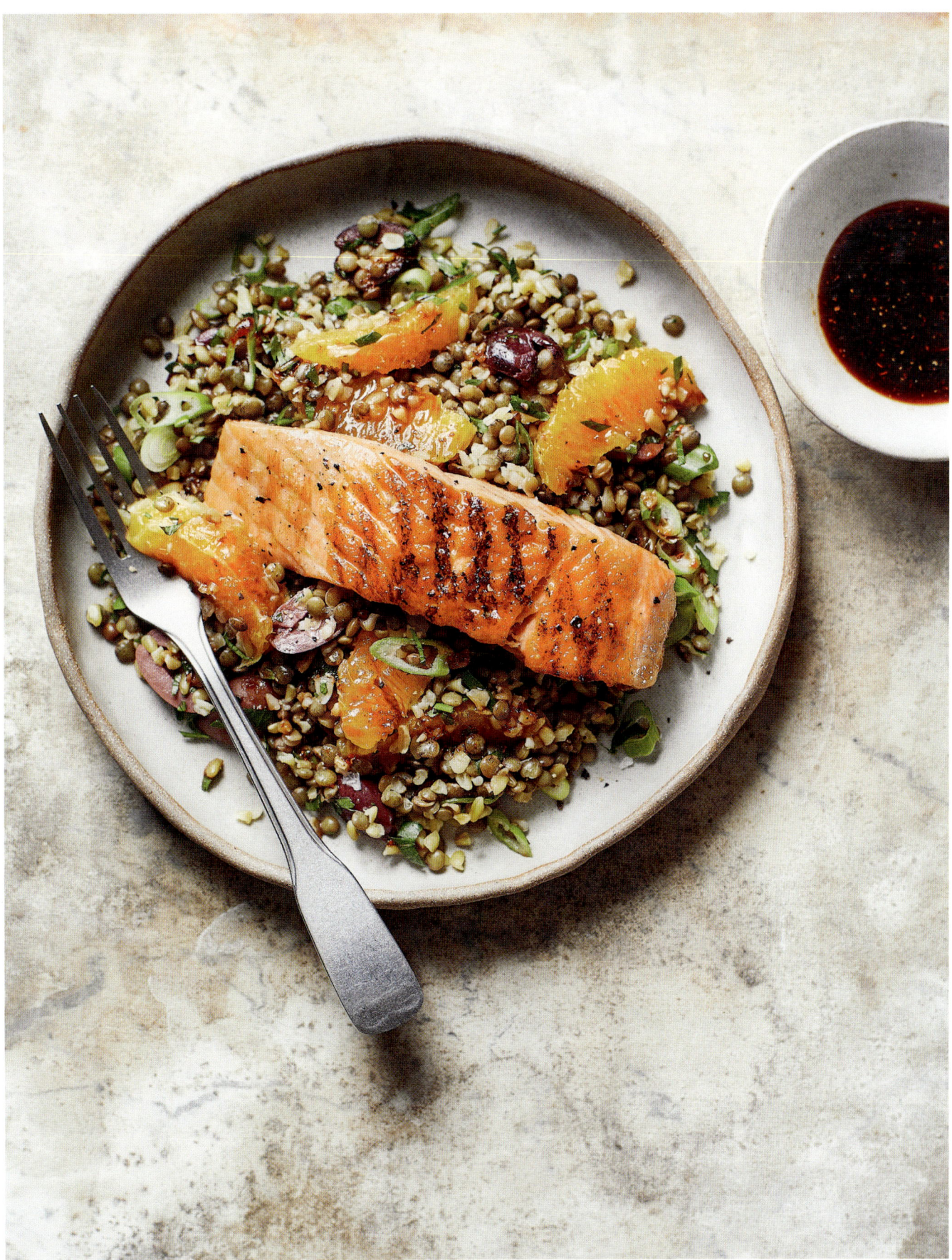

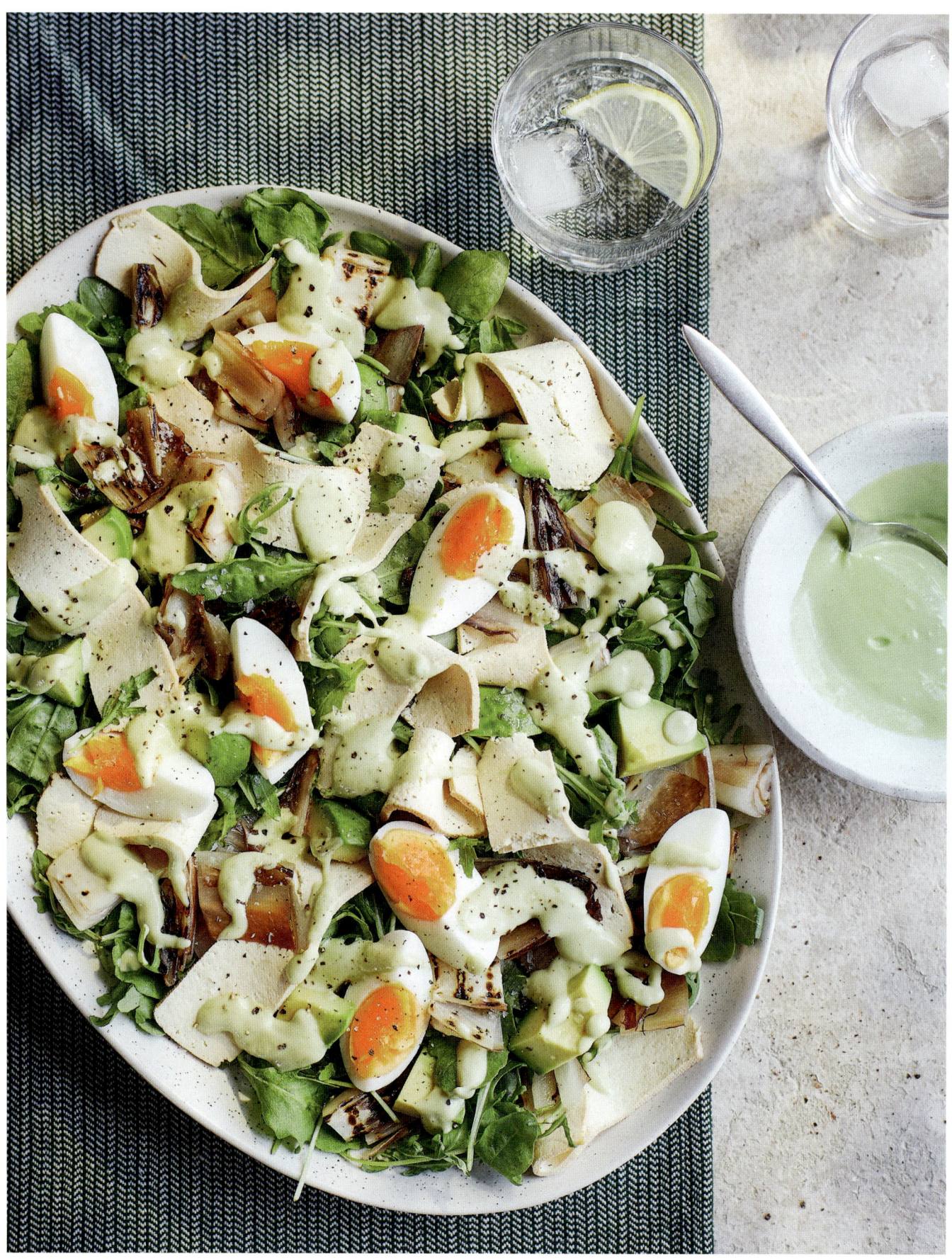

Smoked Tofu, Avocado and Chicory Salad with Mustard Tahini Dressing

Prep 10 minutes
Cook 10 minutes

Serves 2

200g red chicory (Belgian endive), halved lengthways
Olive oil, for brushing
100g rocket leaves
150g smoked tofu, thinly sliced into ribbons
2 hard-boiled eggs, peeled and quartered

For the dressing
2 tbsp tahini
Juice and finely grated zest of 1 lemon
2 tsp Dijon mustard
2 tbsp olive oil
1 avocado, halved, stone removed and cubed

Smoked tofu was a game-changer for me. You can find it in most supermarkets these days, online and certainly in health food shops. It resembles smoked ham when sliced ever so thinly in a sandwich or salad, without the extra processed ingredients that many 'faux meats' contain, with a good amount of protein plus those wonderful gut-supporting, anti-inflammatory phytonutrients from the soya beans. This salad is simple but packed with fresh flavour for a great side or light main meal. Endive also provide a wonderful amount of prebiotic fibre for your gut microbes and I love lightly cooking it to make it sweeter.

Brush the endive with olive oil. Heat a sauté pan or griddle pan over a medium–high heat, add the endive and cook for 5 minutes, turning once, until starting to colour or light char marks appear. Set aside to cool slightly, then slice.

Prepare your dressing by blending the tahini, lemon juice, mustard, olive oil and half the avocado (save the other half for the salad) with 25ml of water in a bullet blender. Add more water, as needed, to get the right consistency – it should be loose enough to drizzle, but thick enough to lightly coat the salad ingredients. Season with salt and pepper.

To build your salad, start with the rocket leaves on the base and top with the warm endive, ribbons of smoked tofu, remaining cubes of avocado, quartered boiled eggs and the delicious tahini-mustard-avocado dressing. Add a little extra lemon juice, the zest and seasoning to taste.

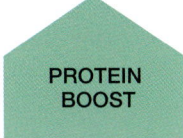

PROTEIN BOOST
Use extra tofu or more eggs.

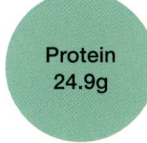

Protein 24.9g | Fibre 8g | Plant Points 4.5

FRESH & LIGHT PLATES

3-INGREDIENT HIGH-PROTEIN SAUCES AND DRESSINGS

You don't automatically think of a sauce as a source of protein, but these easy-to-make, wholesome sauces actually are! They can give a salad a new taste twist, simply sautéed vegetables brightness, and add flavour to any meal. They can also provide extra fibre and inflammation-lowering ingredients such as herbs and spices. They deliver extra polyphenols and beautiful character to a recipe. Have these to hand.

Preserved Lemon and Tahini Dressing

Makes about 120ml

1 preserved lemon (about 30g), cut in half and seeds removed
50g tahini
50ml hot water
10g dill, tough stalks removed, leaves finely chopped

Add all the ingredients, apart from the dill, to a bullet blender with some seasoning and blitz until smooth and creamy. Add the dill and stir.

The dressing should be thick but pourable and it should be able to coat green leaves in a salad or a piece of cooked fish. Add a splash more water if needed.

Soy and Peanut Dressing

Makes about 75ml

2 tbsp smooth peanut butter
1 tbsp light soy sauce
½ tsp mild chilli powder
30ml just-boiled water

Using a small balloon whisk, beat all the ingredients in a bowl, adding more water if needed. The dressing should combine easily and be pourable over, for example, an Asian-inspired salad or on top of simply baked tofu cubes (see page 203).

Miso and Almond Butter Dressing

Makes about 75ml

1 tbsp white miso paste
2 tbsp smooth almond butter
30ml just-boiled water

Using a small balloon whisk, beat all the ingredients together in a bowl, adding more water if needed. The dressing should combine easily and be pourable over, for example, simply baked sea bass fillets, coating the flesh.

Lemon Feta Sauce

Makes about 110ml

Finely grated zest and juice of 1 small lemon
60g feta
20ml water
10g tarragon, tough stalks removed, leaves finely chopped

Add all the ingredients, apart from the tarragon, to a bullet blender with some seasoning and blitz until smooth and creamy. Add the chopped tarragon and stir.

The sauce should be thick but pourable and able to coat, for example, radicchio leaves in a simple salad with walnuts, cucumber and olives. Add a splash more water if needed.

Labneh and Za'atar Sauce

Makes about 110ml

90g labneh
2 tsp za'atar
Finely grated zest and juice of 1 small lemon

Add all the ingredients to a bullet blender with some seasoning and blitz. You may need to add a splash of water.

The sauce should be thick but pourable and it should be able to coat, for example, chopped baby tomatoes, black olives, baked aubergine and crispy baked tofu pieces in a simple salad.

Chilli, Lime and Tahini Dressing

Makes about 120ml

50g tahini
Juice of 1 lime
2 tsp chilli oil
50ml water

Add all the ingredients to a bullet blender with some seasoning and blitz until smooth and creamy.

The dressing should be thick but pourable and able to coat, for example, cooked chicken pieces with pickles, tomatoes and greens. It's perfect for a quick healthy salad bowl. Add a splash more water if needed.

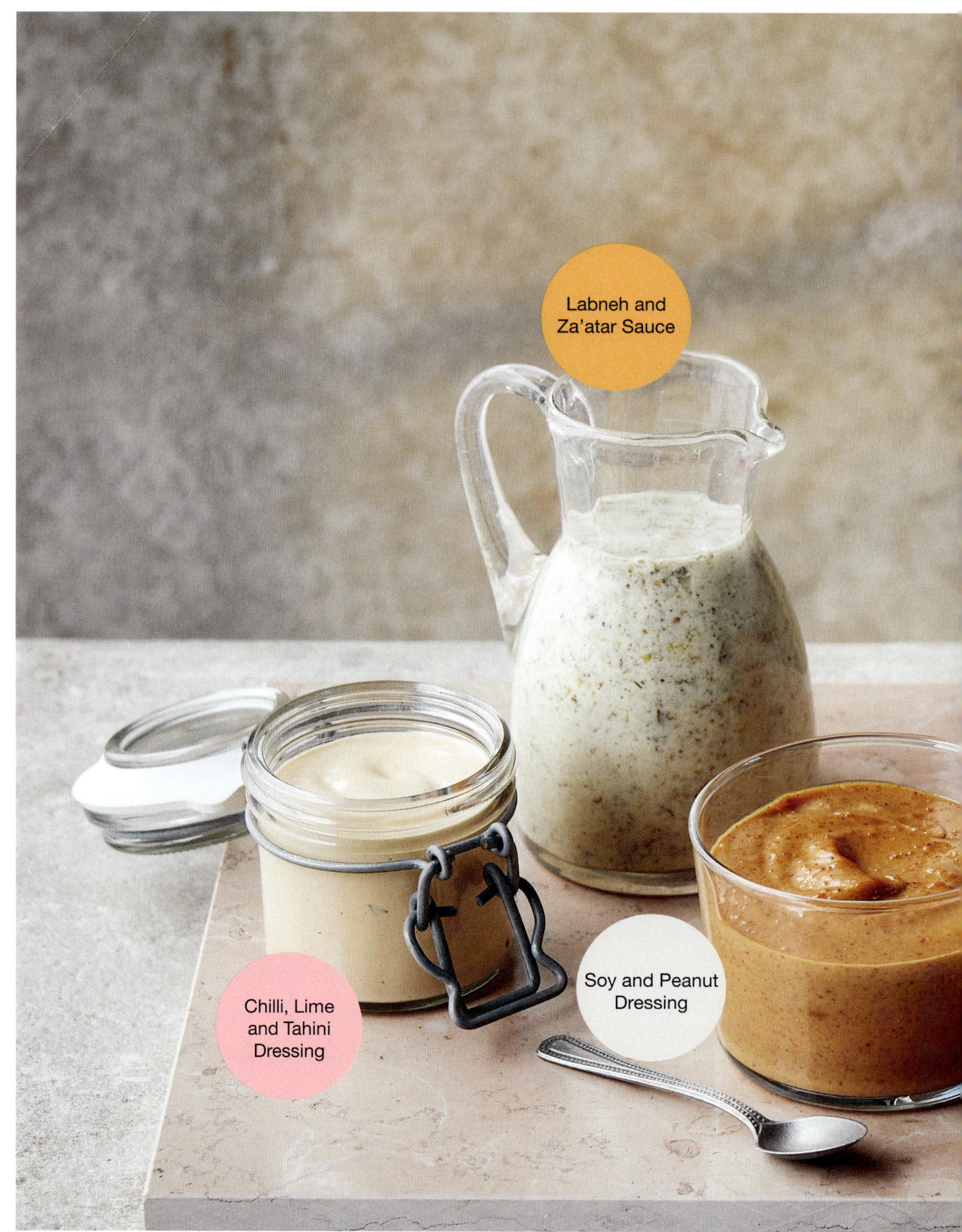

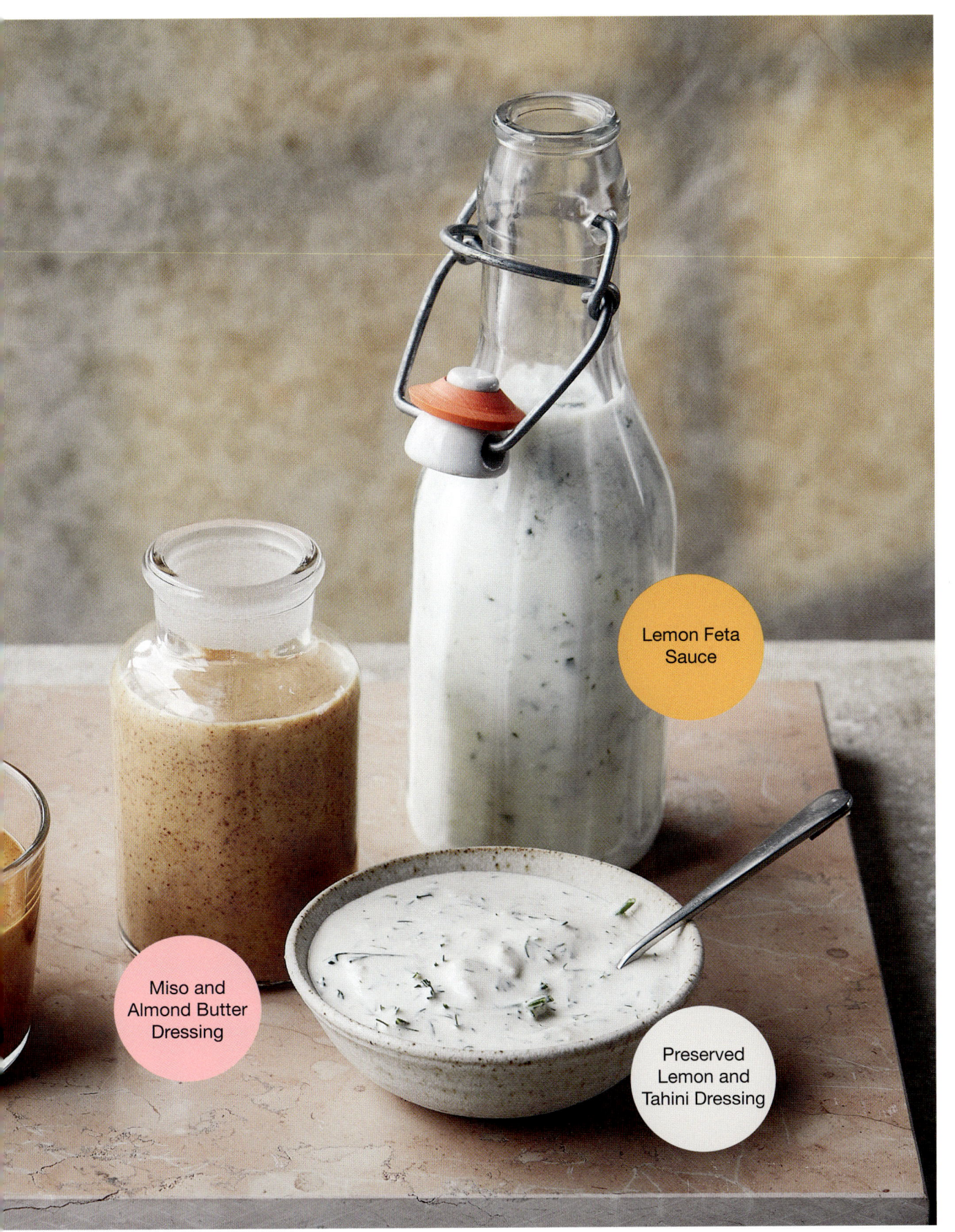

MEAT
-LESS

MID-
WEEK

Miso Mushroom Soba Broth with Crispy Chilli Tofu

Prep 10 minutes
Cook 20 minutes

Serves 2

2 tbsp olive oil
150g spring onions, thinly sliced
3 garlic cloves, grated or finely diced
150g shiitake mushrooms, roughly chopped
150g oyster mushrooms, torn into bite-size pieces
100g edamame beans
700ml boiling water
3 tbsp tahini
2 tbsp white miso paste
150g soba noodles
1 tbsp sesame seeds, lightly toasted, to garnish

For the crispy chilli tofu
300g firm tofu, cut into 2cm thick batons
2 tbsp cornflour
1 tbsp olive oil
1 tbsp crispy chilli oil

I love soba noodles. Their wholesome colour and harder texture are indicative of the extra fibre and nourishment they contain. Sesame paste is a common ingredient in Chinese cooking. Tahini, used in Middle Eastern cooking, generally uses whole, unroasted sesame seeds blended into a paste, and is different to the Chinese variety which uses toasted sesame that delivers a rich flavour. You can absolutely use that variety, but for ease and accessibility I'm using tahini. It still contains the rich nutrients and protein I want to bring to this mushroom broth, plus the miso introduces depth and umami character.

Add the olive oil to a large saucepan over a medium heat and cook the spring onions, reserving a handful for garnish, and garlic for a few minutes. Add the mushrooms and cook for 8–10 minutes, stirring occasionally, until golden. Add the edamame beans and hot water and bring to a simmer. Add more to cover the vegetables if needed.

Put the tahini and miso in a small bowl, then carefully add a few tablespoons of the simmering liquid from the pan and mix together. Continue to add a spoonful at a time until the paste becomes runny. Slowly stir this mixture into the pot and cook for another 4–5 minutes to combine the flavours. Taste for seasoning.

Meanwhile, dust the tofu batons in the cornflour with seasoning. Add the olive oil to a sauté pan over a medium heat and cook the tofu batons for 4–5 minutes on each side until crispy.

Transfer to a plate lined with kitchen paper to soak any excess oil. Remove the kitchen paper and spoon over the chilli oil so the tofu can absorb the flavour.

Prepare your soba noodles according to the packet instructions, then drain and divide between 2 serving bowls. Pour the broth over the top and finish with the crispy chilli tofu batons. Garnish with the reserved spring onion and the sesame seeds.

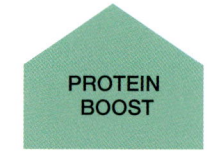

PROTEIN BOOST
Add more tofu batons or cooked edamame.

Protein 49.8g
Fibre 10.8g
Plant Points 9.25

190 MEATLESS MIDWEEK

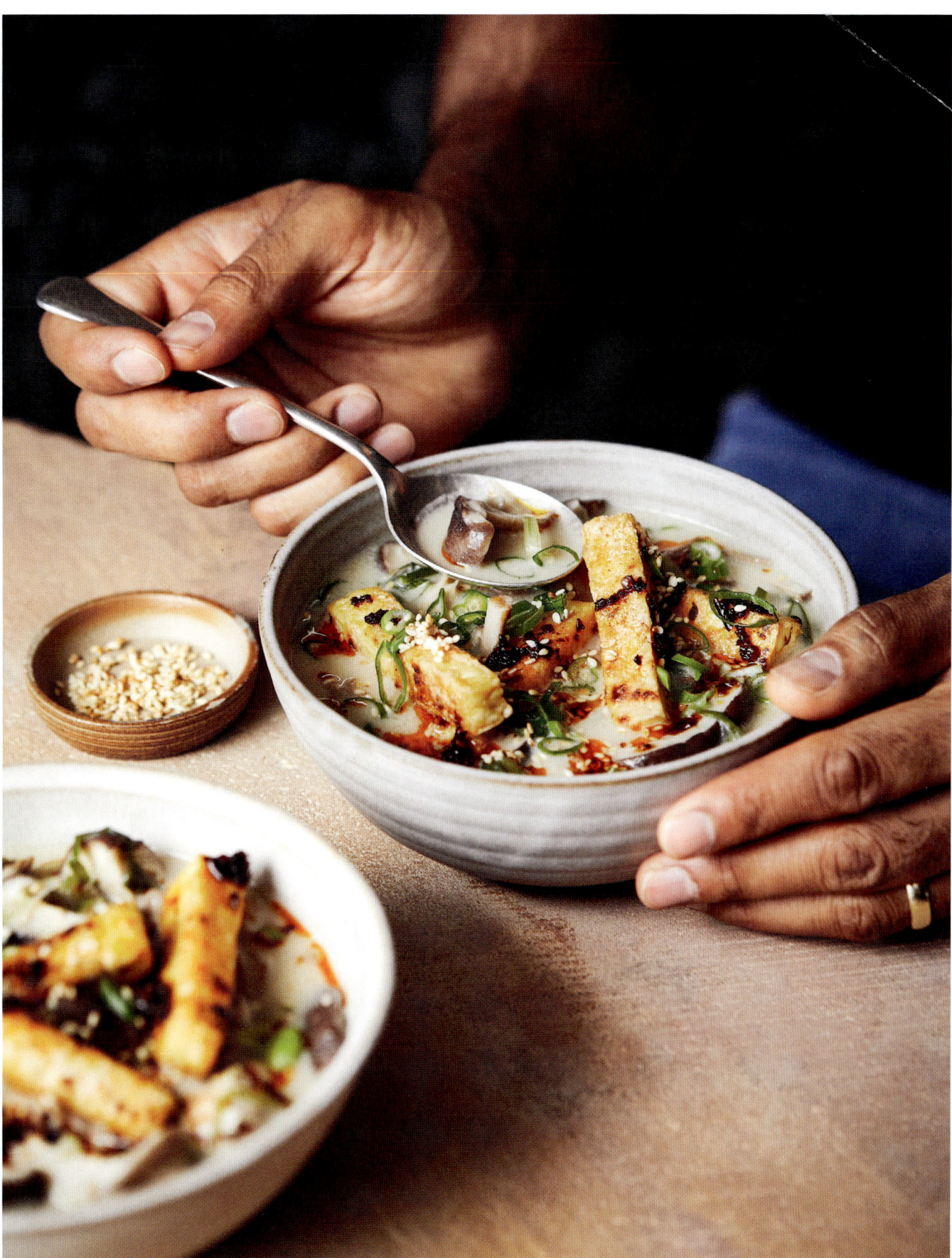

Spicy Thyme Lentil Coconut Curry

Prep 10 minutes
Cook 30 minutes

Serves 4

1 tbsp olive oil
25g fresh root ginger, peeled and coarsely grated
200g courgette, diced
2 sprigs of thyme
2 tsp cumin seeds
2 tsp ras el hanout
1 tsp ground turmeric
2 tbsp tomato purée
1 x 400g can chickpeas
250g cooked beluga or Puy lentils
1 x 400ml can coconut milk
200g baby spinach
Juice of 1 lemon
10g coriander leaves, to finish (optional)

<u>For the crispy tempeh</u>
400g tempeh
1 tbsp olive oil
2 tsp ras el hanout

This gorgeous orange-coloured curry is divine. If you're not a fan of tempeh you can replace it with tofu or even lean beef mince, but I think the body and flavour of tempeh work well with the spices. This is one of my favourite techniques to prepare tempeh and gives extra texture and crunch to what is one of the best ingredients for protein and your gut health. Lemon cuts through the richness of the coconut for a well-balanced dish.

Preheat the oven to 200°C fan.

Coarsely grate the tempeh onto a large baking tray, add the olive oil and ras el hanout, then season and mix everything together with your hands until combined. Bake for 15–20 minutes, turning halfway, until browned and slightly crisp.

Meanwhile, heat the olive oil in a sauté pan or casserole dish over a medium heat. Add the ginger and courgette and cook for 3–4 minutes until slightly coloured. Stir in the thyme, spices and the tomato purée. Stir so the purée doesn't catch and cook for a couple of minutes until it turns dark red in colour, adding a splash of water to loosen the mixture if needed.

Add the chickpeas and their liquid, plus the lentils and stir gently to mix all the ingredients together. Pour in the coconut milk and 50ml of water, if the mixture looks too dry, and simmer over a low–medium heat, stirring occasionally, for 15 minutes until reduced and thickened. Season well with salt and pepper.

Add the spinach and cook, stirring, for about 3 minutes until the leaves cook down in the sauce and soften. Add a good squeeze of lemon to the curry and serve topped with the spiced golden tempeh and a scattering of coriander, if you like.

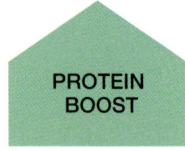

PROTEIN BOOST
Add more tempeh or some nutritional yeast to the sauce.

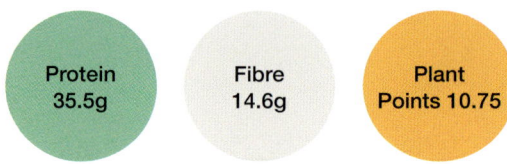

Protein 35.5g
Fibre 14.6g
Plant Points 10.75

MEATLESS MIDWEEK

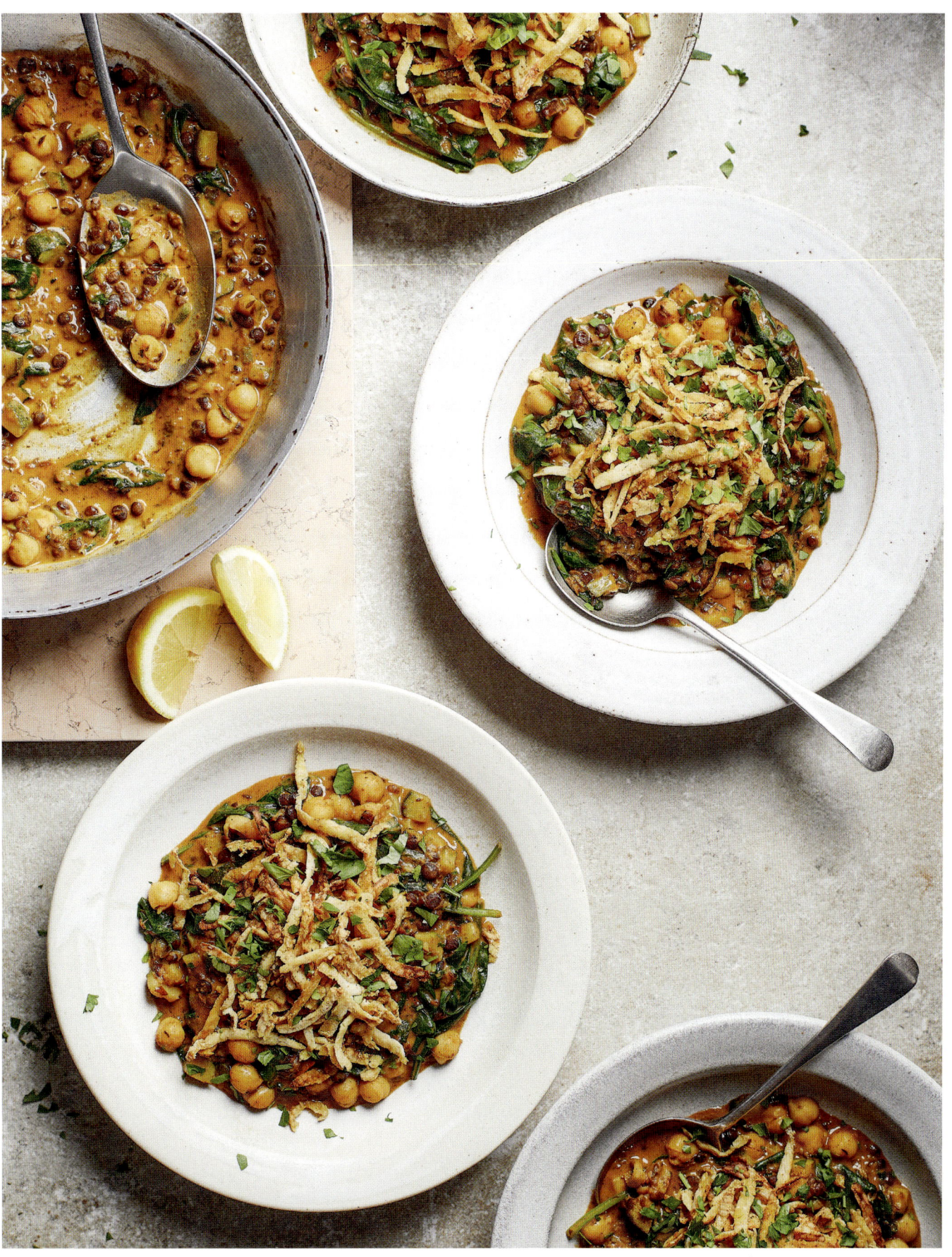

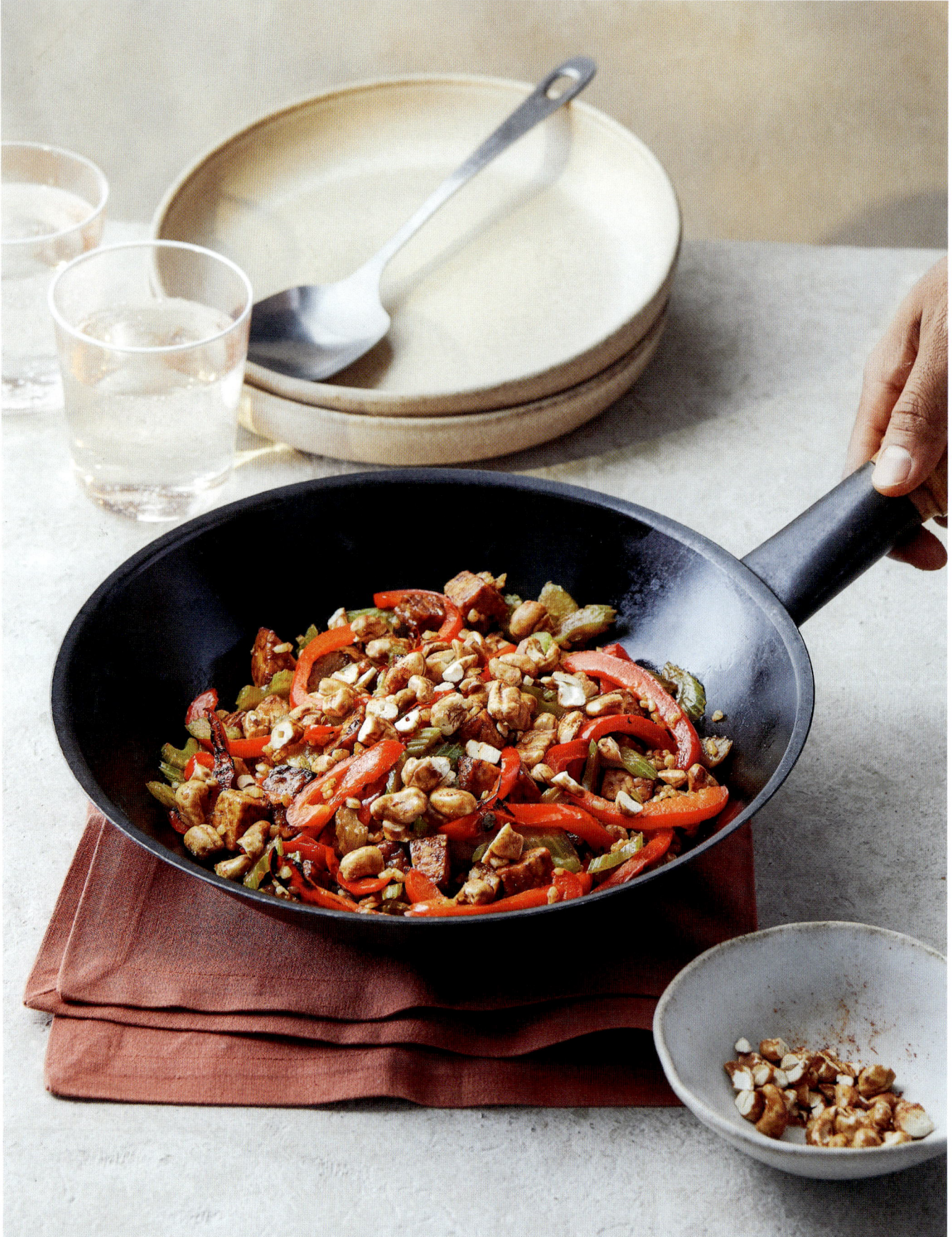

Sweet Chilli Cashew and Celery Stir-fry

Prep 10 minutes, plus
Cook

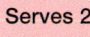
Serves 2

1 tbsp olive oil
200g celery, sliced on an angle into thin pieces
160g red pepper, deseeded sliced into thin slivers
100g cooked short-grain brown rice

For the tempeh
200g tempeh, cut into 1cm cubes
2 tbsp soy sauce, plus extra to serve
2 tbsp oyster sauce or teriyaki
1 tbsp olive oil

For the sweet chilli cashews
3 tsp coconut or soft brown sugar
1 tbsp boiling water
40g cashews, roughly chopped
¼ tsp chilli powder

I love using celery in a stir-fry. Usually reserved for salads, celery completely transforms when stir-fried and adds a delicious light crunch to the dish. Tempeh is one of those special fermented ingredients that will provide your gut microbes with new friends, as well as food to eat. The phytonutrients in the soya beans are anti-inflammatory and heart health-supporting, so they're an ingredient we should learn to love. Combined with the salty, umami flavours of oyster sauce it's a winner.

Add the tempeh to a mixing bowl with the soy sauce, and oyster sauce or teriyaki and olive oil. Mix thoroughly and leave to marinate for at least 10 minutes (the longer the better).

Preheat the oven to 200°C fan.

Spread the tempeh out on a baking tray and bake for 20–25 minutes, turning halfway through.

Meanwhile, to make the sweet chilli cashews, line a baking sheet with baking paper. Scatter the sugar in a dry saucepan over a medium heat and add the hot water. Stir to combine until all the sugar dissolves and begins to caramelise.

Add the chopped cashews and continue stirring into the sugar mixture until combined and the contents become brown and sticky.

Scrape onto the lined baking sheet to cool and sprinkle with the chilli powder and a pinch of salt. Once cooled and solidified (about 10 minutes), roughly chop.

Heat a large wok over a high heat. Add the celery and red pepper and stir-fry for a few minutes until you see some char marks on the vegetables. Add the rice and cook for another 2 minutes until it is piping hot.

Toss in your baked tempeh cubes with some extra soy sauce and black pepper to season. Finish with the sweet chilli cashews to serve.

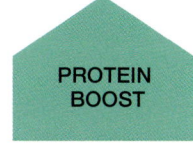
PROTEIN BOOST
Add more tempeh, cashews.

Protein 29g
Fibre 10.7g
Plant Points 5.75

MEATLESS MIDWEEK

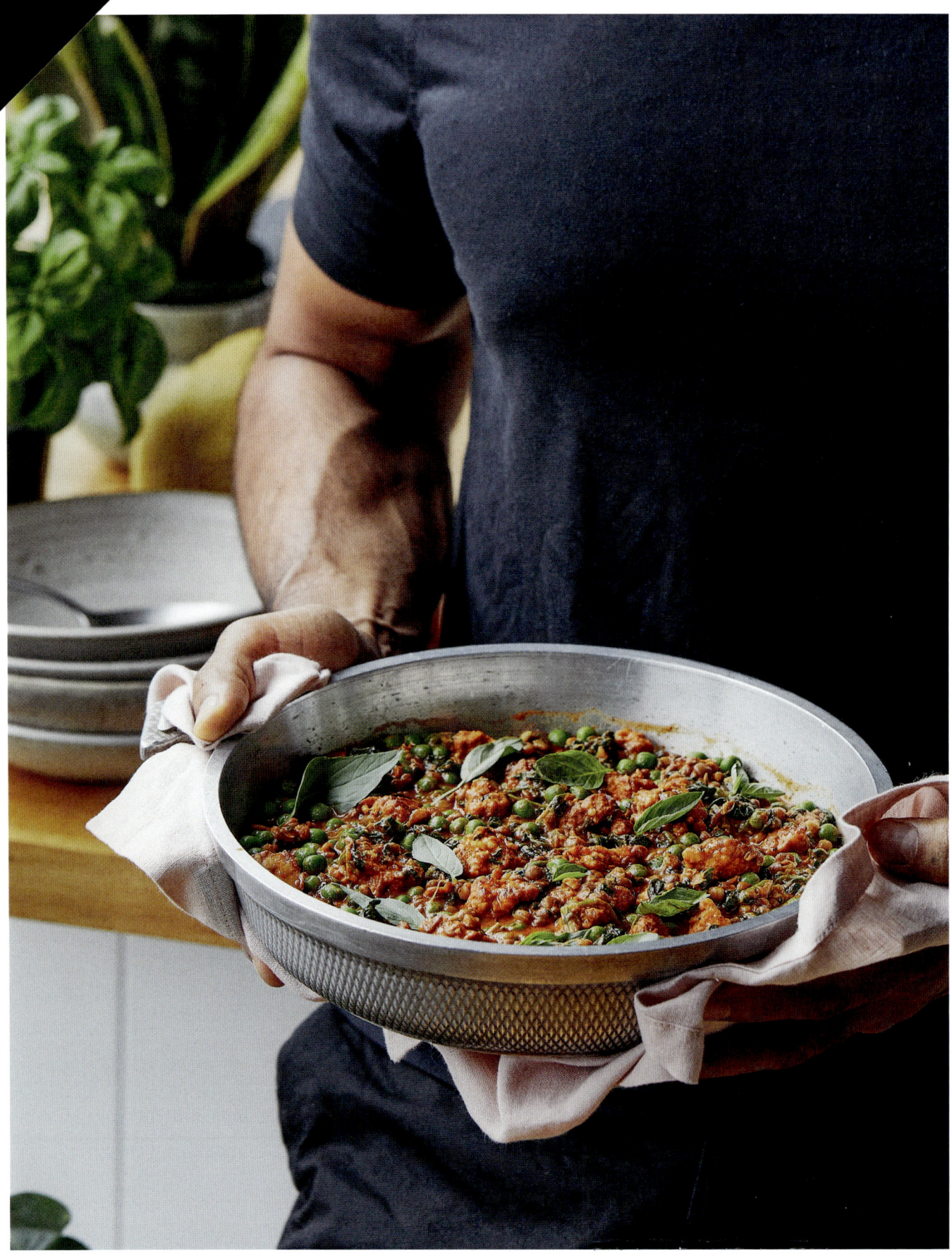

Lazy Ginger and Peanut Thai Curry

Prep 5 minutes
Cook 25 minutes

Serves 2

5cm fresh root ginger, peeled and grated
2 tbsp tomato purée
2 tbsp red Thai curry paste
3 tbsp peanut butter
1 x 400g can brown lentils
150ml boiling water
200g peas (fresh or defrosted from frozen)
100g frozen spinach, defrosted
150g cooked short-grain brown rice, warmed, to serve
10g Thai basil, to garnish

For the crispy tempeh
2 tsp red Thai curry paste
1 tbsp soy sauce
200g tempeh, broken into chunks
2 tsp cornflour
1 tbsp olive oil

This is my version of a lazy curry for when you want something absolutely delicious but are not really up for a long cook. You basically want it all: a healthy, gut-supporting, high-protein recipe that looks after your wellbeing, with minimal effort. And you can have it all with this delicious, easy recipe. The tempeh chunks are flavoured with Thai curry paste and crisp up beautifully with cornflour for a great texture against the buttery, smooth curry.

Preheat the oven to 200°C fan and line a baking sheet with baking paper.

For the crispy tempeh, add the red Thai curry paste to a mixing bowl with the soy sauce and mix together. Throw in the tempeh chunks, dust with cornflour, then drizzle over the oil.

Spread out the chunks on the lined baking sheet and bake for 20 minutes until crispy, turning halfway through.

Meanwhile, to a saucepan over a medium heat add the grated ginger, tomato purée, Thai curry paste, 2 tablespoons of the peanut butter and stir until combined.

Add the brown lentils with their liquid and the boiling water and stir to combine. Bring to a simmer for 10 minutes, stirring often, to infuse all the flavours.

Add the peas and spinach and cook for another 3–4 minutes before adding the crispy tempeh and the remaining peanut butter, seasoning and mixing well.

Serve with the brown rice in bowls with the Thai basil for garnish.

PROTEIN BOOST
Add more tempeh.

Protein 50.3g
Fibre 22.9g
Plant Points 7.75

MEATLESS MIDWEEK 197

Braised Shiitake Mushrooms and Broccoli with Crispy Chilli Yuba

Prep 5 minutes, plus soaking
Cook 35 minutes

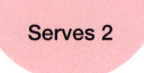
Serves 2

125g tofu knots (yuba)
2 tbsp sriracha sauce
1 tbsp olive oil
1 tbsp tomato purée
1 tbsp soy sauce

For the braised vegetables
30g dried shiitake mushrooms or other wild dried mushrooms
1 tbsp olive oil
20g fresh root ginger, peeled and coarsely grated
150g fresh shiitake mushrooms, roughly torn
2 garlic cloves, coarsely grated
200g Tenderstem broccoli, roughly chopped
1 tbsp soy sauce
1 tbsp oyster sauce (optional)
1 tsp cornflour mixed with 1 tbsp water
1 tbsp rice wine vinegar

Fa gu flower mushrooms bought from Asian supermarkets, would be more traditional in a braised broccoli recipe. But dried shiitake mushrooms pack an incredible depth of flavour, are easy to buy and have a number of anti-inflammatory benefits because of their gut-supporting fibres. You can also use mixed mushrooms or other dried mushrooms.

Put the dried mushrooms in a heatproof bowl, pour over just enough just-boiled water to cover and leave to soak for 20 minutes. When the mushrooms are rehydrated, drain, saving the soaking liquid for later. Roughly chop the mushrooms.

Meanwhile, add the tofu knots to a saucepan of boiling water and cook for 7–8 minutes, then drain well.

Preheat the oven to 200°C fan.

Mix the sriracha, olive oil, tomato purée and soy sauce together in a bowl, add the cooked yuba, then toss until coated in the sauce. Tip the yuba onto a large baking tray and cook in the oven for 20 minutes, turning halfway, until sticky and brown. Remove and set aside.

Meanwhile, for the braised vegetables, heat a lidded wok or sauté pan over a medium–high heat, add the oil and ginger and cook, stirring, for 1–2 minutes to infuse the oil. Add both the rehydrated and fresh mushrooms and stir-fry for 8–10 minutes until browned and starting to crisp. Add the garlic and broccoli and stir-fry for another minute.

Pour 75ml of the mushroom soaking liquid into a bowl and add the soy sauce, oyster sauce, cornflour water and rice wine vinegar. Mix together and pour into the wok, season with pepper and cover with the lid. Reduce the heat down to low and simmer very gently to infuse the flavours for 2–3 minutes. Be sure not to overcook the greens.

Spoon the vegetables into bowls, then top with the crispy sweet and chilli tofu knots. Serve with brown jasmine rice, if you like.

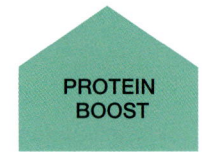
PROTEIN BOOST

Add more yuba. You can also try firm tofu or marinated tofu. If you aren't meat-free, chicken thighs cut into chunks would work well too.

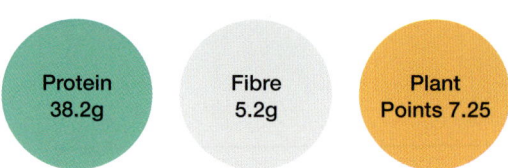
Protein 38.2g
Fibre 5.2g
Plant Points 7.25

198 MEATLESS MIDWEEK

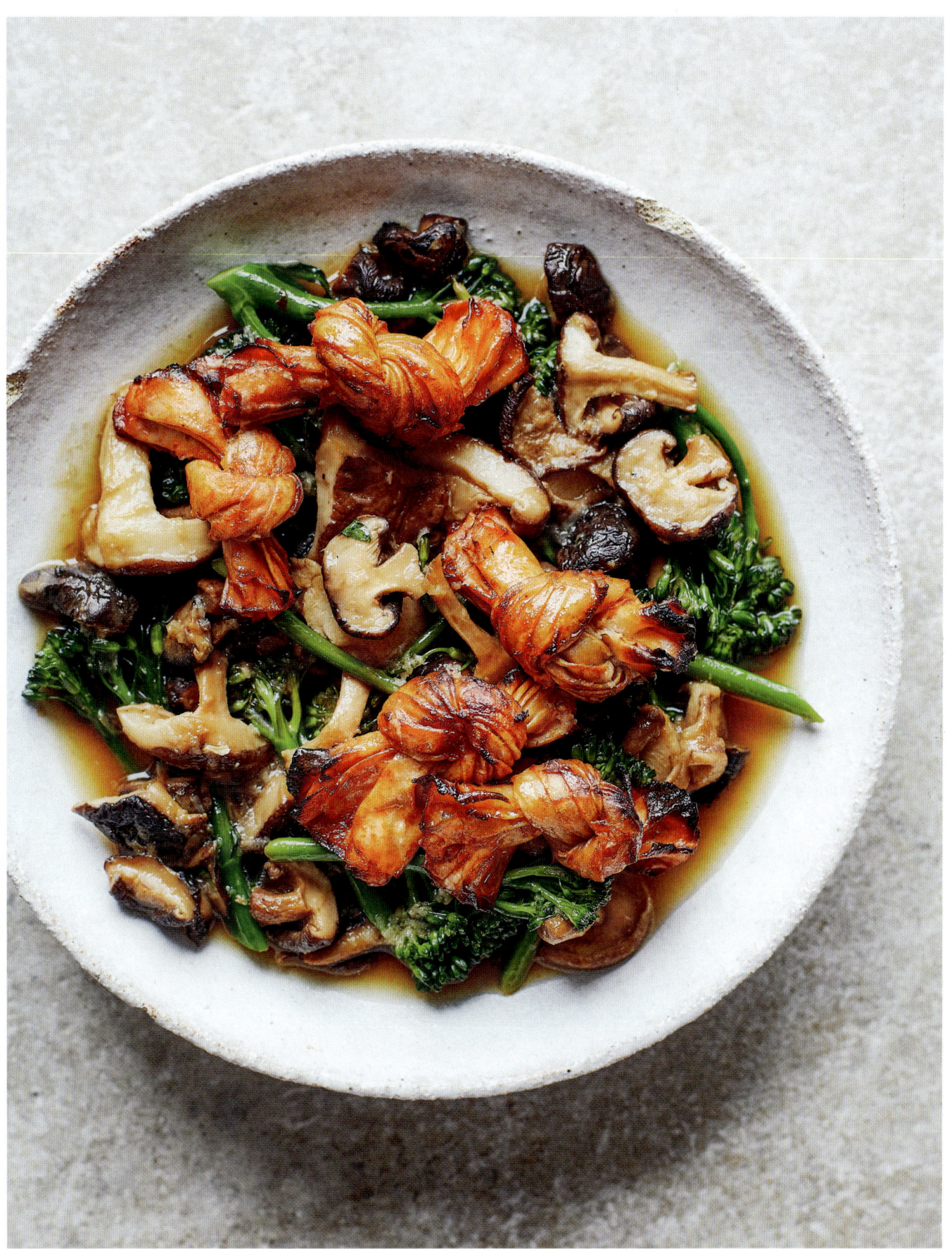

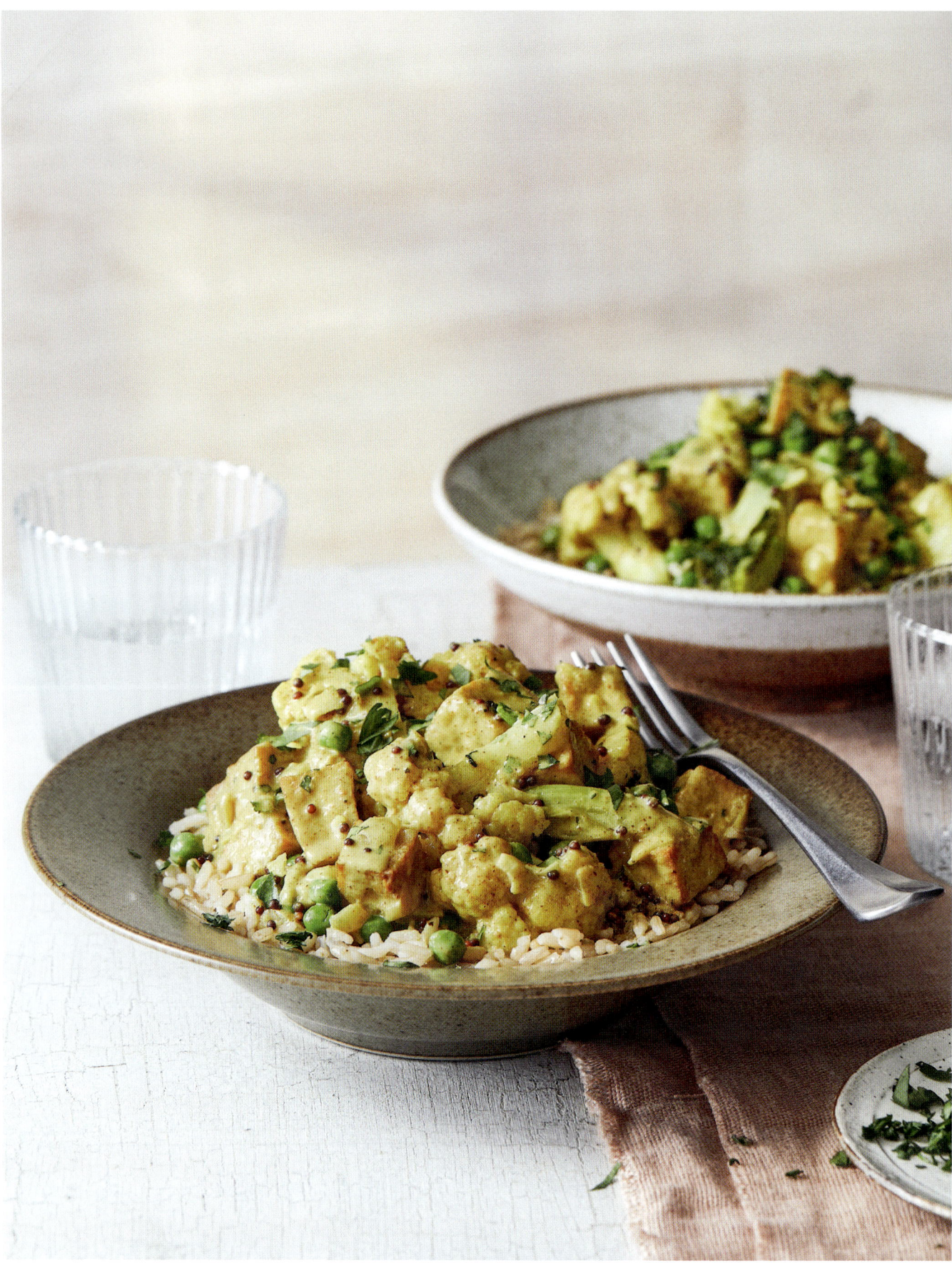

Almond and Cauliflower Curry with Crispy Tofu

Prep 10 minutes
Cook 30 minutes

Serves 2

2 tbsp olive oil
100g onion, diced
2 tsp mild curry powder
2 tsp mustard seeds
1 tsp turmeric
200g cauliflower, florets broken into 2cm pieces, leaves chopped
1 x 400ml can coconut milk
3 tbsp almond butter
100ml boiling water
200g peas (fresh or defrosted from frozen)
10g coriander, leaves and stems finely chopped, to finish
150g brown rice, cooked

For the crispy tofu
250g extra-firm tofu, cut into 2cm cubes
2 tsp cornflour
2 tsp garlic powder
1 tbsp olive oil

Almond butter is a revelation in Indian cooking. I've used ground almonds, other nut butters and whole seeds in the past, but there's something unique about almond butter and its mild sweetness that blends beautifully with the Indian spices in curries. It adds extra protein and fibre, plus the luxurious mouthfeel without the need for cream or butter. I'm using tofu for the bulk of the protein here, but feel free to use paneer instead if you prefer a more traditional ingredient.

Preheat the oven to 200°C and line a baking sheet with baking paper.

First make the crispy tofu. Roll the cubed tofu in a bowl with the cornflour, garlic powder and plenty of seasoning. Place on the lined baking sheet and drizzle over the olive oil. Bake in the oven for 20–25 minutes, turning halfway, until the tofu cubes are crispy.

Meanwhile, add the olive oil and onion to a large casserole dish over a medium heat, seasoning with salt and pepper. Cook for 10–12 minutes until soft and brown. Toss in your spices and stir for another minute.

Add the cauliflower florets and leaves. Stir through the spices so everything is combined, cook for 2–3 minutes and season well.

Add the coconut milk and almond butter with the boiling water. Stir until well combined. Bring the mixture to a gentle simmer for 8 minutes until the cauliflower is cooked through, stirring regularly. Then add the peas and continue to cook for 2 minutes.

Add the tofu cubes and sprinkle over the coriander. Serve with hot brown rice.

PROTEIN BOOST

Add more tofu. You could also add cooked green lentils to the curry.

Protein 35g
Fibre 13.8g
Plant Points 8.25

MEATLESS MIDWEEK

TOFU BASICS

Most people inexperienced with tofu have reservations about this popular soybean-based product. It's bland and they don't know the difference between the various types. I don't blame them. I used to hate the stuff myself, but now I get it into my diet at least every other day.

It has marvellous health benefits, being both high in protein and fibre, but it's also rich in phytochemicals that reduce inflammation and may even have unique anti-cancer and gut health-supporting properties. It's also one of the most versatile foods and one that I use across my culinary repertoire.

From traditional use in Asian dishes, such as China's mapo tofu and Taiwanese sesame noodles, to a meat replacement in a version of Indian butter chicken or an Italian ragu-style sauce, I use this product unashamedly and liberally. Once you master the art of crafting diverse textures – crispy, chewy or soft – and infusing flavour into its neutral taste profile, it can become an exceptional addition to both your diet and cooking.

EXTRA-FIRM TOFU, VACUUM-PACKED (MINIMAL OR NO LIQUID)

No drying or pressing is required for this type of product. It can come plain or flavoured (such as smoked, basil or even sundried tomato) in which case it makes great sandwich fillers when thinly sliced like ham. You can also simply cube it and throw into salads or stir-fries for a fibre-rich protein boost.

EXTRA-FIRM TOFU PACKED IN LIQUID

This requires pressing and drying. Simply drain the water, wrap tightly in kitchen towel and place on a cutting board with a heavy pan on top of it. Ten minutes should get most of the liquid out but some choose a longer pressing time if they need the tofu really dry. I tend to use vacuum-packed extra firm if I need a really dry product for the recipe.

SILKEN TOFU

This is the most liquid of all the tofu types. Do not attempt to dry or press this product. It should only be used cubed or blended into a sauce. It makes a fantastic cream alternative for dishes when combined with hot water and seasoning. It's equally delicious in desserts.

TEMPEH

This is a fermented version of tofu. The soybeans are fermented and pressed into a firm product that has higher protein content as a result of fermentation releasing the amino acids and making them more absorbable. It also has a distinctive flavour that makes it best used in savoury dishes. No drying or pressing are needed for tempeh, it holds it shape very well when cubed and crumbled then sautéed in a bit of oil to get crispy edges. I love it best in an Asian stir-fry with sesame paste, pak choy and tons of chilli oil.

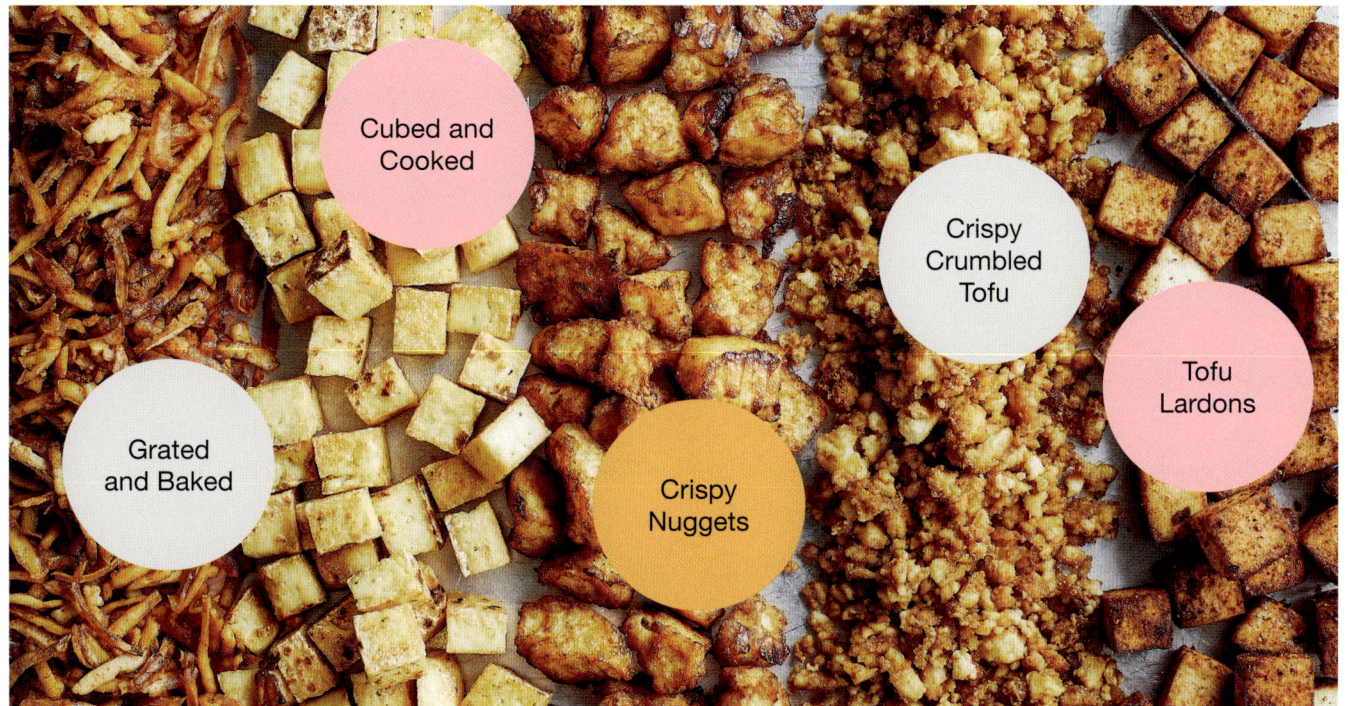

Grated and Baked

Grate **200g extra-firm tofu** (minimal or no liquid) into a baking tray lined with baking paper. Drizzle with **olive oil** and **salt**, **1 teaspoon paprika**, **1 tablespoon soy sauce** and **1 tablespoon maple syrup** and bake at 200°C fan for 20–25 minutes, turning halfway.

Cubed and Cooked

Simply cut **extra-firm tofu** (packed in liquid, dried and pressed) into 3cm cubes, dust in a little corn or rice flour and throw into a pan over a medium heat with **a little olive oil**. Fry on all sides for a couple of minutes until brown and golden, remove and leave to rest on kitchen paper to soak any excess oil. These can be used in any stews or curries to boost the protein and fibre. They'll take on the flavour really well.

Crispy Nuggets

Crumble **200g extra-firm tofu** (either vacuum-packed or packed in liquid, drained and dried) into 2cm chunks with your hands. Douse in **1 tablespoon soy sauce** and then dust in **1–2 teaspoons cornflour or rice flour**. Toss in **a little olive or neutral oil** and bake at 200°C fan for 20–25 minutes. These crispy nuggets of goodness are perfect to throw into a stir-fry, curry or even salad with a delicious dressing.

Crispy Crumbled Tofu

Crumble **200g extra-firm tofu** (packed in liquid, dried and pressed) with your hands into fine pieces, the size of breadcrumbs. Douse in **2 tablespoons soy sauce** and then dust in **1–2 teaspoons cornflour or rice flour**. Toss in **a little olive or neutral oil** and bake at 200°C fan for 20–25 minutes, tossing halfway.

The texture will become crispy and chewy, resembling beef mince. This is perfect to throw into passata with balsamic vinegar and cook down to create a delicious high-protein sauce for pasta.

Tofu Lardons

Cut **200g extra-firm tofu** (packed in liquid, dried and pressed) into 3cm cubes and soak in a mixture of **2 tbsp soy sauce, 1 tbsp balsamic vinegar, 1 tsp sweet paprika, 1 tsp ground black pepper and 2 tbsp maple syrup** for at least 20 minutes, but ideally overnight.

Bake at 200C fan for 20–25 minutes until gloriously chewy, sweet and smoky. Similar to pork lardons, it's great with noodles or pasta.

Butter Bean and Miso Soup with Crispy Tempeh

Prep 5 minutes
Cook 30 minutes

Serves 2

200g tempeh
3 tbsp olive oil
2 tsp sweet paprika
½ tsp ground cinnamon
150g cavolo nero, stalks removed
10g dill fronds, finely chopped
10g chives, finely chopped
2 tsp chilli oil (optional), to finish

For the braised soup
1 tbsp white miso paste
1 x 400g can white butter beans
250ml boiling water
20g nutritional yeast

Silky butter beans with salty miso are one of my favourite combinations. I always have miso lurking in the fridge. It's a fantastic carrier of flavour and white miso has a more delicate, sweeter flavour than darker versions. Typically, you don't think of a soup as 'high protein', but with a tempeh topper, that's about to change. Sweet cinnamon and paprika are a combination that punches into the grated tempeh. You'll start adding this topper to everything.

Preheat the oven to 220°C fan.

Grate the tempeh on a coarse box grater and scatter over a baking sheet. Add 2 tablespoons of the olive oil and some salt. Bake for 15 minutes until the tempeh starts browning.

Remove from the oven and sprinkle with the paprika and cinnamon. Toss the tempeh with a large spoon, drizzle with ½ tablespoon oil and bake for a further 10–15 minutes until crispy.

Meanwhile, blend the ingredients for the soup in a blender or food processor until silky smooth. Pour into a saucepan over a low–medium heat and gently heat through.

Add the cavolo nero to a sauté pan over a medium heat with the remaining oil. Cook gently for 3–4 minutes until the greens are wilted, then remove from the heat.

Pour your soup into shallow bowls. Scatter with half the herbs and add the greens. Top with the tempeh, the remaining herbs and a drop of chilli oil to finish, if you like.

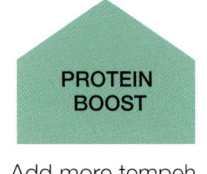

PROTEIN BOOST

Add more tempeh.

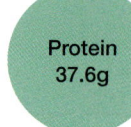

Protein 37.6g Fibre 20.4g Plant Points 4.5

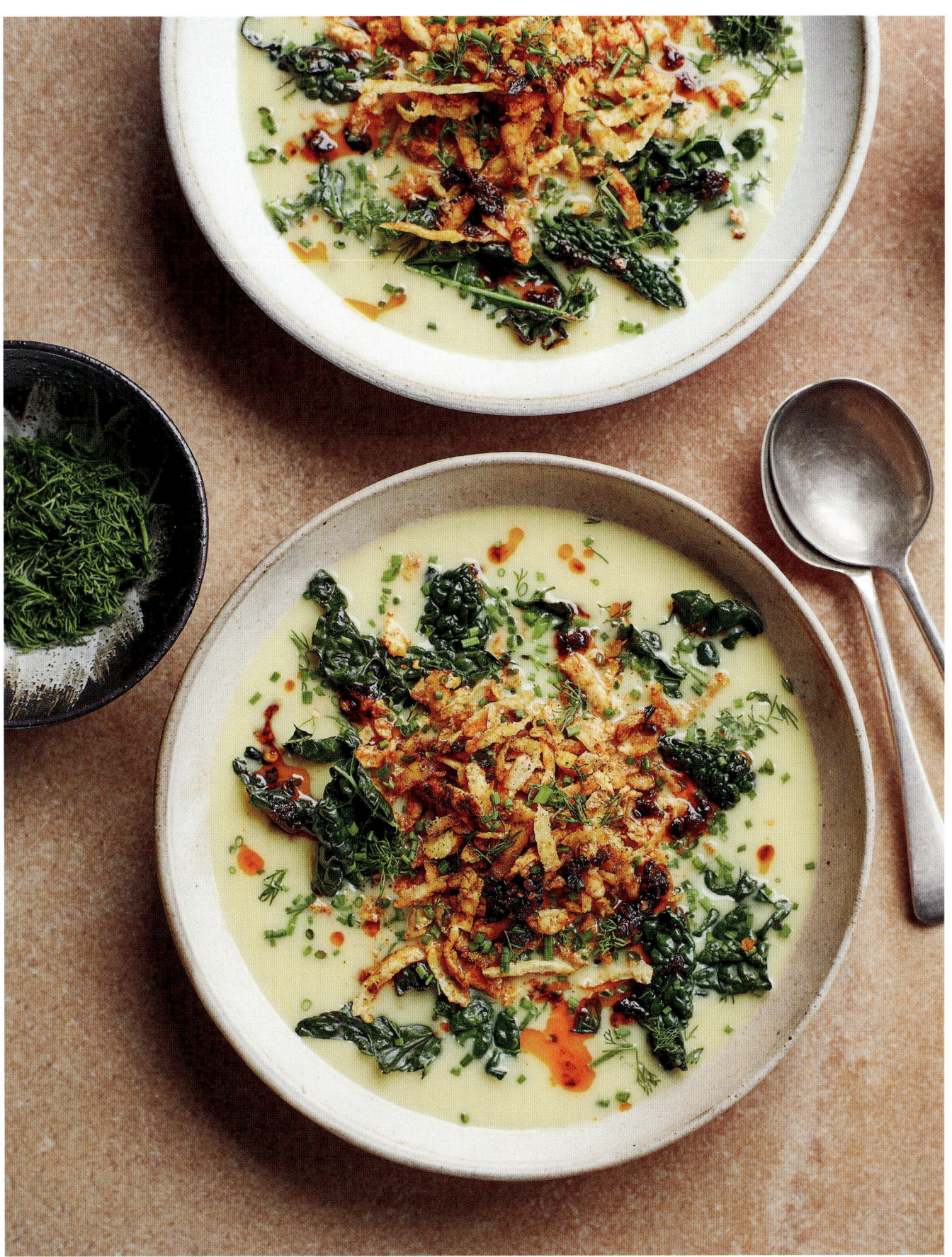

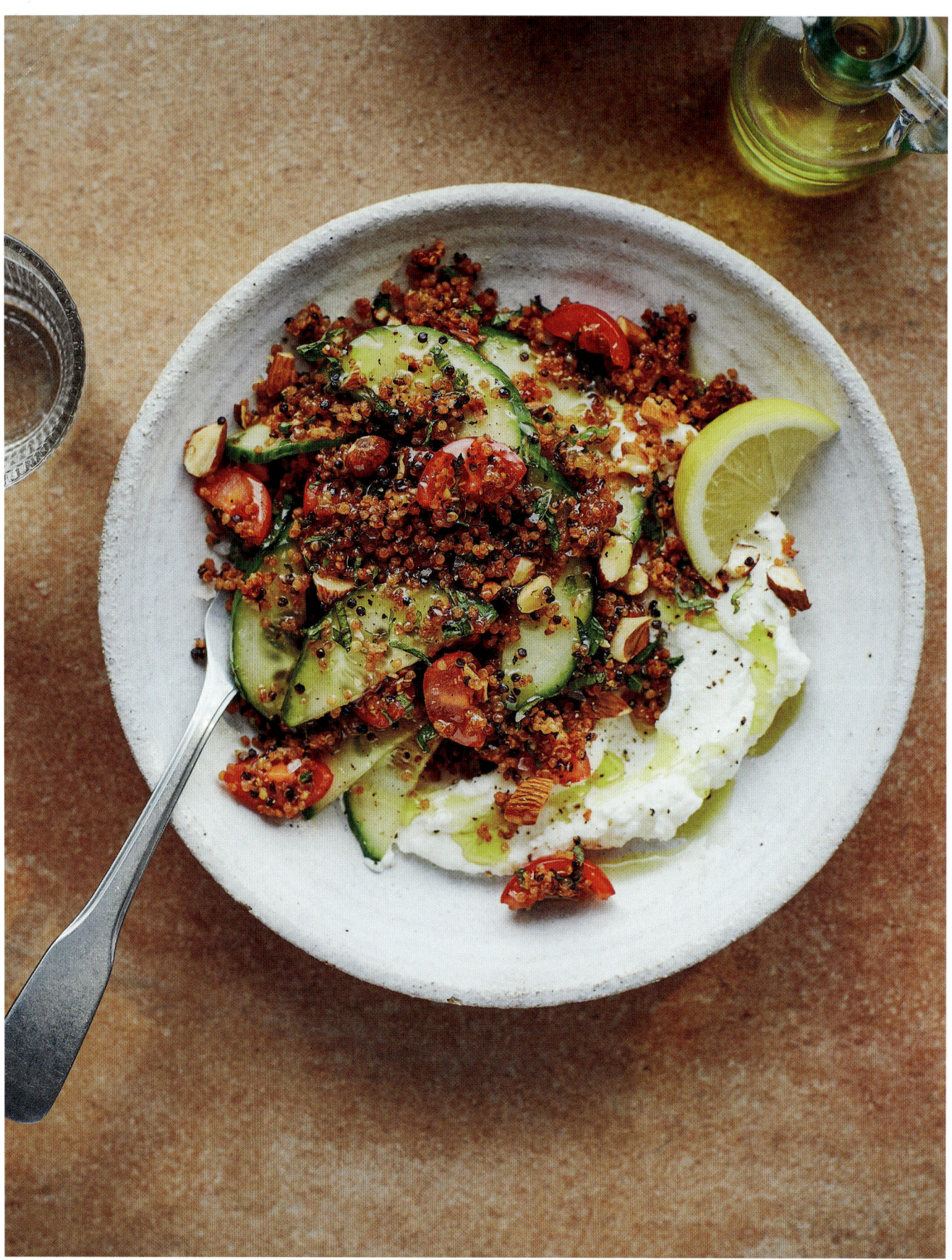

Harissa-toasted Quinoa Salad with Labneh

Prep 5 minutes
Cook 15 minutes

Serves 2

250g cooked quinoa
1 tbsp harissa paste
Olive oil, to drizzle
150g cucumber, halved lengthways and thinly sliced on an angle
100g baby tomatoes, quartered
25g mint leaves, sliced
50g almonds, roughly chopped
100g labneh or cottage cheese
Juice of ½ lemon

Toasting the quinoa in the oven makes a huge difference. It's crispy, flavourful and brings out the natural nutty flavour. In fact, if anyone has an allergy to nuts and wants to mimic the texture and protein content of them, this could be one way to do that. I use harissa for an easy flavour boost and you can also do this in the air fryer, just halve the time. The quinoa, almonds and labneh add most of the protein in this recipe, with plenty of cooling vegetables to tame the spicy harissa and add their anti-inflammatory benefits too.

Preheat the oven to 180°C fan and line a baking sheet with baking paper.

Mix the quinoa and harissa paste with a drizzle of the oil in a large mixing bowl.

Spread out on the lined baking sheet and bake for 8–10 minutes until the quinoa is toasted and slightly crisped up. Keep an eye on it so it doesn't burn.

Meanwhile, add the cucumber, tomatoes, mint leaves and almonds to a large mixing bowl.

Toss the crispy quinoa into the mixing bowl and season. Divide between serving bowls, add the labneh or cottage cheese, drizzle with some olive oil and squeeze over the lemon juice to serve.

PROTEIN BOOST

Add more labneh; almonds. If you aren't meat-free, you could also add smoked fish or cured salmon.

Protein 16.6g
Fibre 5g
Plant Points 5

MEATLESS MIDWEEK

Green Cashew Tofu Curry

Prep 10 minutes, plus soaking
Cook 30 minutes

Serves 2

Soft green herbs and lemongrass are a glorious combination that I love indulging in. The citrus flavour of lemongrass with the anti-inflammatory, sharp plant chemicals found in coriander add a beautiful flavour to this simple curry dish. I've packed this with greens and the soaked cashews give a richness to the curry that mimics heavy cream but with a different collection of fats that are heart healthy and slightly sweet.

1 tbsp olive oil
a bunch of spring onions, thinly sliced
1 lemongrass stick, tough outer leaves removed, and bashed
150g sugar snap peas, chopped
Juice of 1 lime
30g cashews, lightly toasted
150g cooked short-grain brown rice, warmed, to serve

For the crispy tofu
250g extra-firm tofu, cut into 2cm cubes
2 tsp cornflour
2 tsp black peppercorns, freshly ground
1 tbsp olive oil

For the green cashew sauce
120g cashews, soaked for 20 minutes in hot water
30g coriander, roughly chopped, plus extra to finish
15g mint leaves, chopped
1 green chilli, chopped
1 x 400ml can coconut milk
200ml vegetable stock

Preheat the oven to 200°C and line a baking sheet with baking paper.

Roll the cubed tofu in a bowl with salt, cornflour and the black pepper. Place on the lined baking sheet and drizzle over the olive oil. Bake for 20–25 minutes, turning halfway, until the tofu cubes are crispy.

Meanwhile, blend the ingredients for the green cashew sauce in a blender or food processor until smooth. Add a splash of water if needed.

Add the oil to a large casserole pan over a medium heat and cook the spring onions for 2–3 minutes. Then add the green cashew sauce and bring to a gentle simmer.

Add the bashed lemongrass and cook gently for 10 minutes, stirring occasionally, then stir through the sugar snap peas and continue to cook for 10 more minutes. Throw in the tofu pieces for the final bit of cooking to soak up the sauce, season with salt and pepper and stir through half the lime juice.

Finish with some extra coriander leaves, the remaining lime juice and the toasted cashews and serve with the brown rice.

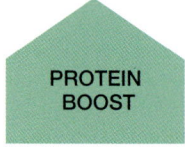

PROTEIN BOOST

Add more tofu. You can also add green lentils to this.

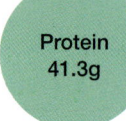

Protein 41.3g

Fibre 9.1g

Plant Points 7.75

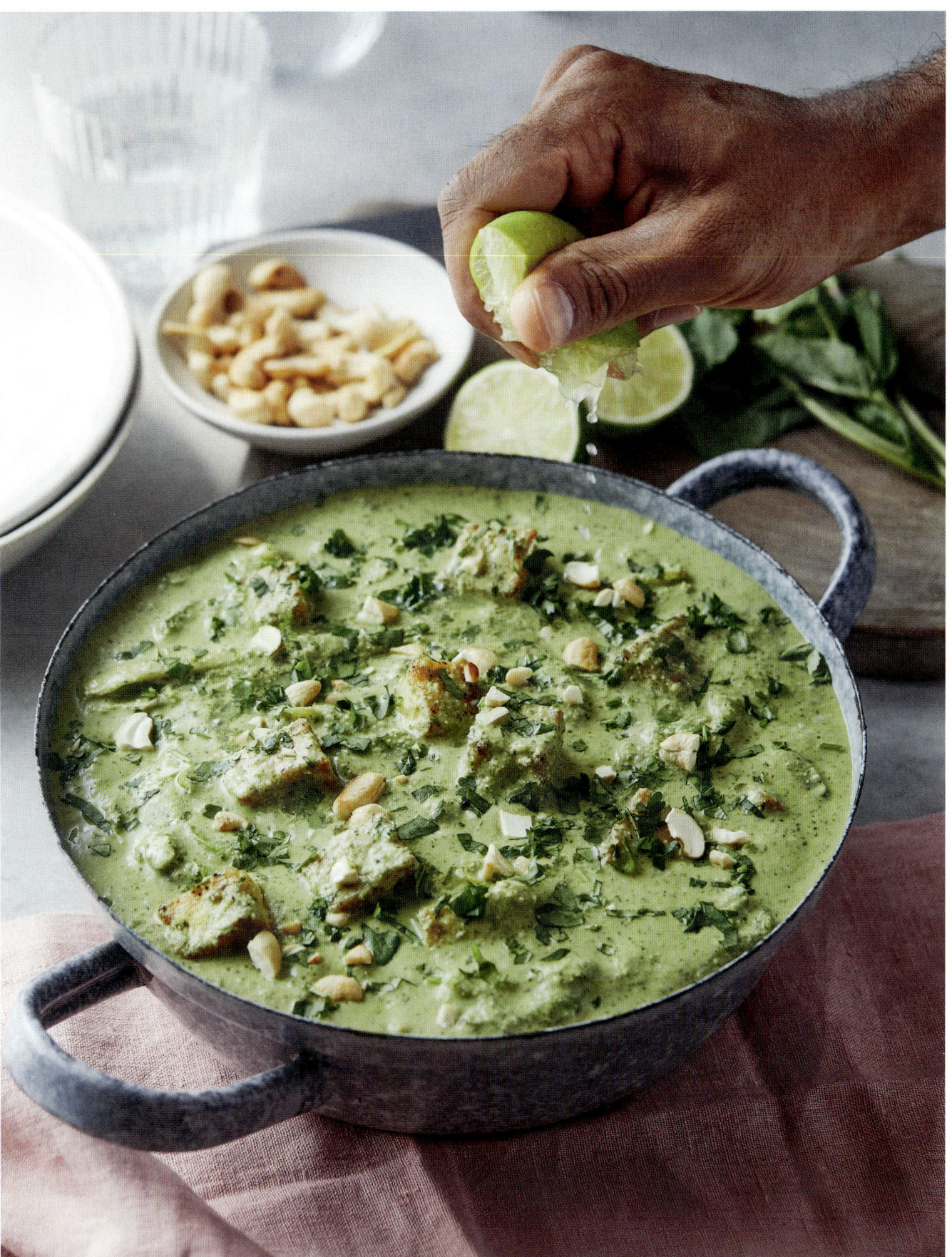

Stir-fried Celery with Sweet and Spicy Yuba

Prep 10 minutes
Cook 20 minutes

Serves 2

125g tofu knots (aka yuba)
1 tbsp olive oil
150g celery, diced
100g spring onion, white and green parts separated, thinly sliced on an angle
10g fresh root ginger, peeled and grated
150g pak choi or gai lan, stalks sliced and leaves chopped
3 tbsp soy sauce
1 tbsp maple syrup
2 tsp Chinese 5 spice

To serve
1 tbsp chilli oil
15g sesame seeds

Yuba, also known as tofu knots, can be found online and in Asian supermarkets. Once you start using them, you'll be hooked. Simply boil for a few minutes and they're ready to be thrown into multiple meals like stir-fries and broths. Packed with incredibly high amounts of protein, they have a delightful chew to them and take on the flavours in this meal wonderfully. Alongside the anti-inflammatory chemicals in the pak choi, 5 spice and ginger, the yuba also have isoflavones that support your immune system and gut health.

Bring a saucepan of water to a rolling boil, add the tofu knots and boil for 7–8 minutes until tender, then drain well in a sieve and set aside to cool slightly.

Heat the oil in a wok or large sauté pan over a medium–high heat, add the celery, white part of the spring onions, the ginger and stalks of the pak choi. Stir fry for 2–3 minutes until they start to colour and soften slightly.

Add the leaves of the pak choi and the cooked tofu knots and stir-fry for another minute.

Now add the soy sauce, maple syrup and Chinese 5 spice, turn up the heat slightly and stir-fry until combined and the sauce is golden and sticky.

Serve in shallow bowls and top with a drizzle of chilli oil, the green part of the spring onions and the sesame seeds.

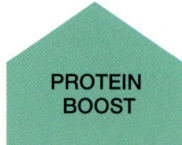

PROTEIN BOOST
Add more yuba. You can also try firm tofu or marinated tofu.

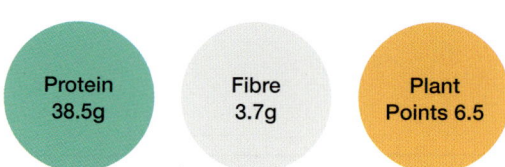

Protein 38.5g
Fibre 3.7g
Plant Points 6.5

210 MEATLESS MIDWEEK

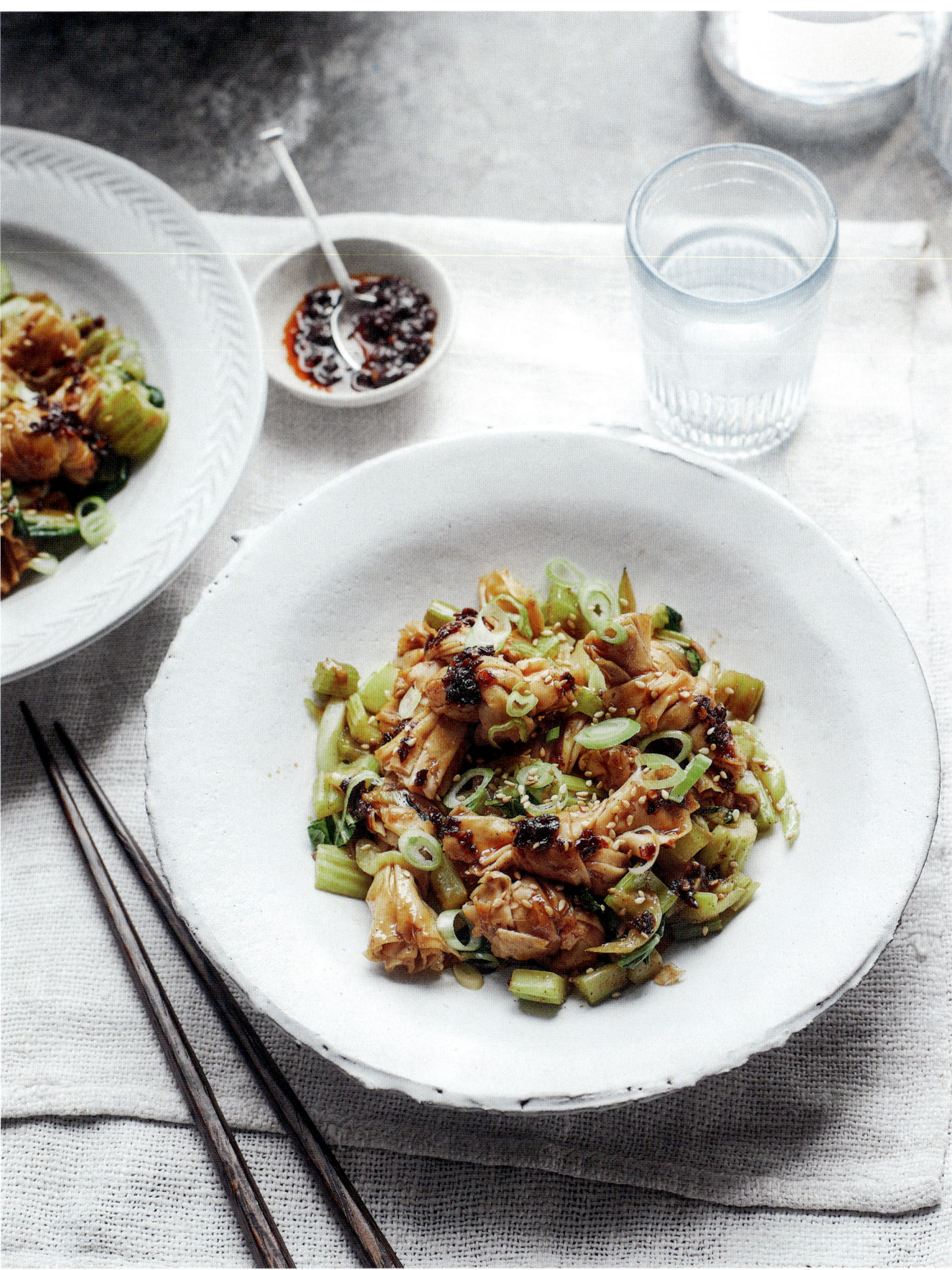

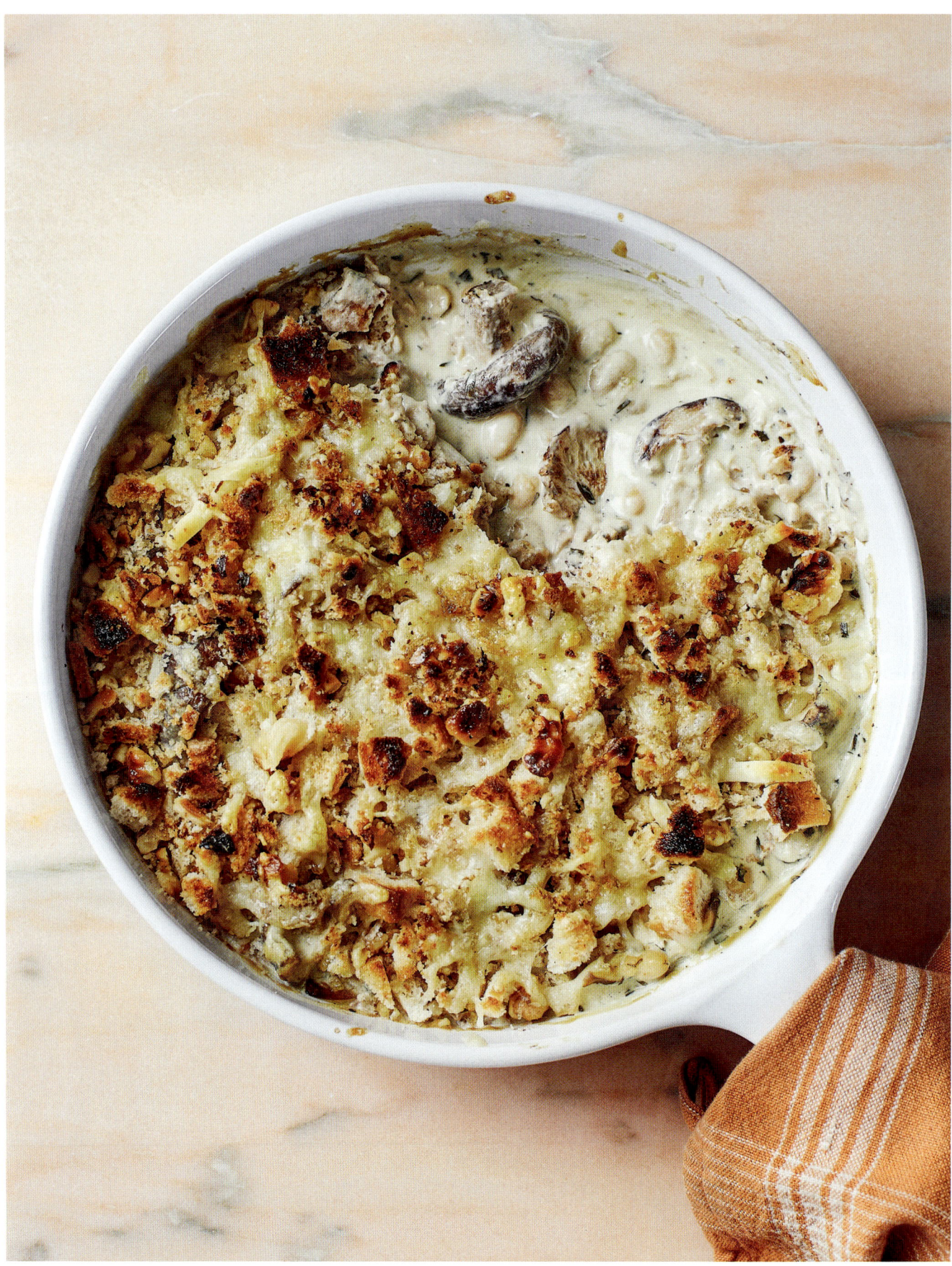

Herby Mushroom and Bean Gratin

Prep 5 minutes
Cook 25 minutes

Serves 2

300g silken tofu
20g nutritional yeast
2 tsp Dijon mustard
1 tsp garlic powder
Juice of ½ lemon
50ml boiling water
2 tbsp olive oil, plus extra to drizzle
300g shiitake mushrooms, roughly torn
1 x 400g can white beans
2 tsp dried tarragon

For the topping
50g walnuts, roughly chopped
50g slightly stale bread
50g Gruyère or Cheddar, coarsely grated

A piping-hot, creamy and cheesy one-pan dish. It's moreish and comforting and you wouldn't guess that it contains tofu. It drastically reduces the heaviness of the dish without skimping on a good dose of cheese to satisfy your cravings. The beans and mushrooms add a fantastic amount of fibre and unique antioxidants to support your immune system during the cold weather, which is when I tend to enjoy these kinds of dishes. You can make the gratin topping gluten free by using oats instead of breadcrumbs.

To make the topping, in a food processor, pulse the walnuts and bread into a coarse crumb mixture and set to one side in a bowl.

Add the silken tofu, nutritional yeast, mustard, garlic powder, lemon juice and hot water to the food processor and blend to a smooth, creamy consistency. Season with salt and pepper and set aside.

Heat the oil in an ovenproof sauté pan over a medium heat, add the mushrooms and fry for about 8 minutes until golden brown.

Add the beans and their liquid to the pan with the tarragon and stir to combine. Stir in the creamy tofu mixture and bring to a gentle simmer to heat through.

Preheat the grill to high.

Scatter the walnut and breadcrumb mix evenly over the mushroom sauce, then top with the cheese. Add a drizzle of olive oil and pop the pan under the grill for a few minutes to toast the top and melt the cheese. Serve piping hot.

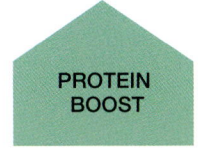

PROTEIN BOOST

Use more silken tofu or walnuts.

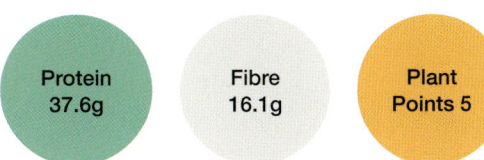

Protein 37.6g
Fibre 16.1g
Plant Points 5

MEATLESS MIDWEEK

Spicy 'Meaty' Tacos with Avo and Lime-soured Cream

Prep 15 minutes
Cook 25 minutes

Serves 2

2 tbsp olive oil
150g onion, finely chopped
250g mushrooms, finely chopped
200g tempeh, coarsely grated
2 large garlic cloves, finely chopped
50g walnuts, finely chopped
2 tsp hot smoked paprika
2 tsp fajita or Cajun spice mix
2 tbsp soy sauce
2 tbsp tomato purée
20g nutritional yeast
3 tbsp soured cream
1 tbsp lime juice

For the slaw
100g red cabbage, thinly sliced
1 tbsp lime juice
1 small red onion, thinly sliced

To serve
4 medium corn tortillas, warmed
1 baby gem lettuce, shredded
1 avocado, halved, stone removed and sliced
30g jalapeños from a jar
1 lime, zested then quartered

I don't use the word 'meaty' lightly. These tacos are really meaty. The blend of umami in the spices, walnut, mushrooms and tempeh in the mixture is phenomenal. And unlike 'meat-like meals', this actually packs a big protein punch that satisfies your body's need for this important macronutrient, rather than just having the texture of meat. A smattering of sharp and fresh ingredients brings this wholesome gut-nourishing meal together. Double up the ingredients to make this family friendly, it's definitely a crowd-pleaser.

Heat the oil in a large sauté pan over a medium–high heat. Add the onion and fry for 5 minutes until starting to turn golden, then add the mushrooms and tempeh and cook, stirring often, for another 8 minutes until there is no sign of any liquid, and everything has browned. Mix in the garlic and walnuts and cook for another 2 minutes, then season with salt and pepper.

Stir the spices into the pan followed by the soy sauce, tomato purée, nutritional yeast and 6 tablespoons water. Turn the heat to low–medium and simmer, stirring occasionally, for 6–8 minutes until cooked through, adding a splash more water to loosen if needed.

Meanwhile, make the slaw. Massage the red cabbage, lime juice, onion and a good pinch of salt in a mixing bowl for a few minutes until the cabbage starts to break down and soften. Set aside while you prepare the rest of the meal.

Mix together the soured cream and lime juice in a small bowl and season with salt, then set aside.

To assemble the tacos, place a warm tortilla on each serving plate and top with the shredded lettuce, the 'meaty' mixture, slaw, avocado, a spoonful of the soured cream mixture and finish with the jalapeños and a squeeze of lime juice with some zest. Serve the tortillas flat or rolled up.

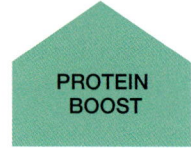

PROTEIN BOOST
Add more tempeh and walnuts.

Protein 41.1g
Fibre 21.1g
Plant Points 12.75

MEATLESS MIDWEEK

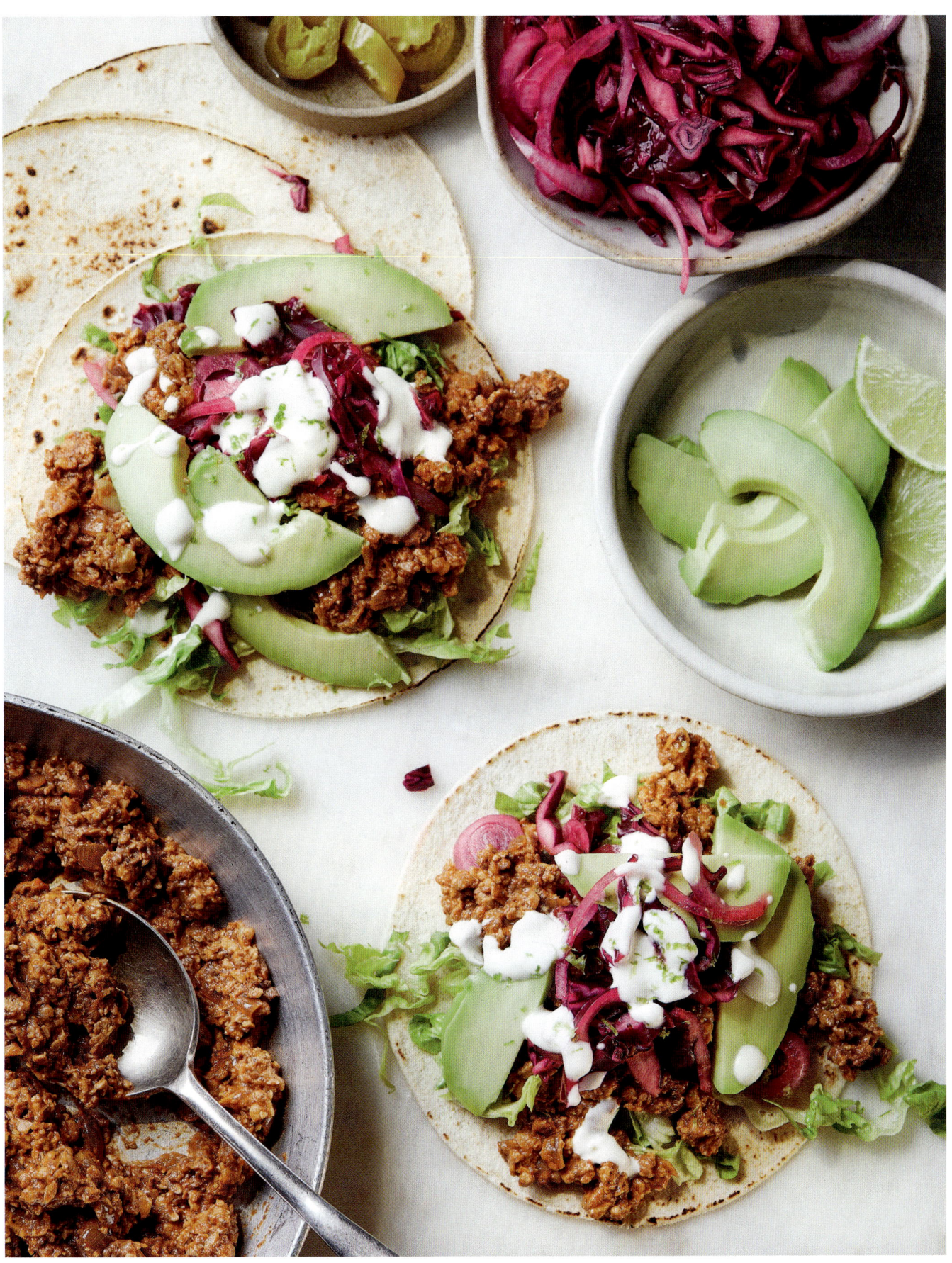

Plant Protein Stir-fry with Greens

Prep 10 minutes
Cook 20 minutes

Serves 2

120g brown rice noodles
2 tbsp olive oil
200g tempeh, cut into 1cm cubes
2 eggs, lightly beaten
3 garlic cloves, finely diced
1 tsp freshly ground black pepper
150g green pepper, deseeded and thinly sliced
150g mangetout, sliced
150g Tenderstem broccoli, roughly chopped
1 lime, cut into wedges, to serve

For the sauce
1 tbsp dark soy sauce
1 tbsp oyster sauce
2 tsp maple syrup
2 tsp chilli oil

Loosely based on a *pad see ew*, but packed with greens and much more fibre, this sweet, salty dish is perfect for those nights when you need a healthy meal in a rush. For the best results, this dish works when the ingredients are cooked separately and then brought together at the end with the sauce. Trust me, it's worth the slight extra effort.

Soak the rice noodles in just-boiled water from the kettle for 8 minutes. Drain and set aside. Don't worry if the noodles break up a bit.

Meanwhile, mix the sauce ingredients together in a bowl and set aside.

Heat a large wok or sauté pan over a medium–high heat and add 1 tablespoon of the olive oil. Add the tempeh cubes and cook for 8 minutes until crispy on all sides, then remove with a slotted spoon and set aside.

Add a splash more oil and the beaten eggs to the wok and scramble for 45 seconds, then remove from the wok and set aside.

Add the remaining oil to the wok and throw in your garlic and black pepper and cook for 30 seconds. Next, add the green pepper, mangetout and broccoli to the wok and cook for 3–4 minutes until the vegetables have softened.

Add half the sauce and stir, before adding the tempeh, scrambled eggs and noodles, toss in the wok and heat through before adding the remaining sauce. Serve with a wedge of lime for squeezing over.

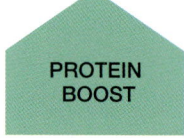

PROTEIN BOOST

Add more tempeh. If you aren't meat-free, this also works well with crispy tofu or chicken.

Protein 39.6g
Fibre 14.2g
Plant Points 6.5

216 MEATLESS MIDWEEK

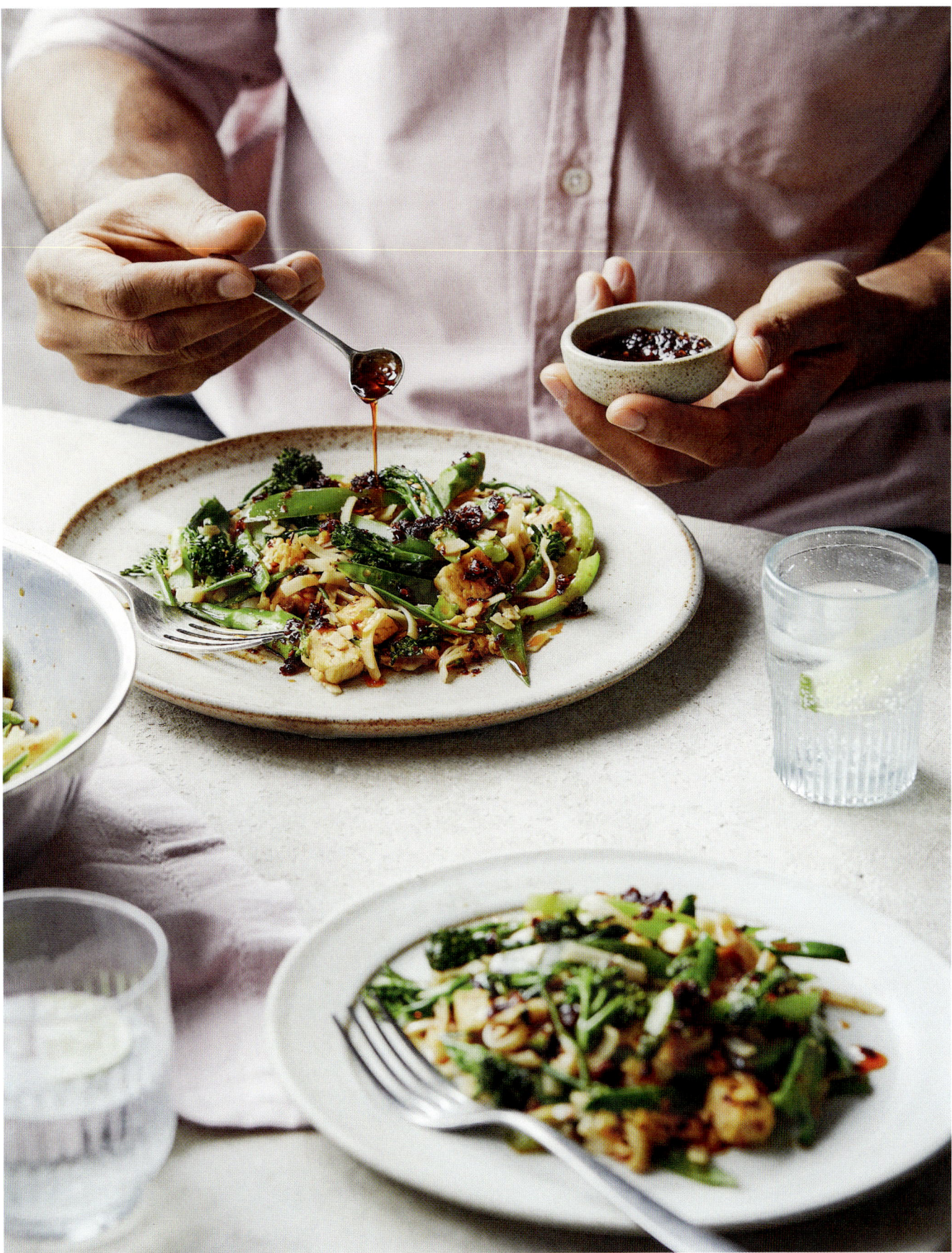

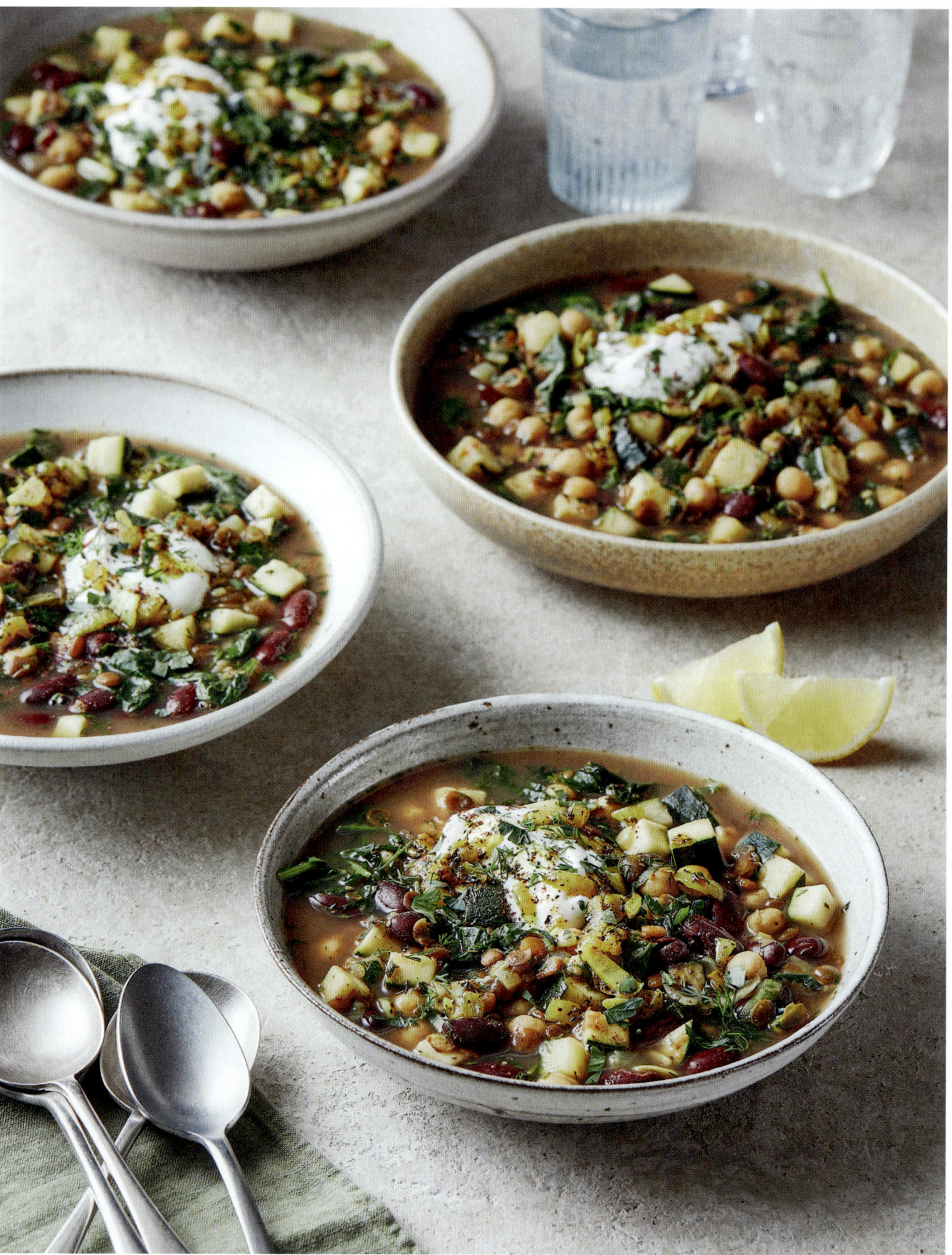

Sumac and Legume Stew with Dried Mint and Garlic

Prep 10 minutes
Cook 25 minutes

Serves 4

1 x 400g can chickpeas
1 x 400g can kidney beans
1 x 400g can green lentils
200g courgette, diced
2 tsp vegetable bouillon powder
4 tsp sumac, plus extra to serve
4 tbsp olive oil
150g white onion, diced
6 garlic cloves, thinly sliced
2 tsp ground turmeric
3 tsp dried mint
2 tsp dried oregano
250g spinach, chopped
30g parsley, chopped
40g dill, chopped
20g fresh mint leaves, chopped

To serve
100g Greek yoghurt
2 lemons, cut into wedges

Inspired by a traditional Persian dish, this legume-heavy stew is a hearty concoction of flavours, proteins and delicious spices. Two of the strongest anti-inflammatory spices in our kitchen cupboards are sumac and turmeric. Studies examining the nutritional value of ingredients show that sumac, the dried ground berries of the vibrant red *Rhus* plant, is one of the highest in antioxidants. Its sharp sour tang is perfect to cut through the rich and heavy legumes and pairs beautifully with the delicate soft green herbs.

Tip the chickpeas, kidney beans and green lentils with their liquid and the courgette into a large saucepan. Pour in 200ml of water and bring to a gentle simmer over a medium heat. Add the vegetable bouillon and sumac, then cook for 10 minutes until warmed through.

Add the olive oil and onion to a sauté pan over a medium heat and fry the onion for 8 minutes until browned. Add the garlic and cook for another 2 minutes until starting to colour. Add the turmeric, dried mint and oregano and stir for 45 seconds before taking the pan off the heat. Transfer half the contents to the saucepan with the chickpeas and reserve the rest to serve.

Add the spinach and half the fresh herbs to the saucepan and stir to wilt for a few minutes before taking the pan off the heat. Season with salt and pepper.

Spoon the stew into serving bowls and top with a dollop of yoghurt and some of the reserved onion and garlic oil. Finish with a sprinkling of sumac and the remaining fresh herbs and serve with lemon wedges for squeezing over.

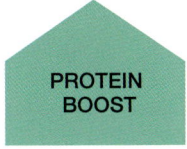

PROTEIN BOOST

If you aren't meat-free, add leftover chicken pieces to make a delicious addition to the pulses or a poached egg.

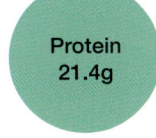

Protein 21.4g

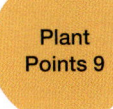

Fibre 16.6g

Plant Points 9

MEATLESS MIDWEEK

Za'atar and Tahini Beans with Crispy Tofu

Prep 15 minutes
Cook 30 minutes

Serves 2

For the crispy tofu
- 2 tbsp soy sauce
- 2 tsp brown sugar
- 1 tsp sweet paprika
- 1 tbsp olive oil
- 200g firm tofu, pressed and dried

For the za'atar and tahini beans
- 1 tbsp olive oil, plus extra to drizzle
- 100g white onion, diced
- 3 garlic cloves, finely grated
- 1½ tbsp za'atar, plus extra to serve
- 1 x 400g can white beans
- 150g spinach, finely chopped
- 30g flat-leaf parsley, leaves and stalks separated, finely chopped
- 4 tbsp tahini
- 150ml just-boiled water
- Juice of 1 lemon (optional)

I love using tahini to add rich creaminess without the heaviness of cream. Little known as a good source of protein, I try and use it in as many ways as possible. You will need to add splashes of hot water to loosen it, and make sure you stir the tahini in the jar properly to prevent clumps in your pan. Although not traditional, the crumbled tofu gives a beef mince-like texture and flavour.

Preheat the oven to 200°C fan and line a large baking tray with baking paper.

For the crispy tofu, mix the soy sauce, sugar, paprika and oil together in a mixing bowl. Crumble the tofu into small pieces, then add to the bowl and stir to coat it in the sauce. Spoon the tofu onto the lined baking tray and spread it out evenly.

Roast the tofu in the oven for 20–25 minutes, stirring halfway, until dark brown, sticky and crisp – it should resemble beef mince.

Meanwhile, heat the olive oil in a large lidded sauté pan over a medium heat. Add the onion and cook for 6–8 minutes until softened and slightly browned. Add the garlic and za'atar and cook for 1 minute to infuse their flavours.

Add the beans and their liquid, the spinach and parsley stalks and leaves, saving some of the leaves to serve, then stir to combine. Mix the tahini into the hot water.

Turn the heat to low, add the tahini mixture and stir until combined. Cover with the lid and gently cook for 5 minutes to allow the greens to wilt and the creamy sauce to thicken slightly.

Season with salt and pepper and add the lemon juice, if using. Serve topped with the crispy tofu, some extra za'atar and the remaining parsley leaves sprinkled over with a drizzle of olive oil.

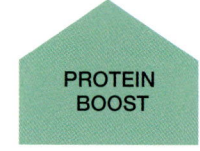

PROTEIN BOOST
More tofu, or use beef mince if you prefer.

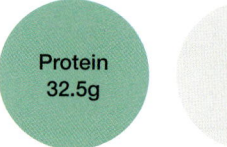

Protein 32.5g | Fibre 18g | Plant Points 8.5

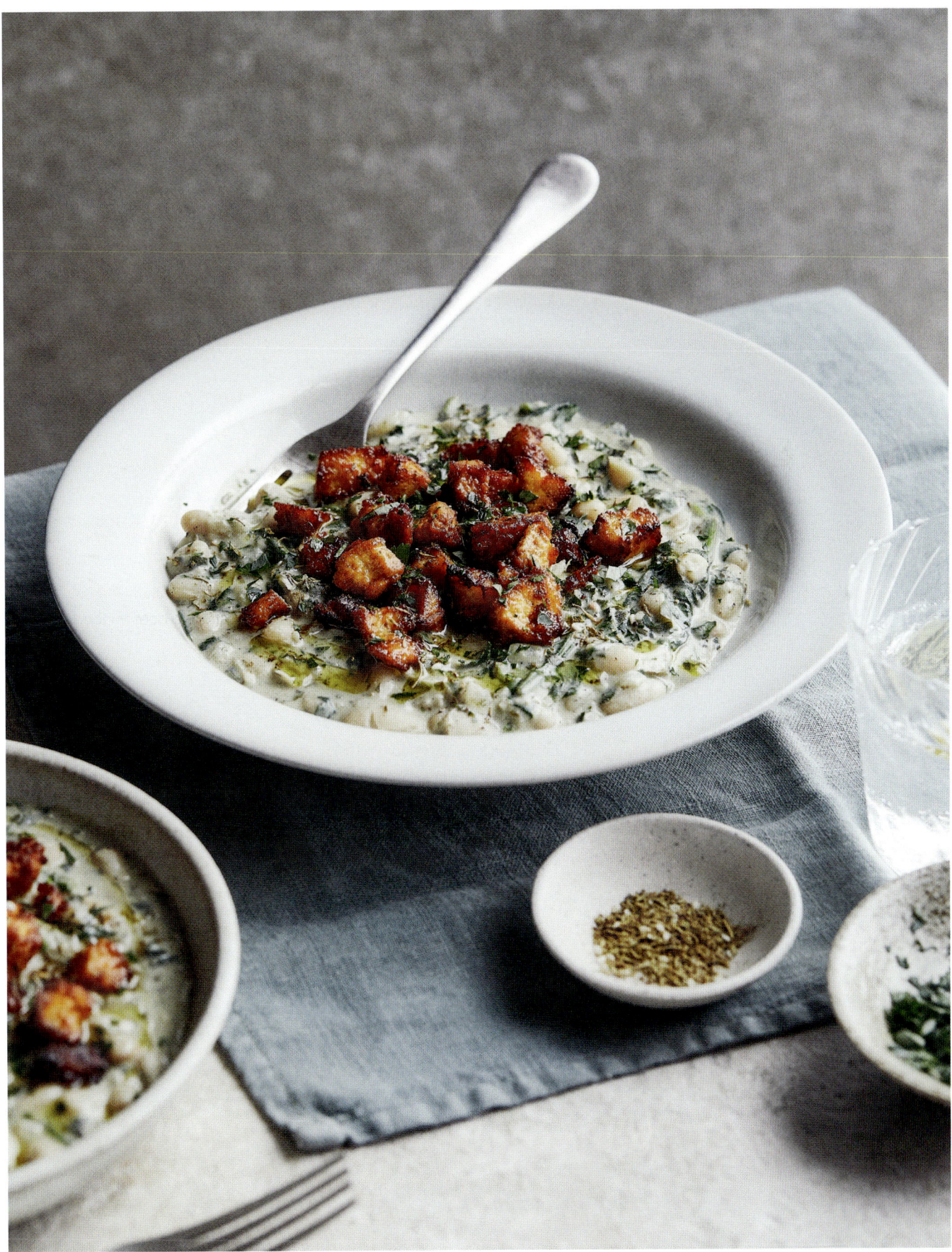

MID-WEEK

MEAT & FISH

Cinnamon and Cumin Curry with Crispy Chicken

Prep 15 minutes
Cook 55 minutes

Serves 4

600g chicken thighs, bone in, skin on
1 tbsp olive oil, plus extra to drizzle
200g frozen spinach, defrosted
150g peas (fresh or defrosted from frozen)
450g jar roasted red peppers (in water or brine), drained
1 vegetable stock cube, crumbled
300ml boiling water
150g white onion, finely diced
30g fresh root ginger, peeled and grated or julienned
2 tsp cumin seeds, crushed
2 tsp coriander seeds, crushed
1 tsp black mustard seeds
1 tsp dried chilli flakes
1 tsp ground cinnamon
1 tsp ground turmeric
30g pitted prunes, roughly chopped
200g dried green lentils, soaked for 20 minutes, drained and rinsed thoroughly
20g coriander leaves, chopped, to finish

A family favourite with its sweet and spicy balance. The rich prunes and sharp coriander seeds are a fantastic pairing with a nod to Middle Eastern cuisine. The dish comes together in one pan making this a great Sunday afternoon affair to set yourself up for a healthy week. It ticks all the boxes for protein, fibre and anti-inflammatory ingredients, yet it has an indulgency to it which is perfect for sharing!

Season the chicken thighs with salt and pepper. Heat the olive oil in a large lidded ovenproof casserole dish over a medium–high heat. Add the chicken, skin-side down and cook for 6–8 minutes until golden and crisp. Then flip and cook for a couple of minutes on the other side and set aside to rest on a plate.

While the chicken is browning, blend the spinach, peas, red peppers, vegetable stock cube and hot water in a blender or food processor and set aside.

Add the onion and ginger to the casserole dish and sauté, stirring regularly, for 5 minutes until softened.

Stir in the cumin, coriander, mustard seeds and chilli flakes and cook for another minute before adding the ground spices, prunes and the soaked rinsed lentils. Stir to coat the lentils in the spices before adding your blended peas, peppers and spinach mixture. Bring to a gentle simmer and cover with the lid. Cook for 15 minutes until the lentils are part-cooked, adding a splash more water if the mixture looks too dry.

Meanwhile, preheat the oven to 200°C fan.

Nestle the chicken, skin-side up, into the lentils, and cook, uncovered, in the oven for 20 minutes until the chicken is cooked through and the lentils are tender.

Serve with a drizzle of oil and sprinkled with coriander leaves.

PROTEIN BOOST

Add more chicken.

Protein 45.6g
Fibre 13.3g
Plant Points 9

MIDWEEK MEAT & FISH

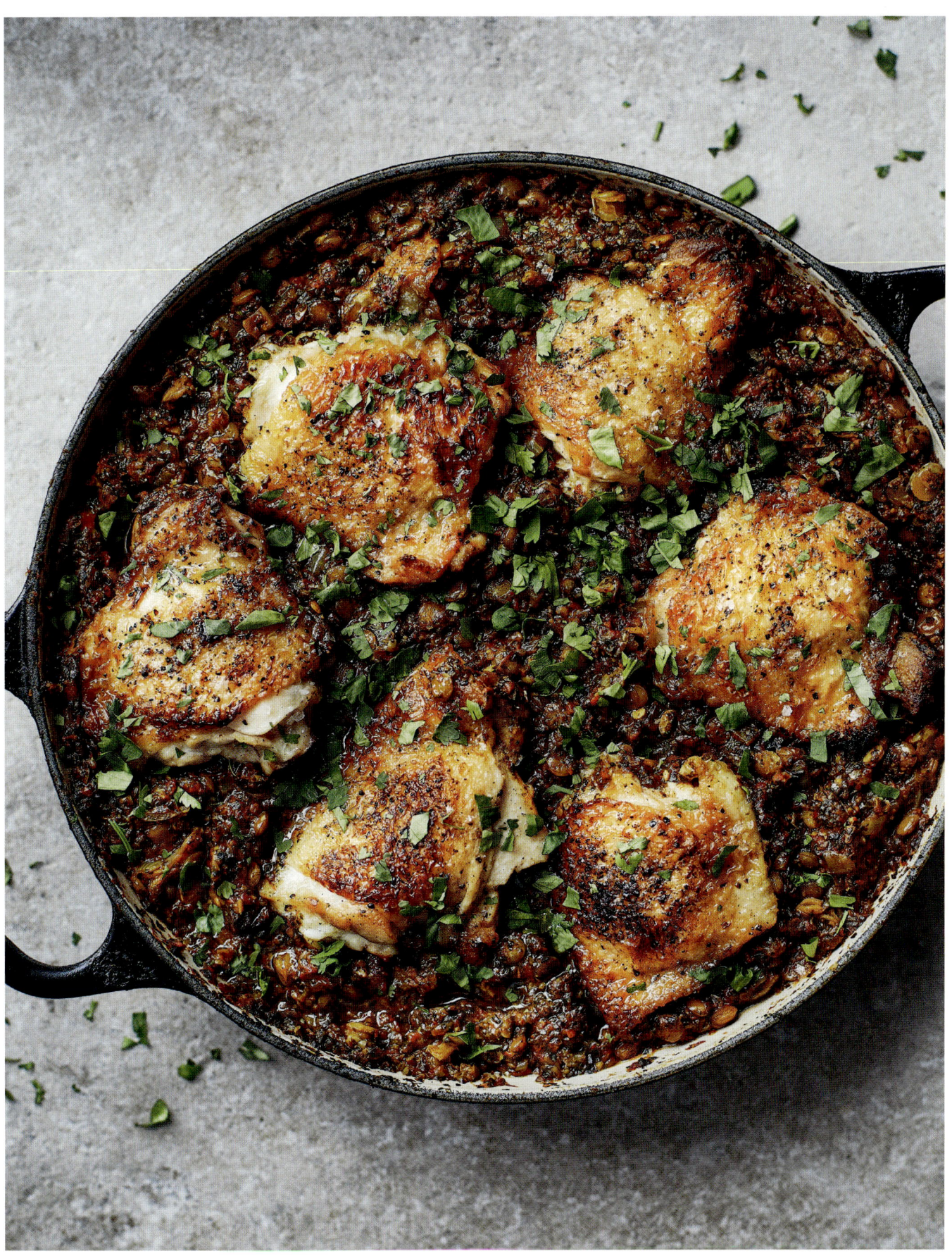

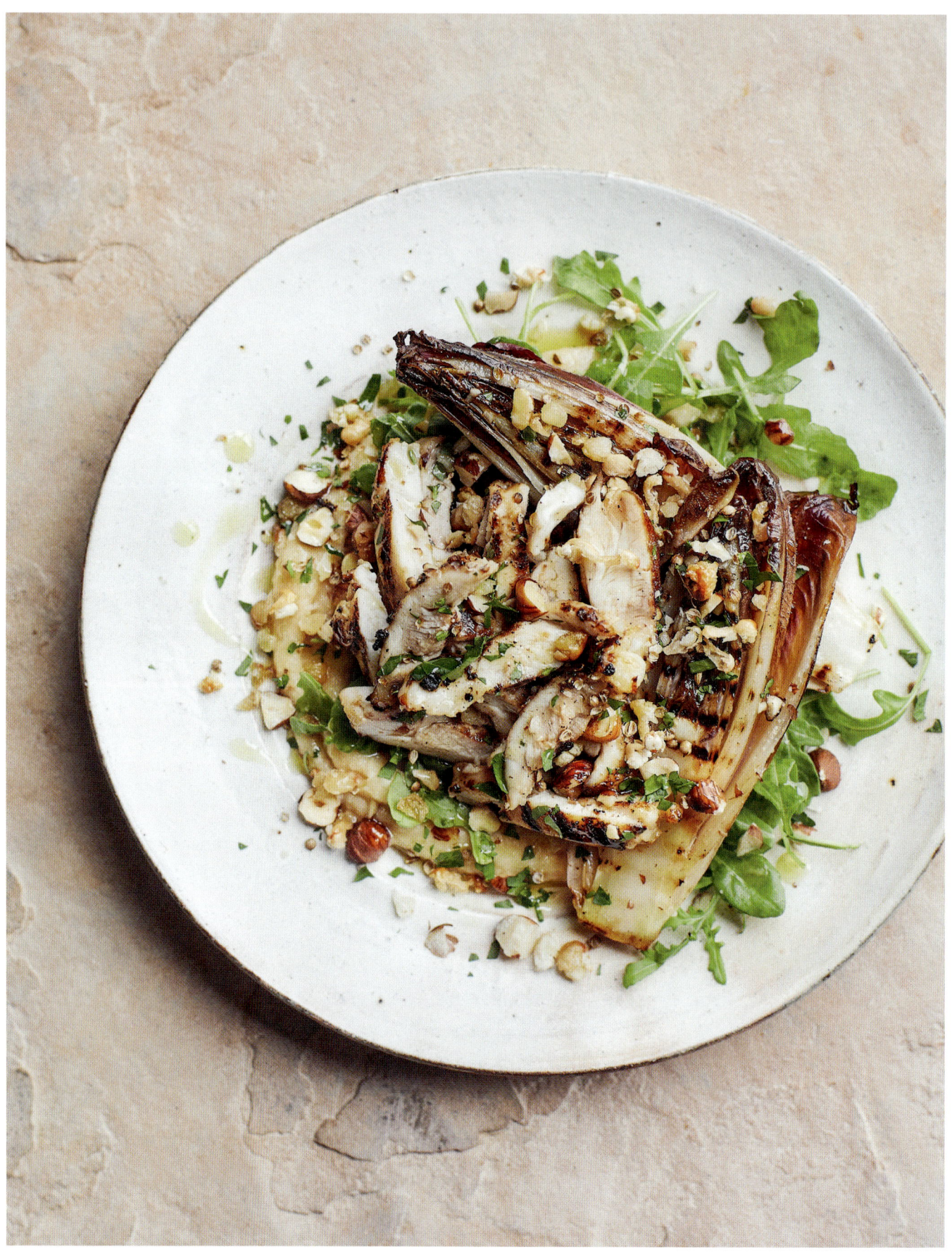

Grilled Chicken Thighs with Miso White Beans, Radicchio and Hazelnuts

Prep 10 minutes
Cook 25 minutes

Serves 2

25ml boiling water
1 tbsp white miso paste
1 x 400g can white beans
2 tbsp olive oil, plus extra to drizzle and finish
2 boneless, skinless chicken thighs, butterflied
2 Treviso radicchio heads, halved lengthways
100g rocket leaves
50g hazelnuts, roughly chopped
2 tsp coriander seeds, lightly toasted and crushed
10g parsley, leaves finely chopped, to finish

The number of things you can do with beans is phenomenal and this recipe showcases two of my favourite ways to prepare them. Smooth, creamy and salty with the miso, and crispy with a little oil and salt from the oven. Radicchio is a beautiful vegetable with bitter notes, rich in gut-boosting polyphenols and it works wonderfully with sweet white miso. See page 156 for how to make crispy beans in the air fryer.

Preheat the oven to 200°C fan and line a baking sheet with baking paper.

Add the boiling water, half of the miso paste and half of the beans plus the whole can's liquid to a blender or food processor. Blend, adding more hot water if needed, to make a warm purée. Set to one side.

Drain and rinse the other half of the beans and dry with some kitchen paper. Add to a mixing bowl with a good pinch of salt, 1 tbsp of olive oil, then scatter onto the lined baking sheet. Roast in the oven for 15–20 minutes until golden and crispy (shaking the baking sheet to turn the beans halfway through cooking).

Mix the rest of the miso paste with 1 tablespoon of the oil and brush over the chicken thighs. Preheat a ridged griddle pan over a medium–high heat and cook the thighs on each side for 5–6 minutes until lightly charred and the juices run clear. Set aside on a plate to rest.

Brush the halved radicchio heads with a drizzle of olive oil and add them to the same pan over a high heat. Cook them cut-side down for 2 minutes until they are lightly charred, then flip and cook for another 2 minutes. Remove and set aside.

Spread the white bean purée over 2 plates, build the rocket leaves and radicchio over them, then slice the chicken thighs and pile on top. Scatter over the crispy beans, chopped hazelnuts and crushed coriander seeds. Finish with the chopped parsley and a drizzle of olive oil to serve.

PROTEIN BOOST

Add more chicken.

Protein 43.4g

Fibre 17.9g

Plant Points 5

MIDWEEK MEAT & FISH

Sage and Garlic Chicken Broth

Prep 5 minutes
Cook 1 hour

Serves 4

500g chicken thighs and drumsticks
4 tbsp olive oil
1 large head of garlic, halved horizontally
200g celery, thinly sliced on an angle
30g sage leaves
1.5 litres boiling water
250g cavolo nero, stalks removed, and roughly chopped
200g spinach, roughly chopped
200g lentil orzo (or regular orzo)

Garlic and sage have strong antioxidant and anti-inflammatory benefits. And the mix of fats and collagen from the chicken bones and skin may also be nourishing for the gut barrier. A number of studies have looked at bone broth in particular for gut-health benefits and, while they aren't all convincing, anecdotally people swear by it for improvements to their gut symptoms. This recipe is warming, wholesome and exactly what I want on an autumnal weekend to power me through the following week. A real nourishing treat.

Season the chicken. Put a very large lidded saucepan over a medium heat and add 3 tablespoons of the olive oil. Add the chicken to the pan and brown the skin for a few minutes, then remove from the pan and set aside.

Add the remaining oil to the pan and add the garlic halves, cut-side down, along with the celery and half the sage leaves and cook for 4–5 minutes until the garlic has browned.

Add the boiling water and cavolo nero. Bring to a simmer and add the chicken back to the saucepan.

Cover with the lid and cook for 40 minutes until the chicken is cooked through and the meat tender.

Remove the chicken from the broth, then remove the skin and shred the meat off the bone. Add the meat back to the saucepan with the spinach, lentil pasta and remaining sage leaves. Cook for 8 minutes, stirring often, until the pasta is cooked. Season with salt and pepper and serve in large bowls.

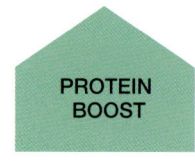

PROTEIN BOOST

Add more chicken.

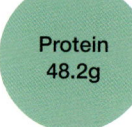

Protein 48.2g

Fibre 8.7g

Plant Points 5.5

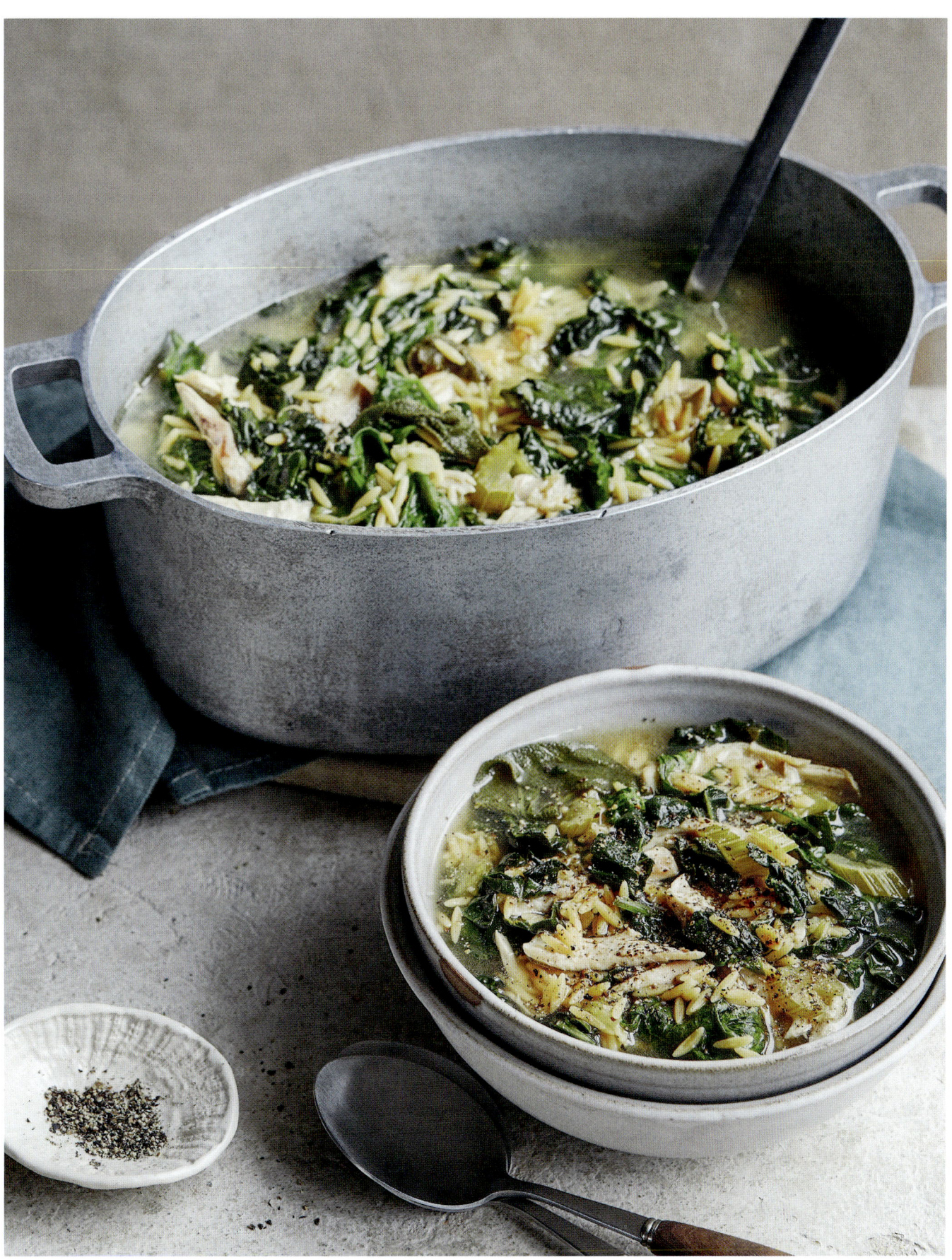

Tahini and Gochujang Noodle Broth with Turkey

Prep 5 minutes
Cook 20 minutes

Serves 2

2 tbsp olive oil
200g lean turkey or chicken mince, or finely chopped boneless thigh or breast
150g shiitake mushrooms, torn into pieces
100g spring onions, sliced on an angle, plus extra to serve
150g mangetout, sliced on an angle
100g ready-to-eat konjac (shirataki), rice vermicelli or udon noodles

For the broth
3 tbsp tahini
3 tbsp soy sauce
1 tbsp gochujang
300ml boiling water

To serve
1 lime, cut into wedges
10g black sesame seeds
2 tsp chilli oil

The creaminess of tahini with the sweet spice of gochujang is a combination I adore. It's not traditional in any way, but it works really well with the mince and crunchy mangetout. Black sesame seeds add an unusual colour contrast, and a slightly deeper flavour but feel free to use regular white sesame seeds that also add extra calcium and protein.

First make the broth. Add the tahini, 2 tablespoons of soy sauce and the gochujang to a large saucepan over a low heat and gradually whisk in the water. Cook gently until heated through, and smooth and creamy. Season with salt and pepper.

Heat 1 tablespoon of the oil in a large sauté pan over a medium–high heat. Add the mince or finely chopped meat and cook for 6–8 minutes, breaking it down into small pieces with a spatula, until browned in places and starting to crisp, then scoop it out with a slotted spoon into a bowl and set aside.

To the same pan, add the remaining oil and the mushrooms and cook over a medium–high heat, stirring often, for 3 minutes until softened and starting to turn golden. Add the spring onions and mangetout and cook for another 2–3 minutes until just tender. Return the meat to the pan and toss through the vegetables with the remaining soy sauce and heat through briefly.

Add the noodles to the pan with the creamy tahini broth, stir to combine with the liquid, then heat through briefly over a low–medium heat. Transfer the hot noodle broth to serving bowls. Spoon the mince and vegetable mixture on top and serve with lime wedges for squeezing over, the extra spring onions, sesame seeds and a drizzle of chilli oil.

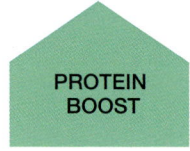

PROTEIN BOOST

Add more turkey or chicken.

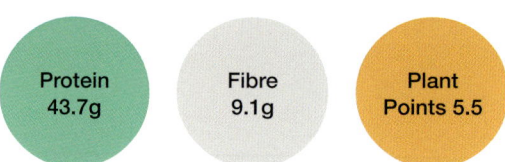

Protein 43.7g
Fibre 9.1g
Plant Points 5.5

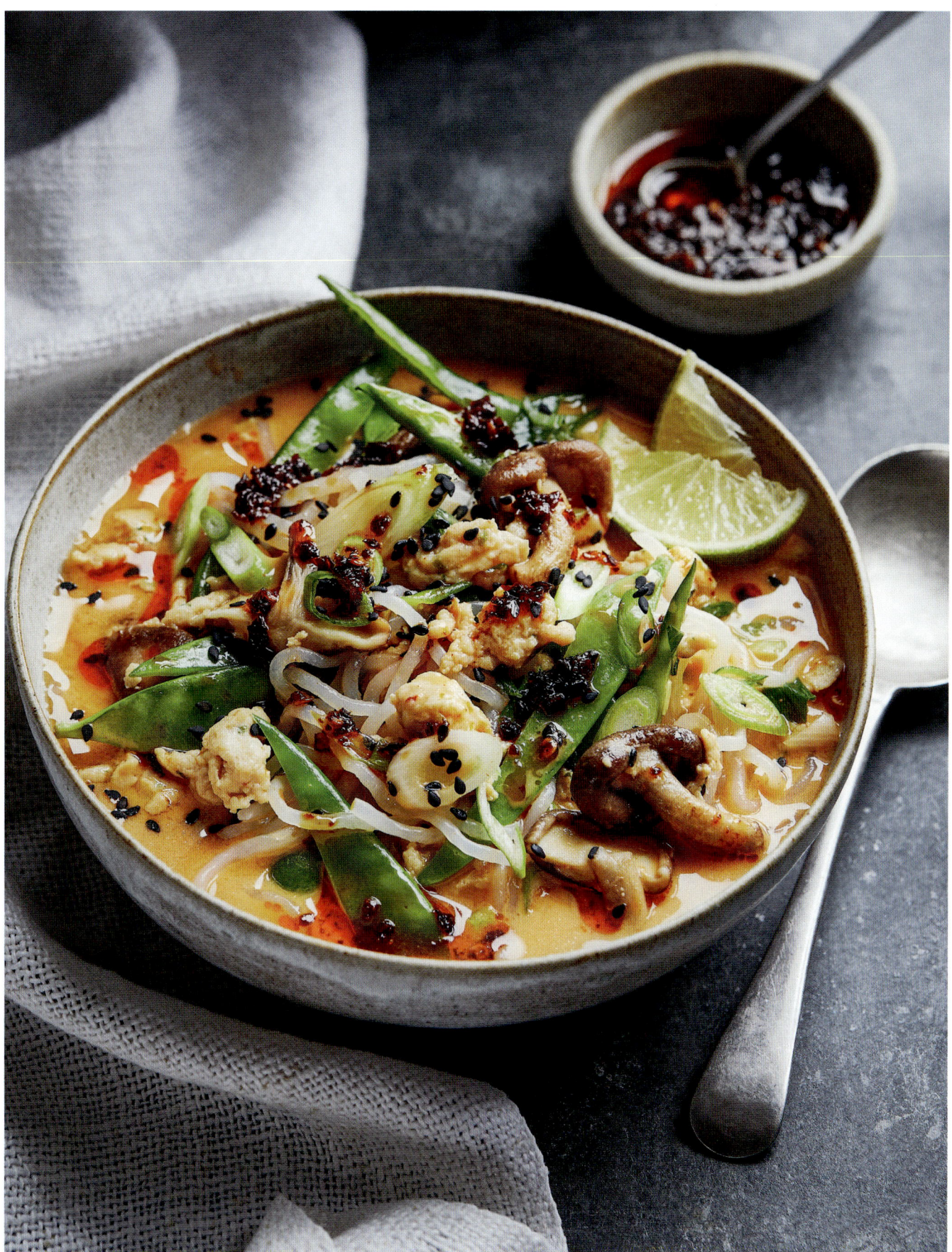

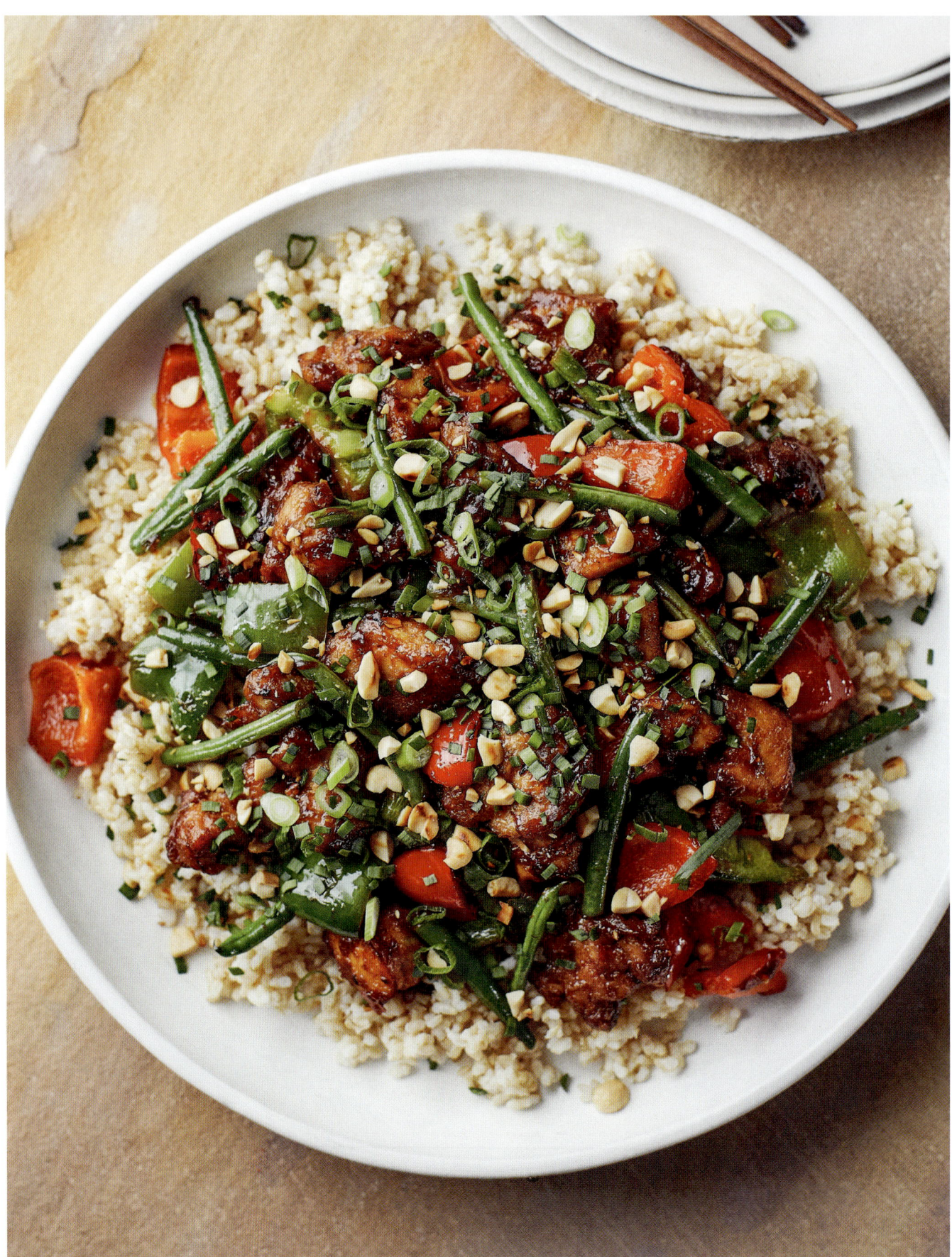

Takeaway-style Chicken

Prep 10 minutes, plus marinating
Cook 25 minutes

Serves 4

2 tbsp soy sauce
500g chicken thighs, skinless and boneless, cut into 3cm chunks
2 tbsp cornflour
2 tbsp olive oil, plus a drizzle for frying
3 garlic cloves, grated
10g fresh root ginger, peeled and grated
200g red pepper, deseeded and cut into 3cm chunks
200g green pepper, deseeded and cut into 3cm chunks
200g green beans or sugar snap peas, halved
80g peanuts, toasted and roughly chopped, to garnish

For the sauce
2 tbsp dark soy sauce
2 tbsp rice wine vinegar
2 tbsp hoisin sauce
1 tbsp cornflour
1 tsp red chilli flakes
½ tsp Sichuan peppercorns, crushed (optional)

To serve
300g cooked short-grain brown rice, warmed
20g spring onions, finely sliced
20g garlic chives, finely chopped

This sticky sweet and salty takeaway-style dish takes minutes. When I want comfort food, it satisfies the craving but it's surprisingly high in fibre, diversity and protein. You could easily swap out the chicken for tofu instead if you prefer to keep it plant based. I generally use whatever vegetables I have in the fridge to toss into a wok, but the classic pairing of peppers and green beans is what I would reach for. This is a crowd-pleasing, flavourful, family-style recipe that has a ton of fibre and plant polyphenols, helping everyone to be healthier with each bite. Boost the protein by adding more meat.

Mix the soy sauce with the chicken in a mixing bowl, dust in the cornflour to coat and leave to marinate for 15–20 minutes.

Add the oil to the chicken, then spread out evenly in a lined air fryer and cook at 200°C for 15 minutes until crispy and cooked through. Alternatively, bake in the oven at 200°C fan for 20–25 minutes.

Mix the sauce ingredients with 4 tablespoons of water and set aside.

Heat a large wok over a medium–high heat, add a drizzle of olive oil and cook the garlic and ginger for 30 seconds before adding the peppers and green beans or sugar snap peas and stir-frying for 3–4 minutes.

Add the chicken to the wok, then add your sauce and give everything a good mix. The sauce will reduce and thicken quickly so make sure to keep the ingredients in the wok moving.

When the sauce has thickened, remove from the heat. Serve on a platter with the warm rice, spring onions and garlic chives. Garnish with the toasted peanuts.

Protein 44.3g
Fibre 7.5g
Plant Points 8.25

MIDWEEK MEAT & FISH

Cinnamon and Lentil Chicken Soup

Prep 10 minutes
Cook 45 minutes

Serves 4

- 3 tbsp olive oil
- 300g boneless, skinless chicken thighs, cut into bite-size chunks
- 300g celery, sliced on an angle
- 2 tsp ground cinnamon
- 2 tsp ground ginger
- 1 tsp turmeric
- 3 tbsp tomato purée
- 1 x 400g can green lentils
- 1 x 400g can chickpeas
- 1 x 400g can peeled whole tomatoes
- 700ml boiling water
- 1 vegetable or chicken stock cube
- 100g dried orzo pasta
- 25g parsley, leaves and stalks, finely chopped
- 25g coriander, leaves and stalks, finely chopped
- Juice of 1 lemon

Medicinal turmeric and lentil soup is a recipe I always have to hand when I need to support my immune system or recover from a long week. I tend to make this as a big-batch cook that I can enjoy over the following few days or simply freeze for the next time I need a quick meal. The mixture of pulses adds a wealth of fibres for optimal gut health and orzo offers add a touch of comfort.

Heat the oil in a large saucepan over a medium heat, add the chicken pieces and cook for 6–7 minutes until well coloured all over. Remove and set aside.

Add the celery to the same pan and fry, stirring regularly, for 5 minutes before adding the spices and tomato purée and cooking for another 2 minutes.

Tip in the lentils and chickpeas with the liquid from the cans, the tomatoes (squeeze them with your hands before putting them in the pan) and hot water and crumble in the stock cube. Bring to the boil, then turn the heat down to low and simmer for 10 minutes.

Return the chicken to the pan with the orzo and cook, stirring occasionally to stop the pasta sticking, for another 10 minutes until the orzo is tender. Stir in three-quarters of the herbs and the lemon juice and season with salt and pepper.

Spoon into large bowls and serve topped with the remaining herbs.

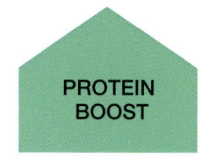

PROTEIN BOOST
Add more chicken.

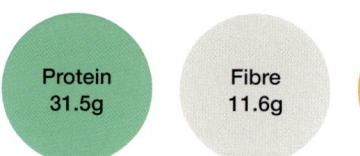

Protein 31.5g
Fibre 11.6g
Plant Points 6.75

MIDWEEK MEAT & FISH

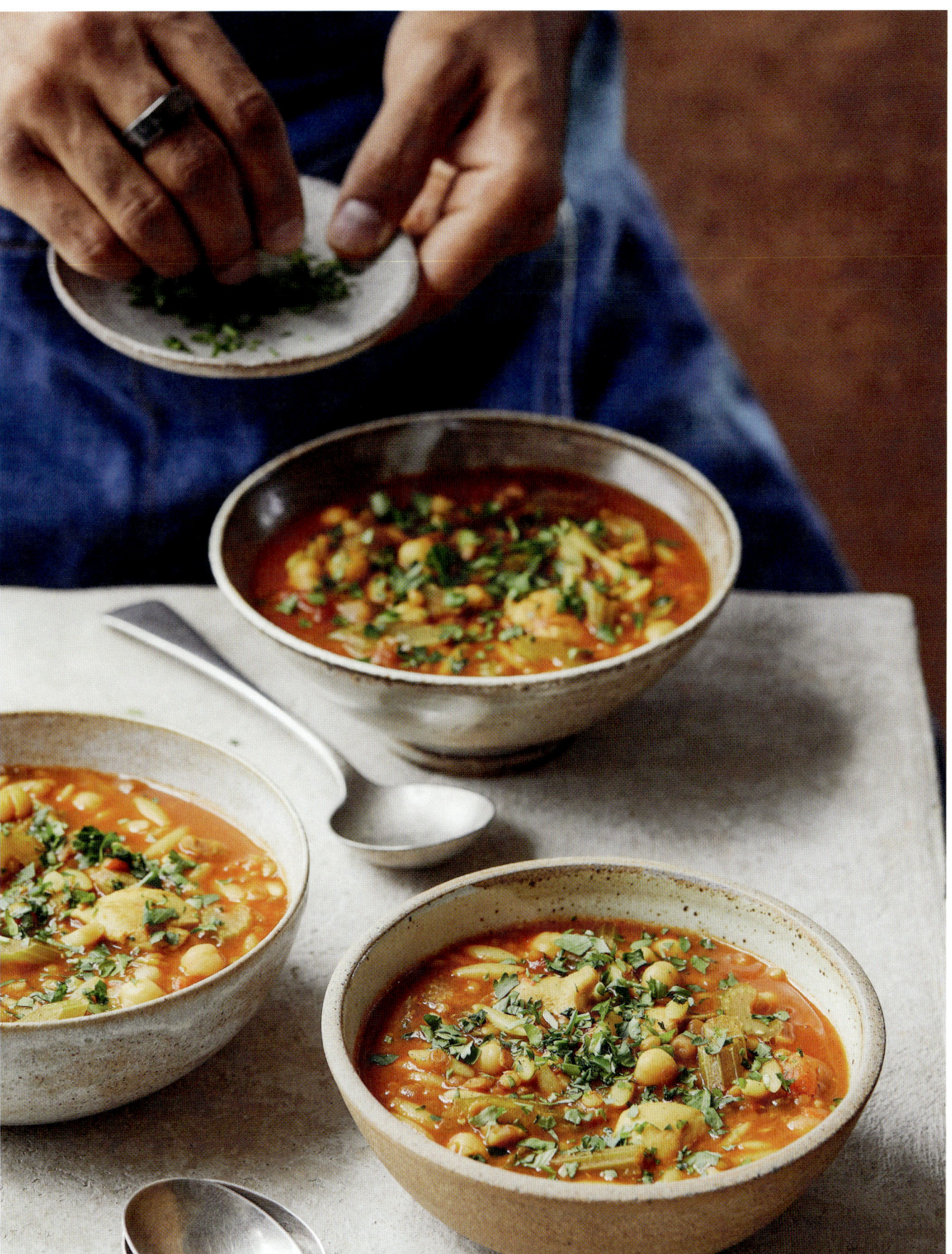

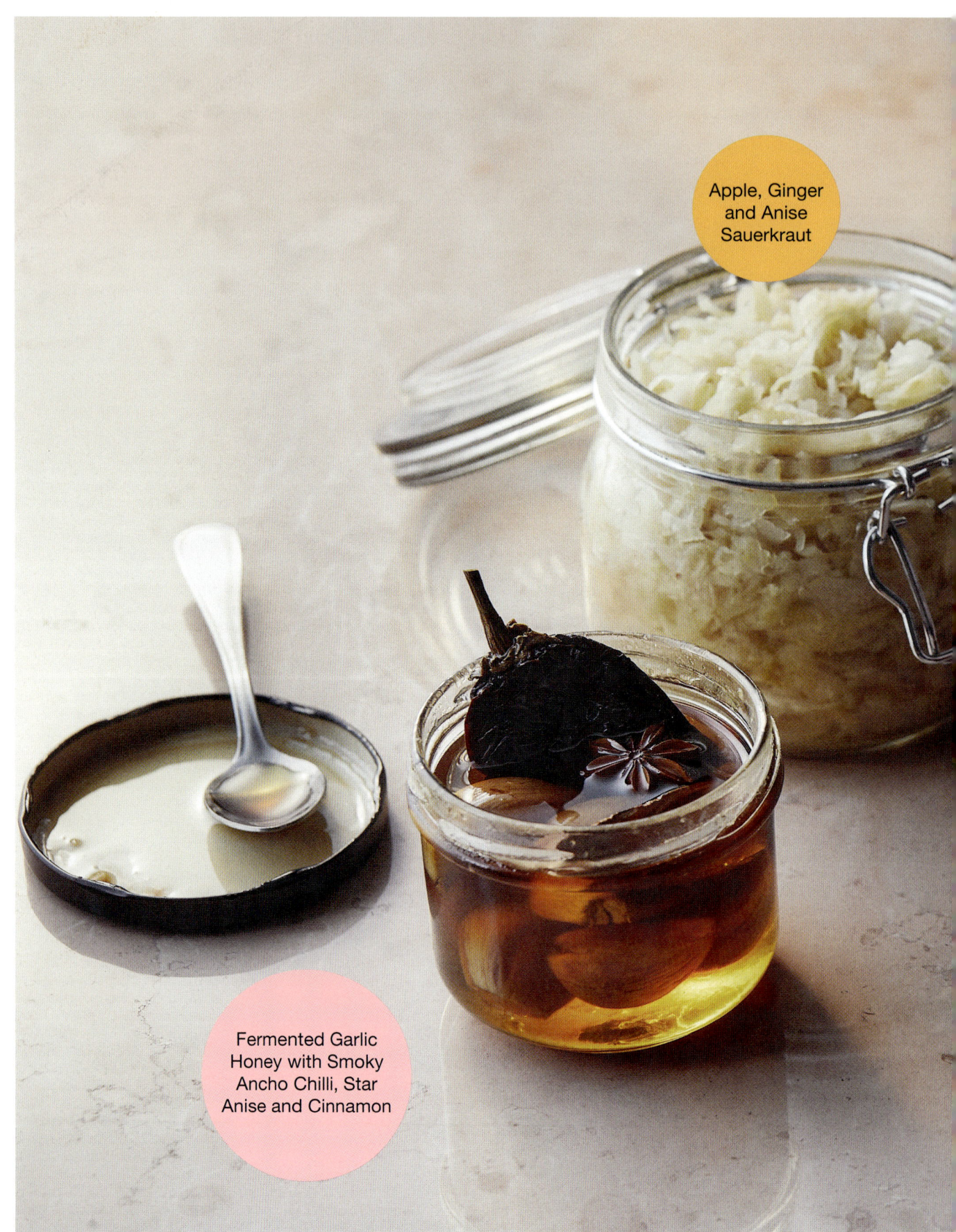

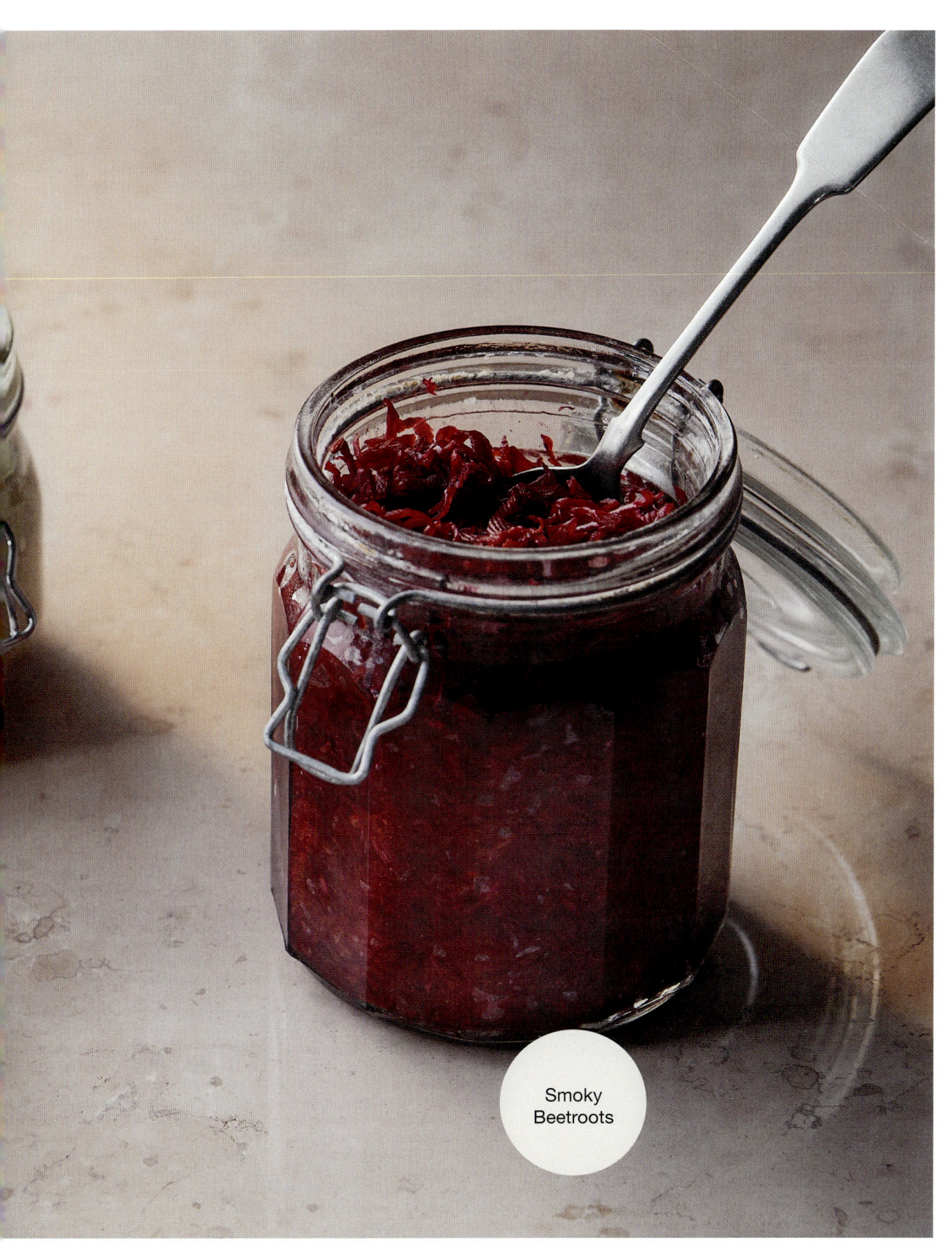
Smoky Beetroots

KRAUT CORNER: FERMENTS

Because I'm a simple kind of home cook, I use a 2% lactic acid, wild-ferment method to make a selection of very basic probiotic rich ferments. It provides you with a safety net to make sure you are preparing the food in the healthiest and safest way possible, while leaving plenty of room for experimentation.

My rough formula is to use something sweet (like apple, pear or carrot) with an aromatic spice (say cinnamon, clove, fennel or star anise) and something sharp (such as onion or ginger). But there are multiple combinations to play around with when making your own ferment, as long as you follow some basic steps.

- Measure the ingredients you're using and add 2% salt.
- Ensure that the vegetables are submerged beneath the brine where oxygen cannot spoil the ingredients.
- Other than that, make sure you 'burp' your ferment regularly (depending on how warm your kitchen is, this could mean daily or every other day) for a couple of weeks and when you can taste that characteristic sour tang of beautifully fermented vegetables, you can transfer them to the fridge and keep for at least 3 months.

I also adopt this fermenting technique to use up scraps that I save when prepping vegetables. This recipe will work with common veg scraps such as broccoli stalks, radishes, cauliflower stalks, parsnips, onions and beetroots.

Fermented Garlic Honey with Smoky Ancho Chilli, Star Anise and Cinnamon

I was taught this simple recipe by world-renowned 'fermentista' and co-author of *Fermented Vegetables*, Kristen Shockey, in the Doctor's Kitchen studio. It's painfully simple and absolutely gorgeous as a condiment for everything ranging from simple eggs or to finish a quiche, to add a spicy sweet zing to a stir-fry or simply to mix with hot water when you have a cold.

300g jar of raw honey
1 star anise
1 cinnamon stick
5 garlic cloves, lightly bashed
1 dried ancho chilli

Add to the jar of raw honey the remaining ingredients and allow to become engulfed in the honey. Keep in a cool, dark place, turn upside down once a day and 'burp' the ingredients by gently opening the lid of the jar and allowing the gas to escape.

It should take around 2 weeks and you'll be rewarded with a smoky, sweet spicy honey for lots of uses!

Apple, Ginger and Star Anise Sauerkraut

1 red onion, thinly sliced
2 star anise
20g fresh root ginger, peeled and coarsely grated
1 white cabbage, outer leaves resserved, thinly sliced or shredded
Salt
2 apples, cored and thinly sliced

Weigh the total amount of the ingredients (onion, ginger and cabbage) in grams and multiply that by 0.02 to get the amount of salt required. For example, if your total ingredients weighed 1200g, multiple that by 0.02 and you're left with 24g of salt to be added.

Add all the ingredients, apart from the apple, to a large bowl. Firmly massage the salt into the ingredients until a brine forms in the bowl and your ingredients are limp and wet. Add the apple and mix thoroughly to combine.

Start packing your fermenting vessel. I use a large, airtight clip-top jar for ferments.

Pour over the brine from the bowl. It should cover the ingredients fully when you pack them down to the bottom of the jar.

Cover the ingredients in the jar with an outer cabbage leaf and place a small weight on top. This could be a smaller jar filled with water that you place inside your large clip-top jar to keep the ingredients submerged in the liquid. You must make sure that the shredded ingredients are completely submerged, as anything left exposed to air could grow mould.

Close the lid and transfer to a cool, dark place (the back of a kitchen cupboard is ideal). You can taste the sauerkraut as soon as you like, but it will probably take at least 7–10 days. Release any built-up gas in the container every other day by gently opening and closing the lid, or pulling the plastic seal of the clip-top.

It is ready when you think it tastes delicious, sour and tangy. At that point, decant the contents into smaller, sealed containers. The sauerkraut will keep in the fridge for at least 3 months.

Smoky Beetroots

1 red cabbage, outer leaves reserved, thinly sliced or shredded
2 candy-striped beetroots or regular beetroots, coarsely grated or thinly sliced
1 garlic clove, grated
Salt
1 tsp smoked paprika
½ tsp ground turmeric
1 tsp fennel seeds

Add the red cabbage, beets and garlic to a large mixing bowl. Weigh the total amount of the ingredients (cabbage, beetroots and garlic) in grams and multiply that by 0.02 to get the amount of salt required.

Add all the weighed ingredients to a large bowl. Firmly massage the salt into the ingredients until a brine forms in the bowl and your ingredients are limp and wet. Add the spices and mix thoroughly to combine.

Start packing your fermenting vessel, following the method for the previous recipe.

After the same 7-10 days of fermenting, and when you think it's ready, decant the contents into a smaller container and place in the refrigerator. You can keep in the fridge for at least 3 months.

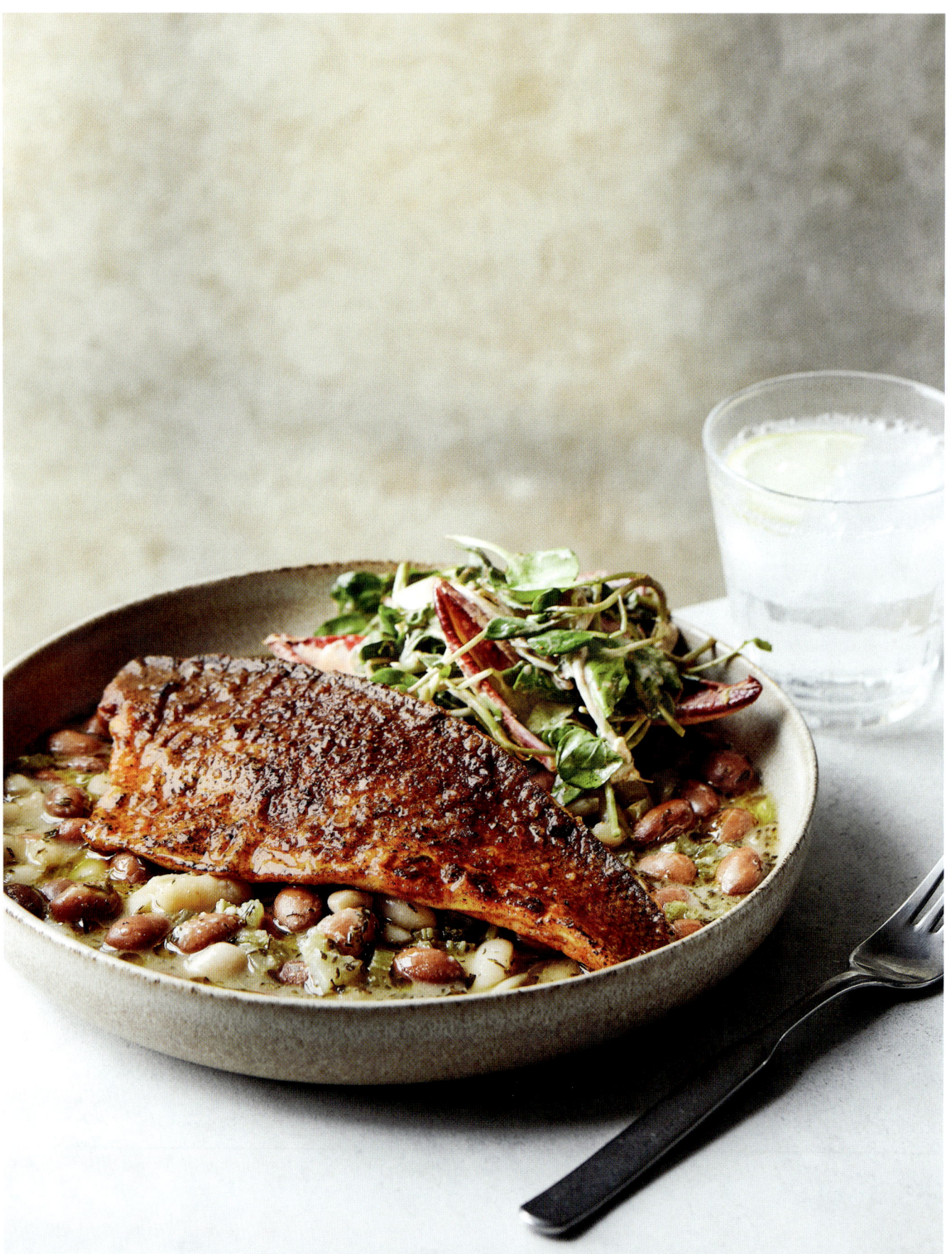

Tarragon and Thyme Beans with Spicy Sea Bass

Prep 15 minutes
Cook 30 minutes

Serves 4

For the beans
- 1 tbsp olive oil
- 150g celery, finely diced
- 2 tsp dried tarragon
- 2 tsp dried thyme
- 1 tbsp butter
- 250ml fish stock
- 1 x 400g can cannellini beans, drained and rinsed
- 1 x 400g can borlotti beans, drained and rinsed
- 150g peas (fresh or frozen)
- 1 tsp white miso paste

For the spicy sea bass
- 1 tbsp plain or gluten-free flour
- 1 tsp ground cumin
- 1 tsp sweet paprika
- ½ tsp ground cinnamon
- 2 tbsp olive oil
- 4 sea bass or bream fillets or red snapper

For the radicchio salad
- 2 tbsp mayonnaise
- 1 tbsp apple cider vinegar
- 1 tsp paprika
- 200g radicchio, roughly torn
- 100g watercress, roughly torn

For a dinner party or when I want to prep a couple of meals ahead, I use this gut-friendly, super-easy recipe. The fish stock-miso combination is gloriously simple, delivering a deep flavour, and I love combining different beans in the same dish. If I can find red snapper at the fishmongers, even better, but more readily available bass or bream work really well. It's packed with a diversity of powerful anti-inflammatory herbs, multiple fibre types to keep it gut friendly and plenty of protein per serving.

Start with the tarragon and thyme beans. Heat the olive oil in a large lidded casserole pan over a medium heat. Add the celery and sauté for about 6–8 minutes until translucent and softened.

Add the tarragon, thyme and butter and cook for another 2 minutes before adding the fish stock and bring to a gentle simmer.

Turn the heat to low–medium, stir in the beans, peas and miso paste and bring back to a gentle simmer, cover with the lid and cook for another 5 minutes.

To prepare the fish, tip the flour into a shallow dish, stir in the spices and season with salt and pepper. Heat the olive oil in a large frying pan over a medium–high heat. Coat the fish fillets in the spice mix and place them, skin-side down, in the pan. You may need to do this in batches, depending on the size of the pan. Cook the fillets 80% of the way through, about 3–4 minutes depending on their thickness, then turn them and cook for another minute before transferring to a plate to rest.

Meanwhile, prepare the salad. Add the mayonnaise, vinegar, paprika and a splash of water to a clean jar and shake thoroughly to combine. Toss the leaves together in a large serving bowl, season well and drizzle over the dressing.

Serve the bean mixture in shallow bowls with the fish on top and the salad on the side.

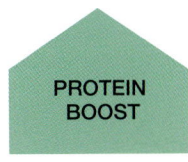

PROTEIN BOOST

Add more fish.

Protein 36.5g

Fibre 14.9g

Plant Points 8.75

MIDWEEK MEAT & FISH

Coconut, Prawn and Pineapple Curry

Prep 10 minutes
Cook 30 minutes

Serves 2

For the paste
- 2 red chillies, seeds removed, roughly chopped
- 120g onion, roughly chopped
- 3–4 makrut lime leaves, chopped
- 6 garlic cloves
- 5cm piece of fresh root ginger, peeled and roughly chopped
- 1 lemongrass stick, tough outer leaves removed and inside chopped
- 1 tsp ground turmeric

For the curry
- 1 tbsp coconut oil
- 1 x 400ml can light coconut milk
- 1 tbsp tamarind paste
- 200g pineapple, cut into bite-size chunks
- 150g pak choi, white part thinly sliced and leaves roughly chopped
- a bunch of spring onions, green and whites separated, sliced
- 100g bean sprouts
- 200g raw king prawns, peeled and deveined

Inspired by a delicious Nyonya dish I experienced in Penang, this spicy prawn curry balanced with the sharp sweetness of pineapple is such an unusual but successful combination. Its citrus tang, lemony notes and sour tamarind are beautiful marriages for the heat of this curry with the sweet fruit. Packed with inflammation-lowering spices and tons of polyphenols from green vegetables that your gut will love.

Blitz the paste ingredients in a blender or food processor with a little water to get it going.

Heat the coconut oil in a large lidded sauté pan over a medium heat. Add the paste and fry for 4–5 minutes until darker in colour. Stir in the coconut milk to combine.

Add the tamarind paste and pineapple chunks, the white part of the pak choi and the white part of the spring onions and bring to a gentle simmer. Cook, covered with the lid for 4–5 minutes, stirring occasionally, until the vegetables soften, and the pineapple infuses its sweet flavour into the sauce. Season with salt and pepper.

Add the pak choi leaves and bean sprouts, stir to coat them in the sauce and cook for 2 minutes. Add the prawns to the simmering mixture and cook for another 3–4 minutes, turning halfway, until pink and cooked through. Remove the pan from the heat and serve sprinkled with the green part of the spring onions.

PROTEIN BOOST

Add more prawns. You can also add some finely diced tofu or beancurd to the curry.

Protein 25g

Fibre 6.2g

Plant Points 7.5

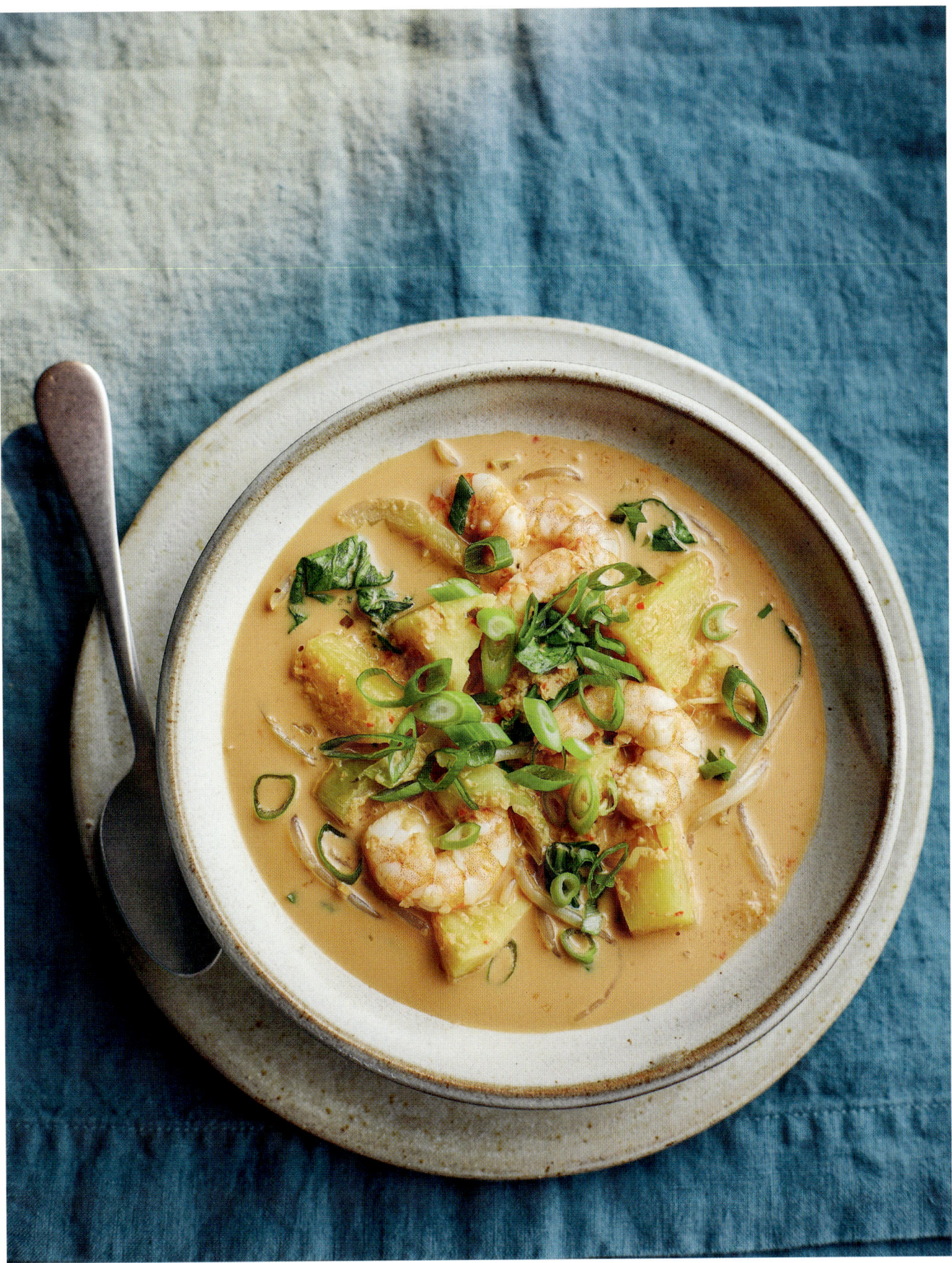

Spinach and Masala Cod with Spicy Fennel Oil

Prep 5 minutes
Cook 20 minutes

Serves 2

1 tbsp olive oil
20g fresh root ginger, peeled and grated
100g peas (fresh or defrosted from frozen)
100g frozen spinach, defrosted
1 x 400g can large butter beans
½ vegetable stock cube
50ml boiling water (optional)
2 tsp garam masala
300g skinless cod fillets
10g coriander leaves, finely chopped, to finish

For the spicy fennel oil
3 tbsp olive oil
1 tsp fennel seeds
½ tsp chilli flakes

The spiced oil in this dish is worth the extra effort to elevate the cod and greens. The fennel and chilli are a simple but effective pairing for the fish. You can also try adding a mild curry powder instead of garam masala for less aromatics and more earthy, spicy cumin notes. Either way, you'll be effortlessly introducing more anti-inflammatory spices in essentially a one-pan dish.

Heat the olive oil in a large lidded sauté pan over a medium heat, add the ginger and cook for a minute.

Add the peas and spinach to the pan, then tip in the butter beans with their liquid and crumble in the stock cube. Bring to a gentle simmer and cook for 5 minutes, adding the hot water if it's too dry. Stir in the garam masala and season with salt and pepper.

Place the cod fillets in the pan on top of the vegetables and cook, covered with the lid, for 5–6 minutes until they are just cooked through.

Meanwhile, make the spicy fennel oil. Add the oil and spices to a small sauté pan over a low heat and gently warm for 2 minutes to infuse the oil. Avoid smoking the oil or burning the spices. Remove the pan from the heat and season.

Serve the cod with the vegetables, topped with a spoonful of the spicy fennel oil and finished with coriander leaves.

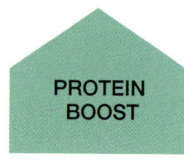

PROTEIN BOOST

Add more fish.

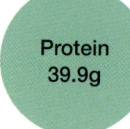

Protein 39.9g | Fibre 12.3g | Plant Points 5.25

MIDWEEK MEAT & FISH

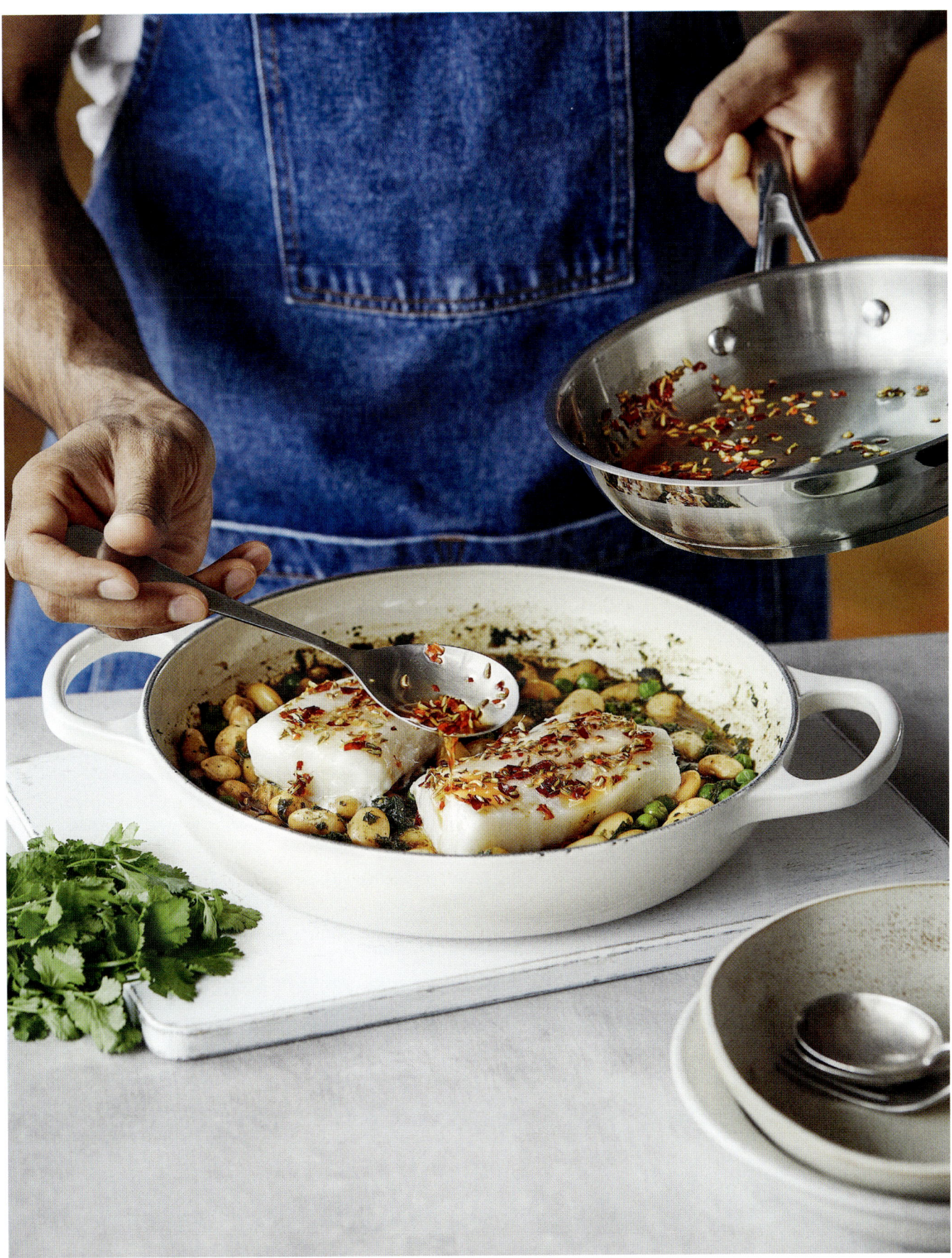

Grilled Mackerel with Roasted Radish and Chilli-pea Pesto

Prep 15 minutes
Cook 40 minutes

Serves 2

100g French beans, cut into thirds on an angle
100g Swiss chard, stalks removed, leaves massaged
1 tbsp olive oil
2 mackerel fillets, skin on

For the roasted vegetables
200g Pink Fir or Charlotte potatoes, quartered lengthways
1 red onion, cut into thick wedges
1 tbsp olive oil, plus extra if needed
200g radishes, halved if large
2 garlic cloves, crushed
2 tsp cumin seeds
2 tsp coriander seeds

For the chilli-pea pesto
25g basil
10g oregano sprigs, leaves picked
10g flat-leaf parsley
100g peas (fresh or defrosted from frozen)
125g pine nuts
1 tbsp olive oil
Juice of 1 lemon
20g Parmesan, finely grated
½ tsp chilli flakes

This effortless dish looks so impressive, making it perfect for date nights. Massaging the chard leaves breaks down their cell walls and makes them easier to eat raw. You also get a higher dose of the vitamin C and other phytonutrients that are reduced by cooking. You can use salmon here if you find mackerel too strong a flavour. Boost the protein by adding more fish.

Preheat the oven to 200°C fan.

Blanch the French beans in a small amount of boiling water for 3 minutes, then drain. Put the beans in a bowl, add the massaged leaves, then drizzle with a little of the olive oil and season. Set aside.

For the roasted vegetables, par-boil the potatoes for 6 minutes, drain and leave to steam-dry in the pan briefly. Tip onto a baking tray.

Add the onion to the baking tray. Drizzle over the oil, season with salt and toss until everything is combined. Roast in the oven for 15 minutes until the potatoes start to colour. Stir, then add the radishes, garlic and spices, and drizzle over a little more oil if needed. Roast for another 15 minutes until the potatoes are crisp and golden. The onions and garlic should catch in places and the radishes soften.

Make the pesto by roughly blending the basil, oregano, parsley and peas in a food processor – it should be a little rough. Season well with salt and pepper. Add the pine nuts, olive oil and half the lemon juice and pulse a few extra times until combined. Scrape into a bowl and stir in the Parmesan and chilli flakes until combined. Set aside.

Rub the mackerel fillets with a little oil and seasoning. Cook in a griddle pan over a medium–high heat, skin-side down, for 3–4 minutes, until crisp. Flip over and cook for another 1–2 minutes to cook through.

To serve, spread the chilli-pea pesto over the base of a platter. Top with the French beans and chard and the roasted vegetables. Place the mackerel on top. Add an extra squeeze of lemon to finish.

Protein 40.9g
Fibre 13.7g
Plant Points 9.25

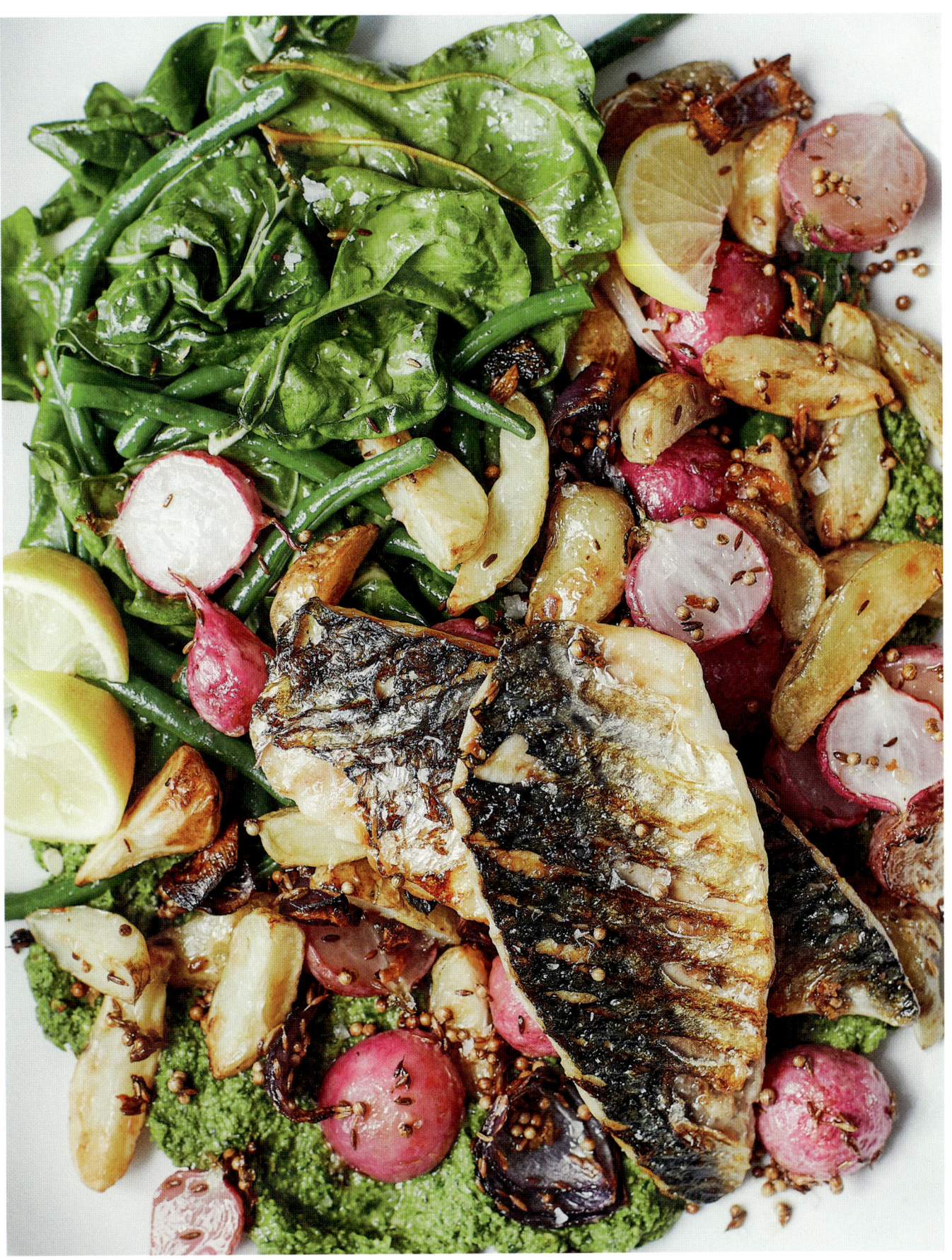

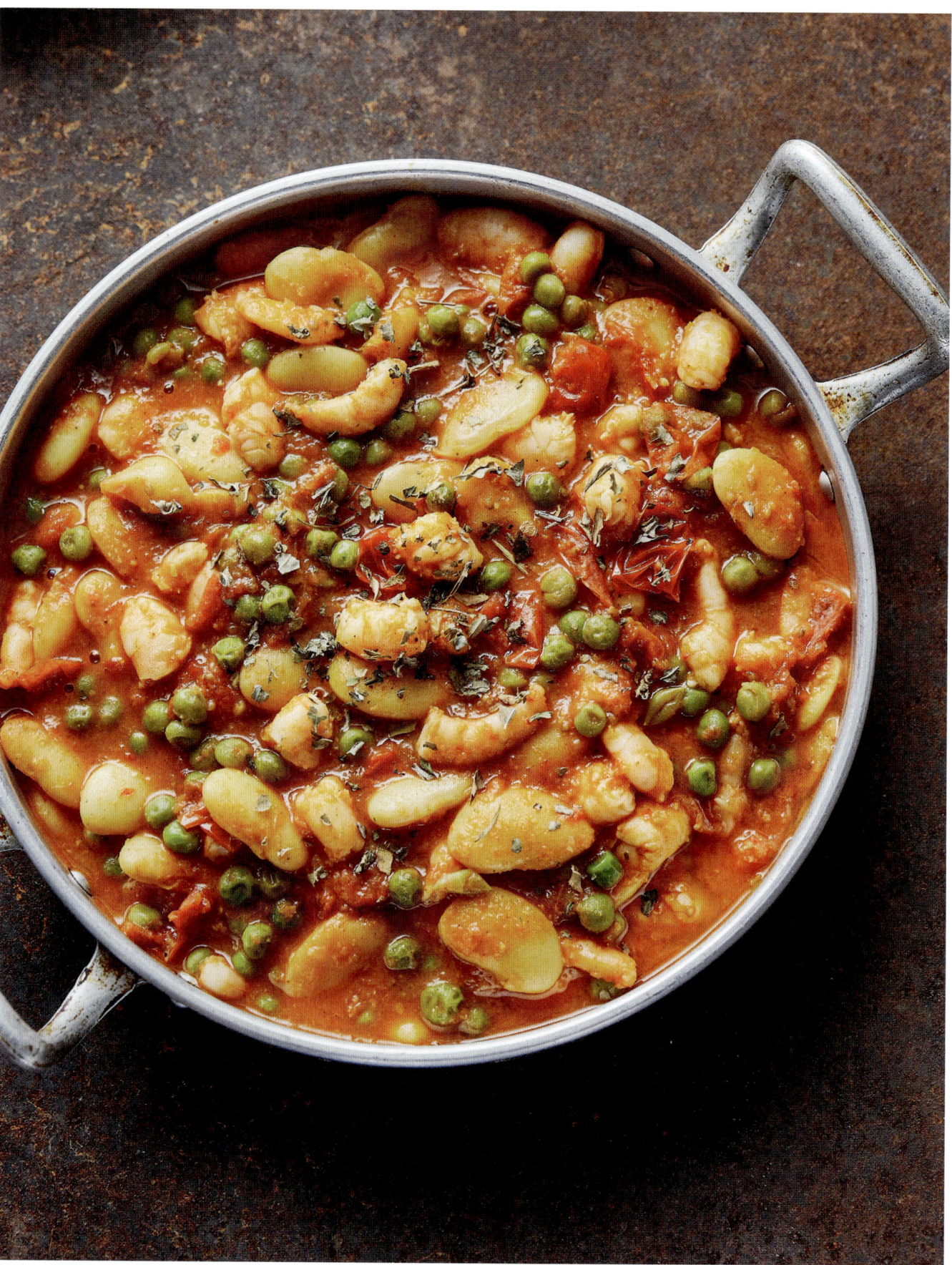

Easy Tomato Curry with Prawns and Peas

Prep 10 minutes
Cook 25 minutes

Serves 2

For the paste
- 2 garlic cloves, roughly chopped
- 5cm piece of fresh root ginger, peeled and roughly chopped
- 50g white onion, roughly chopped
- 1 small red chilli, seeds removed and roughly chopped
- 1 tbsp coconut oil
- 2 tsp mild curry powder
- 2 tbsp tomato purée

For the curry
- 1 tbsp coconut oil
- 200g raw king or tiger prawns, peeled and deveined
- 200g baby tomatoes, halved
- 1 x 400g can butter beans
- 150g peas (fresh or defrosted from frozen)
- 1 tsp dried fenugreek leaves, to serve (optional)

This curry paste is really simple to make. Once you get into the habit, you'll only use store-bought pastes when you're feeling super lazy. That's totally fine, I do it all the time, but the flavour of your own paste is unmatched. Plus, you have complete control over the quality of the ingredients and ready-made pastes tend to come with excessive sugar, additives and ingredients that have no place in your kitchen. Cooking down the tomatoes in this way creates a lovely light sauce and dried fenugreek is a perfect ending to this high-protein, gut-supporting recipe packed with an anti-inflammatory spice paste.

To make the paste, blend all the ingredients with a splash of water in a blender or food processor.

Heat a little of the coconut oil in a large lidded frying pan over a medium heat, then add the prawns. Cook for 2–3 minutes on each side (depending on size) until pink and cooked through. Set aside.

Heat the remaining coconut oil in the same pan, add the paste and cook, stirring, for 3–4 minutes over a low heat until darkened and slightly reduced. Season well.

Add the baby tomatoes and stir through the paste with a splash of water. Cover with the lid and continue to cook over a low–medium heat for 10–12 minutes until the tomatoes start to break down and create a sauce. Remove the lid and gently mash the tomatoes with the back of a spoon or fork.

Add the butter beans with their liquid and simmer for 5 minutes until heated through. Add the peas and continue to cook for another few minutes.

Roughly chop the prawns and stir them through the curry to warm them through. Stir in some of the fenugreek and sprinkle the rest on top, if you like.

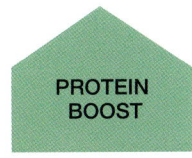

PROTEIN BOOST
Add extra prawns or beans.

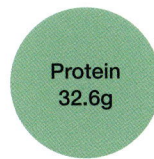

Protein 32.6g | Fibre 15g | Plant Points 5.5

MIDWEEK MEAT & FISH

Asparagus and Wild Garlic Green Orzo with Salmon

Prep 10 minutes
Cook 20 minutes

Serves 2

- 1 x 400g can white beans
- 100g spinach, roughly chopped
- 25g wild garlic or basil, stalks and leaves chopped (if using basil, add 2 crushed garlic cloves)
- 2 tbsp olive oil
- 150g asparagus, roughly chopped
- 125g dried orzo
- 325ml vegetable stock
- 20g Parmesan, grated
- Zest and juice of 1 lemon
- 300g salmon fillets, skin on
- 10g basil leaves, torn, to garnish

The beans blended with the greens add a ton more fibre and body to the orzo, which is otherwise a fairly refined carbohydrate to use. I love adding extra ingredients to mitigate against the blood sugar-spiking potential of white flour pasta, while still being able to enjoy the delicate texture that is otherwise lacking in wholegrain pasta varieties. The salmon adds protein and anti-inflammatory fats to the dish, and a flourish of Parmesan with lemon zest at the end completes this simple but delicious meal.

Place the beans with their liquid, spinach, wild garlic or basil and garlic cloves, and a pinch of salt and pepper in a blender or food processor and blend into a green sauce. Add a splash of boiling water if needed to loosen it. Set aside while you cook the orzo.

Add 1 tablespoon of the olive oil to a large sauté pan over a medium heat and sauté the asparagus with plenty of seasoning for a minute. Add the orzo and stir through the asparagus before adding the vegetable stock.

Bring to a simmer and cook for 7–9 minutes, stirring every so often to make sure the orzo does not stick to the bottom of the pan. Add a little more water if needed to cook the orzo until al dente.

Add the green sauce to the orzo once it's cooked al dente. Then add half the Parmesan and half the lemon juice. Stir thoroughly to combine.

Meanwhile, in another sauté pan over medium heat, heat the remaining olive oil and cook the salmon fillets, skin-side down, for 5–6 minutes. Flip and cook for another minute.

Serve the salmon on top of the asparagus orzo with the remaining lemon juice and the zest, remaining Parmesan and the basil leaves.

PROTEIN BOOST
Add more salmon.

Protein 58.4g
Fibre 15.8g
Plant Points 4

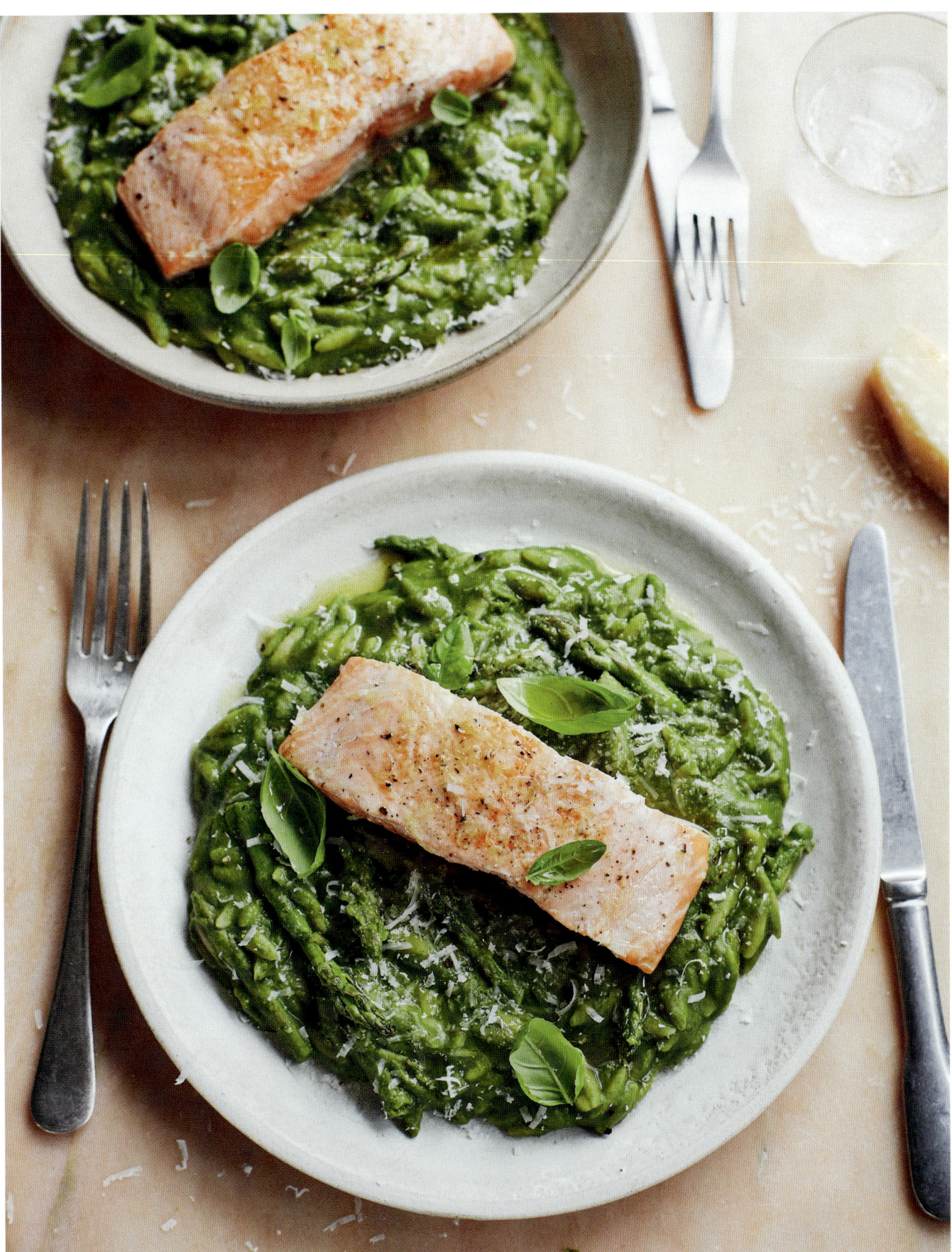

Masala Sea Bass Nuggets with Spiced Vegetables

Prep 15 minutes
Cook 25 minutes

Serves 2

For the spiced vegetables
30g desiccated coconut
1 tbsp olive oil
50g shallots, diced
2 tsp mustard seeds
10–12 fresh curry leaves
150g carrot, diced
150g celery, diced
150g broccoli florets separated and stalks roughly chopped
30g raw unsalted peanuts, toasted and roughly chopped
Juice of 2 limes, to serve

For the masala sea bass
1 tbsp plain or gluten-free flour
1 tbsp garam masala
300g sea bass, cut into 4cm chunks
1 tbsp olive oil
1 tbsp butter (optional)

Fresh coconut, mustard seeds and curry leaves are all I need to transport me back to Colombo, Sri Lanka. The combination of these flavours transforms humble celery, carrot and broccoli into a dish wildly more exotic. This is meant to be a dry curried dish with plenty of flavour injected into the crispy sea bass nuggets. It contains a good dose of polyphenols to keep your gut microbes happy and plenty of protein to support bone health and keep you full. I like to serve this with a simple cucumber salad, lime and mango pickle or even a sauerkraut.

First toast the desiccated coconut in a large, dry sauté pan, tossing frequently, until starting to turn golden. Tip into a bowl and set aside.

Heat the olive oil in the same pan, add the shallots and cook for 5 minutes over a medium heat until lightly browned. Add the mustard seeds and curry leaves and stir for 1–2 minutes until the seeds pop.

Add the carrot, celery and broccoli stalks and toss for 3–4 minutes until softened. Add the florets and cook for a further 4–5 minutes until all the vegetables are just tender. Toss in half the toasted coconut and peanuts, season with salt and pepper and set aside.

Mix together the flour and garam masala in a wide shallow bowl with seasoning. Toss the sea bass chunks in the spiced flour mixture until lightly coated.

Heat the olive oil and butter, if using, in a large frying pan over a medium heat. Add the sea bass, skin-side down, and fry for 3 minutes until the skin browns and crisps and the white flesh becomes opaque. Flip and cook for a further minute before placing on a plate lined with kitchen paper to remove any excess oil.

Spoon the spiced vegetables into 2 serving bowls, top with the sea bass and scatter over the remaining coconut and peanuts. Squeeze over the lime juice to serve.

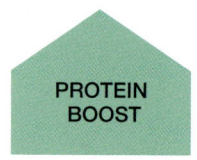

PROTEIN BOOST
Add more fish. Try this with cooked brown lentils.

Protein 42.6g
Fibre 10.5g
Plant Points 7.25

MIDWEEK MEAT & FISH

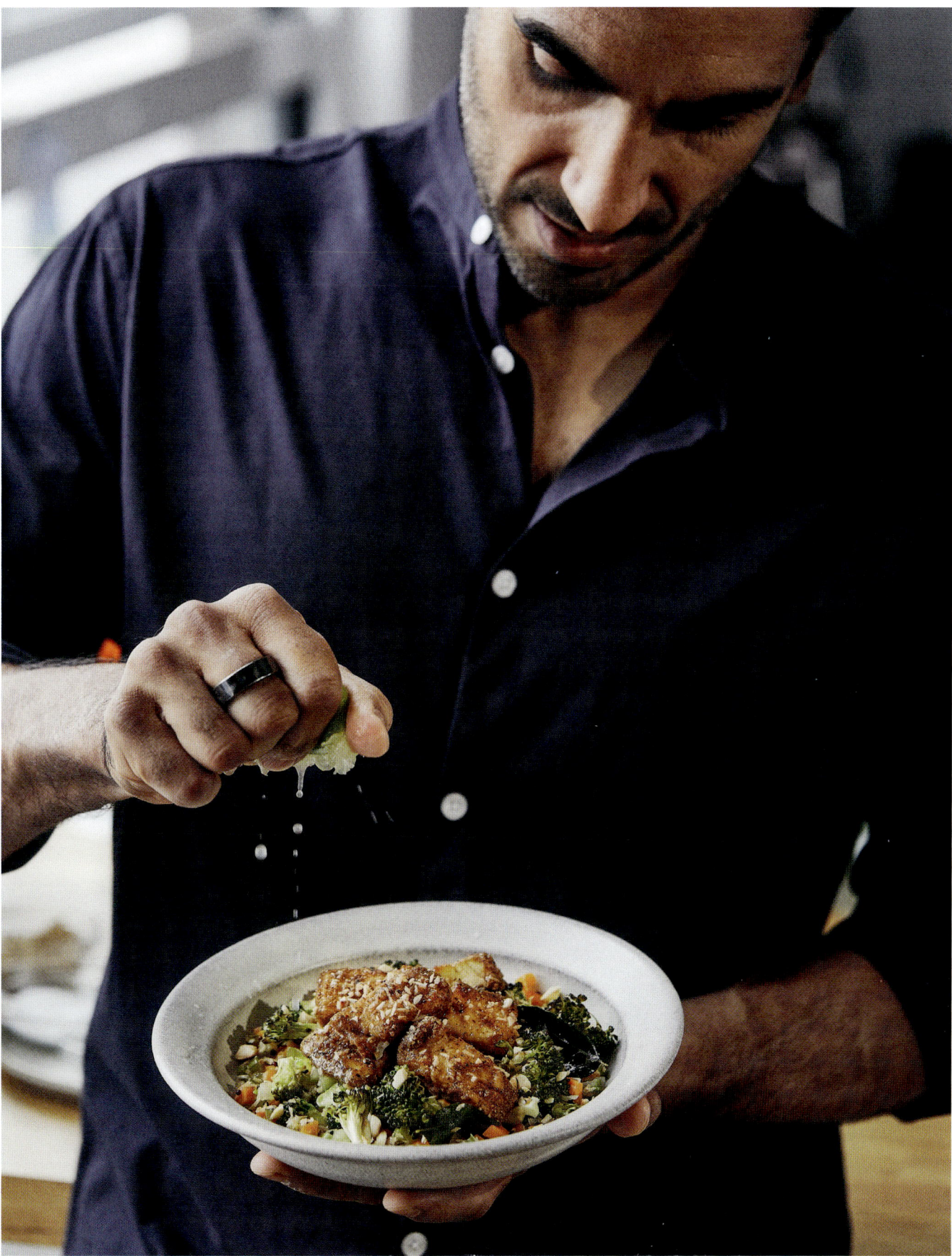

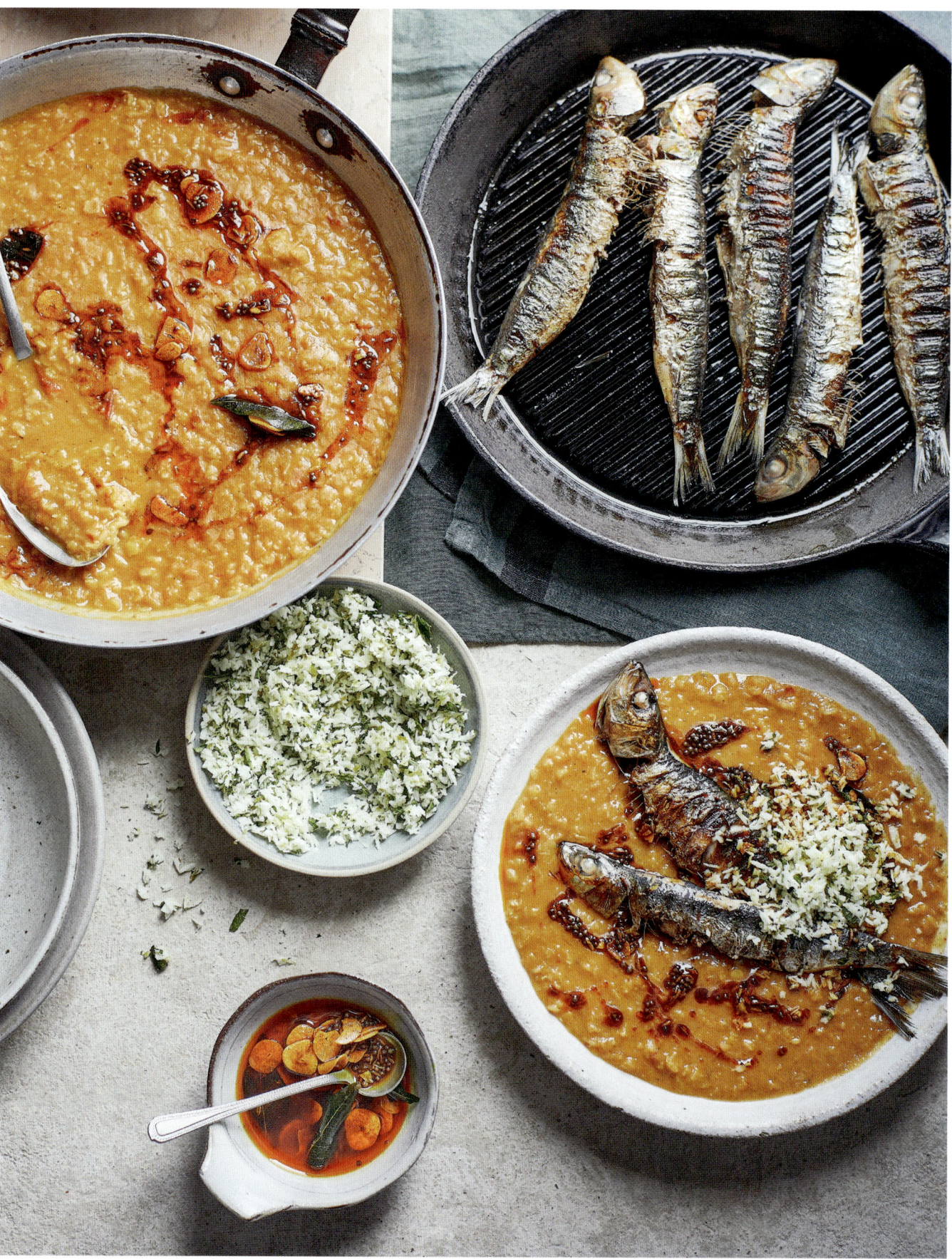

Sri Lankan-style Coconut Lentils with Griddled Sardines

Prep 15 minutes
Cook 35 minutes

Serves 4

12 fresh sardines
Olive oil, for rubbing

For the coconut lentils
1 tbsp coconut oil
10g fresh root ginger, peeled and grated
200g split red lentils, soaked for 20 minutes, then rinsed
3 tsp mild curry powder
250g tomatoes, chopped
400ml boiling water
1 tsp vegetable bouillon powder
1 x 400ml can light coconut milk

For the coconut chutney
50g desiccated coconut
15g mint leaves, finely chopped
Finely grated zest and juice of 2 limes

For the spiced oil
3 tbsp coconut oil
4 garlic cloves, thinly sliced
2 tsp mustard seeds
6 curry leaves
1 tsp cumin seeds
1 tsp ground turmeric
1 tsp Kashmiri chilli powder or sweet paprika

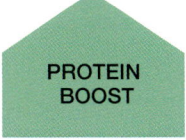

PROTEIN BOOST
Add more fish or lentils.

If you can find Sri Lankan-style curry powder please use it. It uses slightly different ratios of similar spices and some also contain more exotic ingredients, but regular mild curry powder also works well. If you can source fresh curry leaves for the oil, do use those as well; they make a world of difference. The lentils, tomatoes and incredible mix of spices deliver a wealth of antioxidants that support balanced inflammation, plus the sardines deliver both protein and anti-inflammatory fats.

To make the coconut lentils, heat the coconut oil in a large lidded saucepan over a medium heat and add the grated ginger. Stir for a minute to infuse the oil, then add the lentils, curry powder and tomatoes. Cook for 2 minutes before adding the hot water and vegetable bouillon powder. Bring to a simmer, then reduce the heat to low, part-cover with the lid and cook for 15 minutes until the lentils are tender. Stir in the coconut milk.

Meanwhile, make the coconut chutney. Mix together all the ingredients in a small bowl with seasoning and set aside.

To make the spiced oil, add the coconut oil to a sauté pan over a medium heat. Add the garlic and cook for 2–3 minutes until light golden. Add the mustard seeds, curry leaves and cumin seeds and cook for another minute, then stir in the turmeric and chilli powder or paprika. Take the pan off the heat after 3–4 minutes and set aside.

When the lentils are tender, mix in half of the spiced oil and save the rest to serve.

Rub the sardines with a little oil and salt. Heat a griddle or sauté pan over a medium–high heat and cook the sardines in batches on both sides for a few minutes. Transfer to a warm plate while you cook the rest.

Serve the sardines on top of the lentils in bowls, drizzled with the garlic-spiced oil and a good spoonful of the coconut chutney.

Protein 45.2g
Fibre 7.7g
Plant Points 7.25

Radishes, Caraway and Chard with Baked Salmon

Prep 5 minutes
Cook 20 minutes

Serves 2

1 lemon, sliced
300g salmon fillets
2 tbsp olive oil
3 garlic cloves, grated
200g radishes, halved or quartered if large
200g Swiss chard, stalks and leaves separated, chopped
2 tsp caraway seeds
30g pitted Kalamata olives, quartered
1 x 400g can white beans, drained and rinsed

To serve
30g pickled cucumbers or gherkins, thinly sliced or with a mandoline
30g flaked almonds, toasted

Sautéing radish is a novel use for this antioxidant-rich, peppery-tasting vegetable. Typically found raw in salads or pickles, the oil mellows its flavour and the combination with chard and caraway seeds adds a gorgeous warm flavour that works beautifully with the garlicky salmon roasted in a hot oven. You can also use trout or sardines in place of salmon for a delicious simple twist.

Preheat the oven to 200°C fan.

Lay the slices of lemon on a baking sheet. Place the salmon fillets on the lemon slices and smother in 1 tablespoon of the olive oil and half the grated garlic. Add plenty of seasoning. Bake for 10–12 minutes until the salmon is cooked through and slightly golden on top.

Meanwhile, heat the remaining oil in a sauté pan over a medium heat. Add the radishes and a pinch of salt and cook for a few minutes until slightly browned. Add the chard stalks, caraway seeds, olives and remaining garlic and cook for another minute.

Add the chard leaves, turning them for 2 minutes so they wilt, and then tip in the beans. Stir gently to ensure all the ingredients come together and heat through, adding a splash of water, for another minute. Season with salt and pepper.

Serve the salmon with the vegetable mix, topped with the pickled cucumbers or gherkins and flaked almonds.

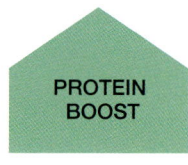

PROTEIN BOOST
Add more fish.

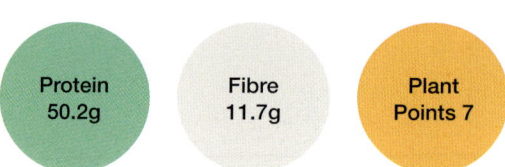

Protein 50.2g
Fibre 11.7g
Plant Points 7

MIDWEEK MEAT & FISH

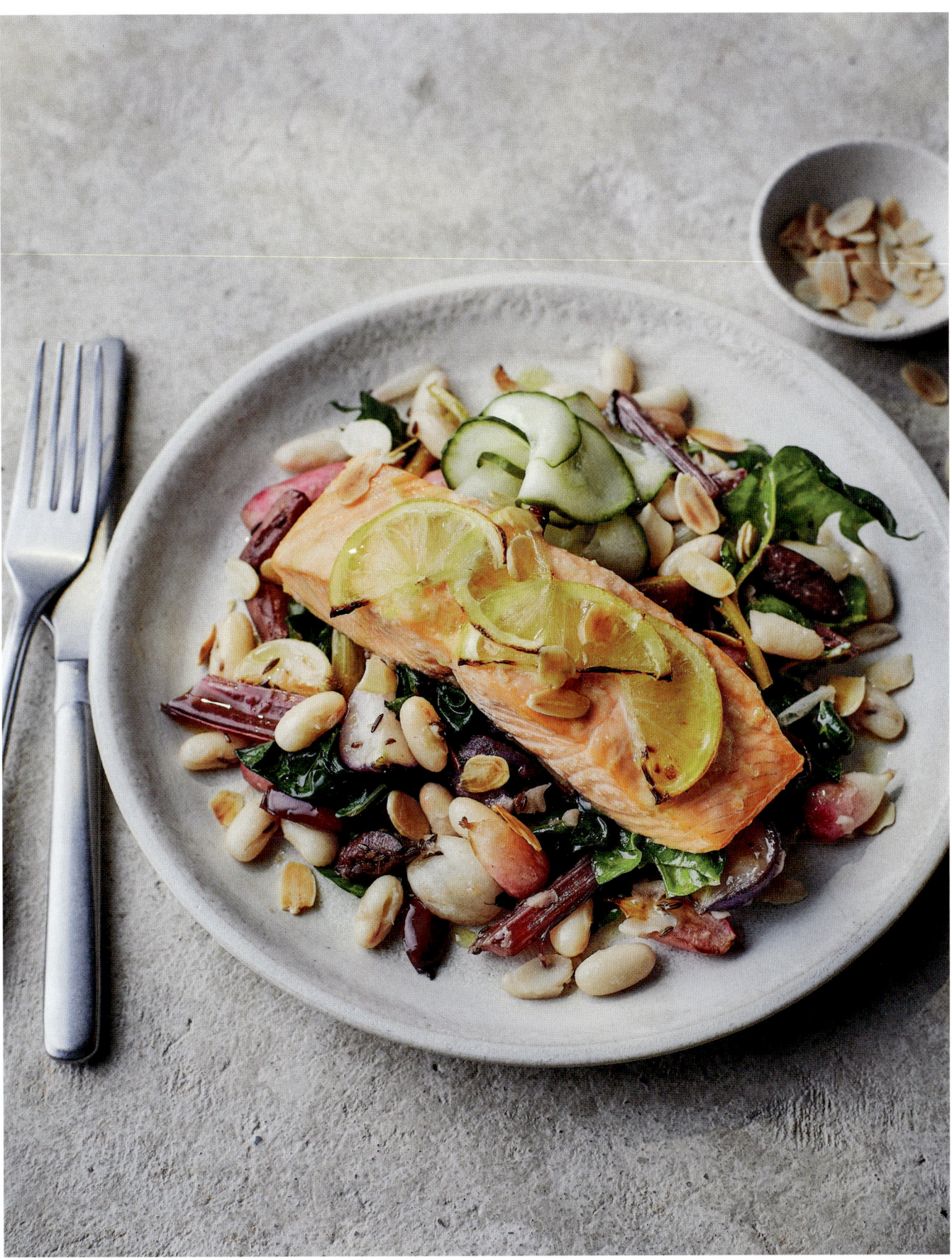

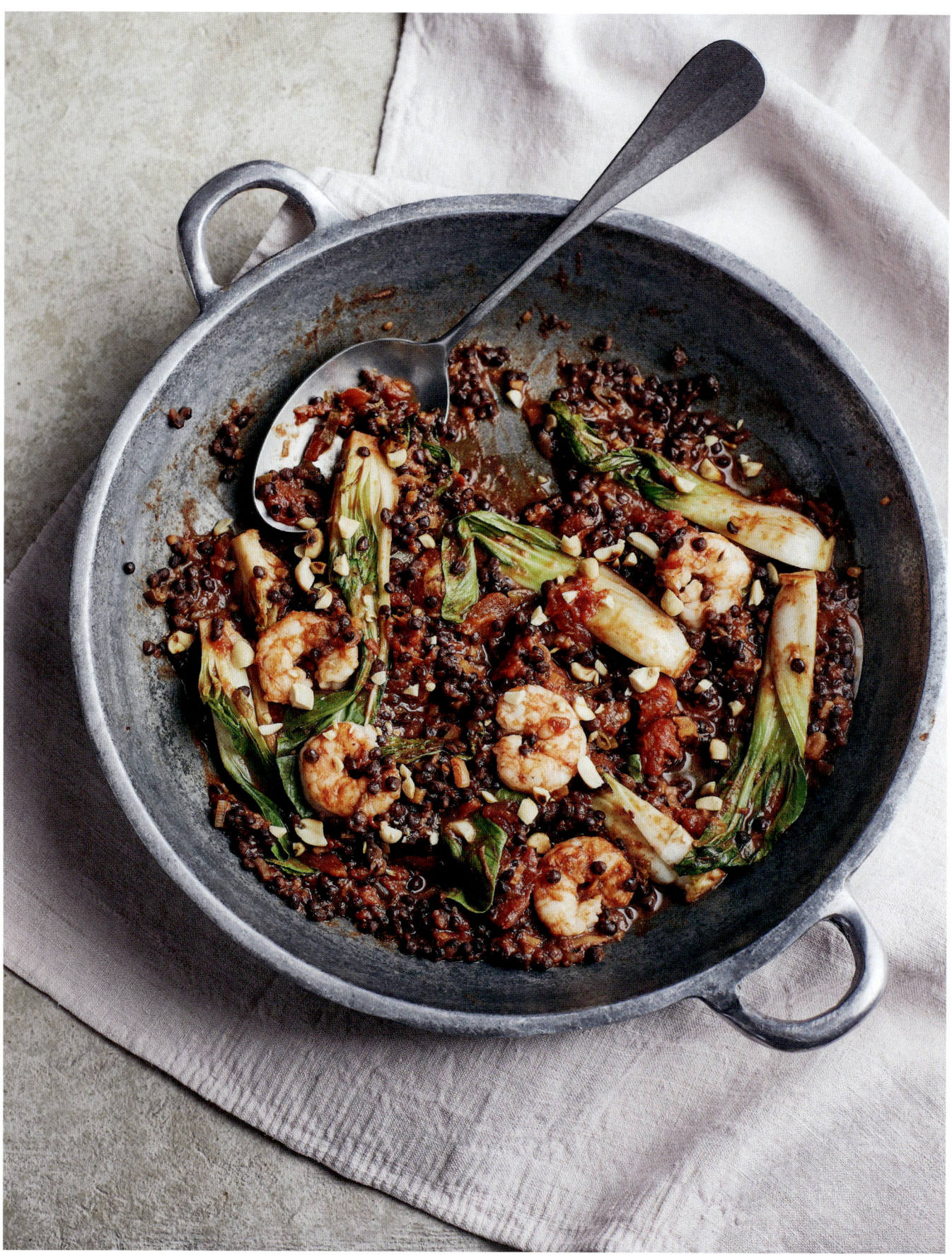

Ginger, Miso and Tamarind Prawns with Beluga Lentils

Prep 10 minutes
Cook 25 minutes

Serves 2

2 tbsp olive or coconut oil
50g spring onion, thinly sliced
20g fresh root ginger, peeled and finely diced
6 garlic cloves, finely diced
1 x 400g can whole peeled tomatoes
1 heaped tbsp white miso paste
1 heaped tbsp tamarind paste
250g cooked beluga lentils
150g baby pak choi, quartered
200g raw king prawns, shelled and deveined

To serve
10g Thai basil, chopped
10g coriander, chopped
Juice of 1 lime
20g peanuts, crushed

I love using one pan to concentrate flavours and minimise washing up. This is my go-to midweek meal when I want something nourishing, gut supporting and easy. The combination of ginger, miso and tamarind injects plenty of flavour and the anti-inflammatory nutrients in tomatoes, along with garlic and onion, work harmoniously to make this meal both healthy and delicious. You also have plenty of protein from the prawns and lentils, which work beautifully together.

Add the oil to a large but shallow lidded pan and add the spring onion, reserving a little to garnish, ginger and garlic. Sauté the ingredients over a low–medium for 2–3 minutes until lightly browned.

Add the tomatoes, breaking them up with the back of a spoon and stir in the miso and tamarind pastes. Bring to a gentle simmer, cover with the lid and cook for 10 minutes.

Remove the lid, add the lentils and stir them through, then add the pak choi and cover with the lid again for 4 minutes to allow them to gently wilt.

Remove the lid and lay the prawns onto the simmering ingredients. Turn up the heat slightly and cook the prawns for 5–6 minutes until they are pink and cooked through. Flip them halfway through to make sure they evenly cook.

Garnish with the herbs, lime juice and peanuts and dig in.

PROTEIN BOOST
Add more prawns or lentils.

Protein 38.4g
Fibre 10.3g
Plant Points 7

MIDWEEK MEAT & FISH

SNACKS, TOPPERS

& DRINKS

Fennel, Oregano, Chia and Pumpkin Seed Crackers

Prep 5 minutes
Cook 1 hour 10 minutes

Serves 8

35g chia seeds
100g pumpkin seeds
125g sunflower seeds
1 tsp fennel seeds
2 tsp dried oregano
½ tsp chilli flakes

These easy crackers are great for snacking, topping with cheese or yoghurt or even snapping into smaller shards to make a crunchy topper for salads. They're so easy to make, deliver plenty of anti-inflammatory fats and are high in protein from chia and pumpkin seeds.

Preheat the oven to 120°C fan. Line a baking sheet with baking paper.

Mix together the chia seeds and 240ml of water in a mixing bowl and leave for 5 minutes. The liquid should become thick and gelatinous with the chia. Add the rest of the ingredients and thoroughly combine. Season well with salt and pepper.

Spread over the lined baking tray and place another sheet of baking paper on top. Roll out to around 2mm thickness. Remove the top sheet of baking paper and sprinkle with extra salt.

Place in the oven and bake for 1 hour.

Remove from the oven and break into roughly 5cm squares. Flip over and return to the oven for another 10 minutes to cook off any moisture. Allow to cool completely on a wire rack and store in an airtight container for up to 30 days.

Protein 4.6g | Fibre 2.3g | Plant Points 3.75

Serves 4

100g edamame beans
100g peas (fresh or defrosted from frozen)
100g tahini
Juice of 1 lemon
1 tsp chilli oil, plus extra to drizzle

EDAMAME AND PEA DIP WITH CHILLI OIL Prep 2 minutes

Add all the ingredients to a blender or food processor with seasoning and blitz until it comes together. Add a little water if it needs to be smoother.
Drizzle some extra chilli oil on top. This is perfect on rye bread or on the side of a main meal for a little dip with crudités. It'll keep in the fridge for a few days at least.

Protein 13.2g | Fibre 7.1g | Plant Points 3.25

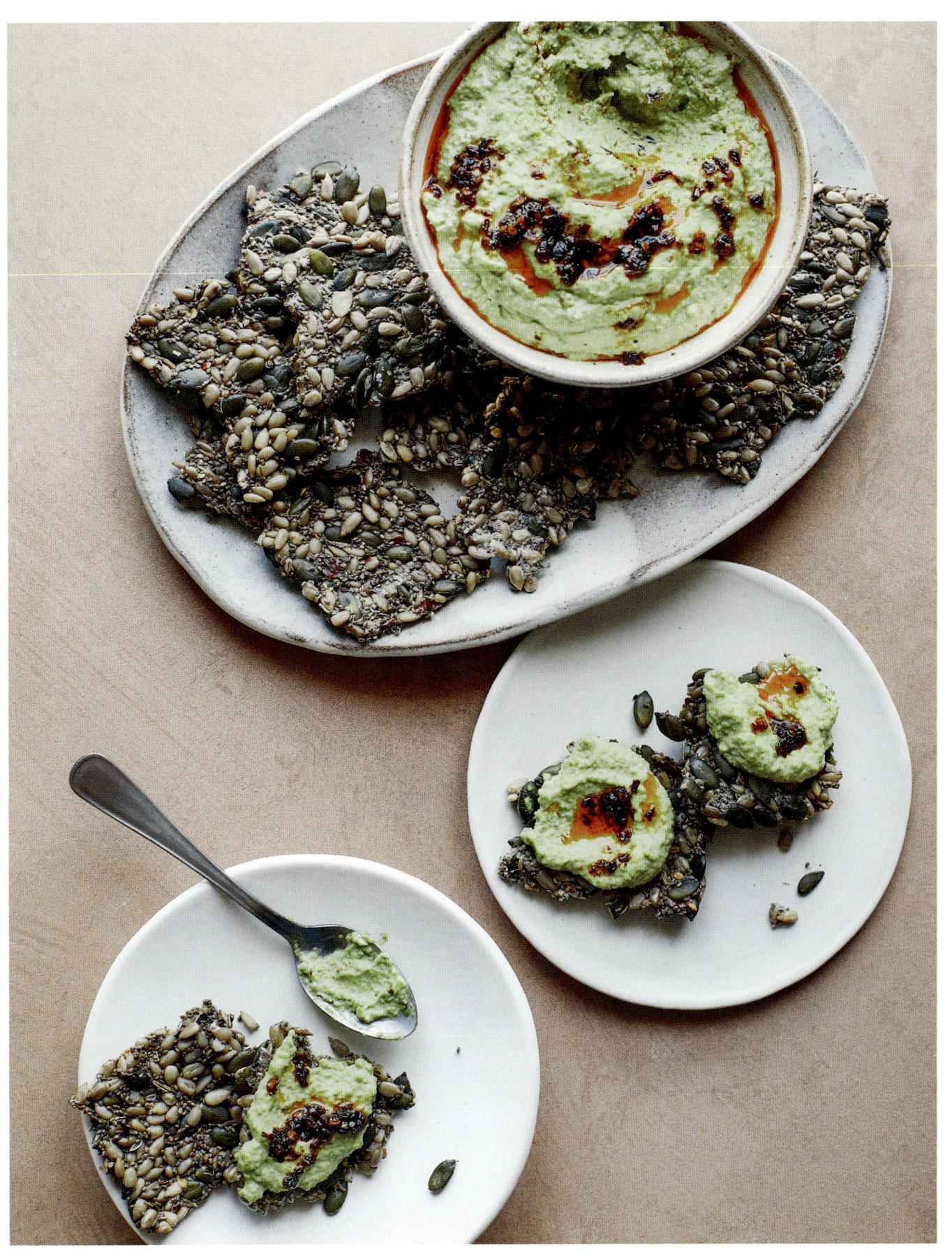

Frozen Yoghurt, Peanut and Berry Bark

Prep 10 minutes, plus freezing

Serves 6

150g frozen blackberries or mixed berries
50g dark chocolate, 75% cocoa solids, roughly chopped
250g authentic Greek yoghurt
50g hazelnuts, crushed
50g smooth peanut butter
1 tsp ground cinnamon
3 tbsp date syrup or raw honey

We always have some of these to hand as a little mid-afternoon snack for the weekends or a sneaky dessert midweek. Sweet enough to feel indulgent, healthy enough to keep you on track for your goals.

Line a baking tray with baking paper. You may need multiple baking trays that fit your freezer.

Add all the ingredients, apart from the date syrup or raw honey, to a mixing bowl and gently swirl together with a wooden spoon.

Spoon out the mixture onto the lined baking tray(s) and spread into a layer no thinner than the height of a berry. Drizzle over the date syrup or honey and freeze for at least 2 hours to harden.

Once hardened, you can break into pieces and keep them in a box in the freezer. Allow them to come to room temperature for 5 minutes to melt slightly before enjoying.

Protein 6.8g Fibre 3.3g Plant Points 4.25

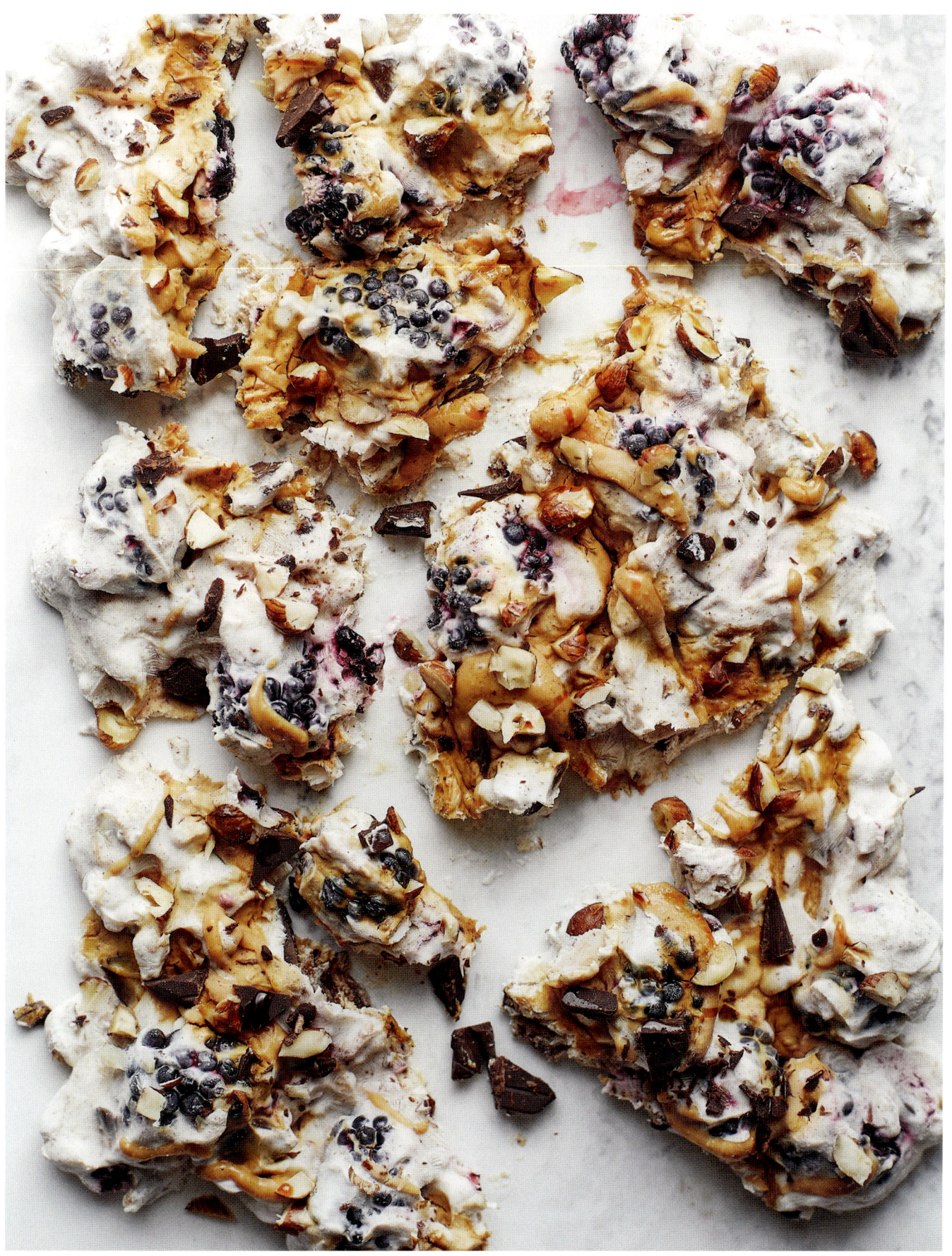

Curried Hemp Seeds

Prep 1 minute
Cook 5 minutes

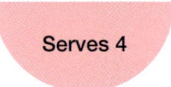
Serves 4

100g shelled hemp seeds
1 tsp mild curry powder

I throw these into salads, or over a curry for a nice spicy hit. You can also use gently crushed sunflower seeds or pumpkin seeds as an easier-to-source alternative.

Add the seeds and curry powder to a sauté pan over a medium heat. Move around the pan with a spoon until you see the seeds slightly toast and the spices release their aromas.

Take off the heat, season well and add straight to your meal or cool and store in an airtight container.

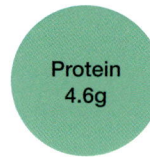

Protein 4.6g | Fibre 0.7g | Plant Points 1.25

Crispy Chilli Edamame

Prep 2 minutes
Cook 25 minutes

Serves 4

150g edamame beans
1 tbsp chilli oil
Salt

Note
You can also do this in an air fryer at maximum heat for 10 minutes.

This is a super-simple snack or salad topper that you can do with other beans such as butter beans or chickpeas. The aromas in chilli oil are delicious and instantly add flavour to the crispy legume without any work.

Line a baking tray with baking paper and preheat the oven to 200°C fan.

Mix the edamame and chilli oil together in a bowl. Spread out the edamame evenly on the lined baking tray and sprinkle with salt.

Bake for 20–25 minutes until golden and crispy. Allow to cool slightly before enjoying as a snack or topping salads with it.

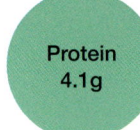

Protein 4.1g | Fibre 1.9g | Plant Points 1

SNACKS, TOPPERS & DRINKS

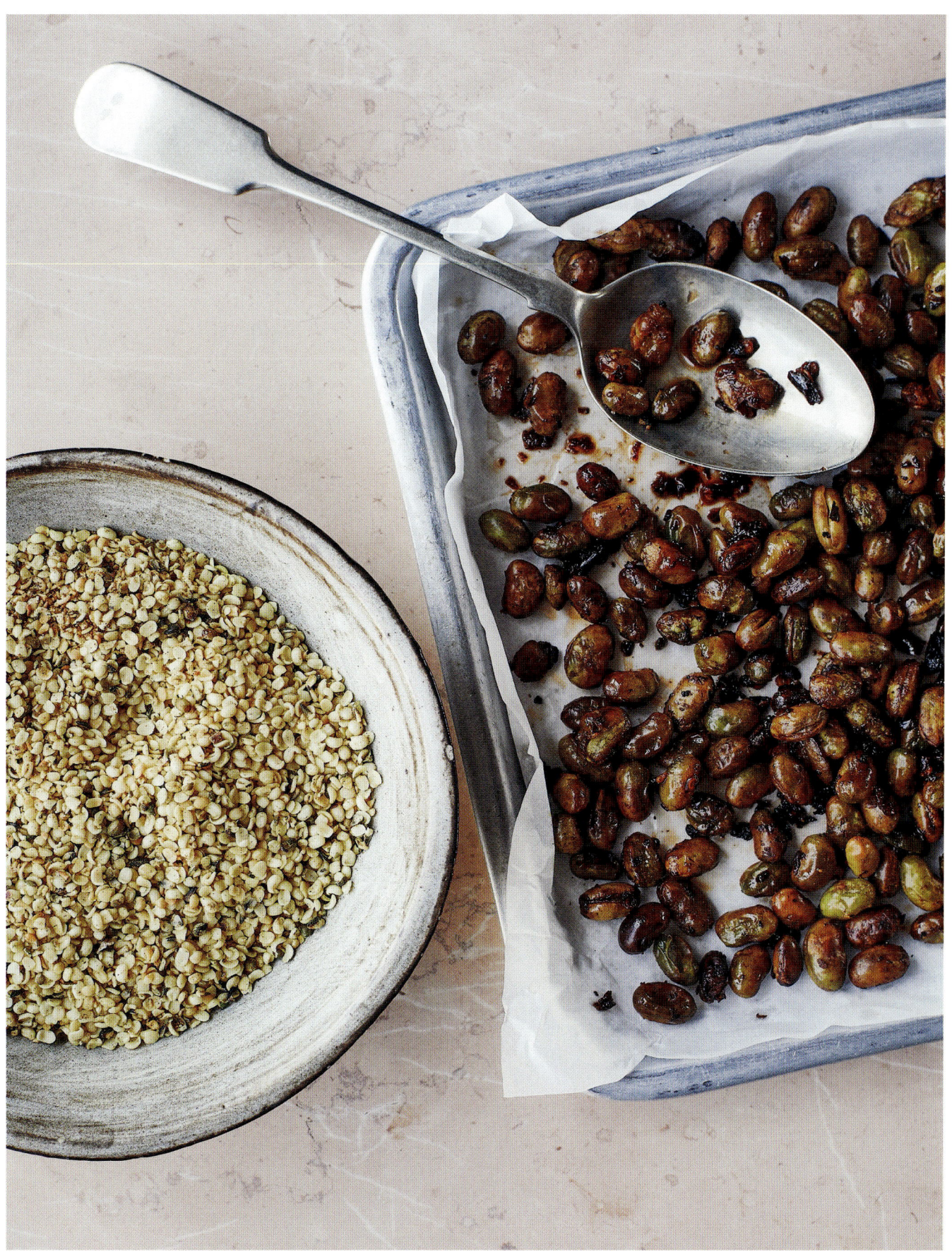

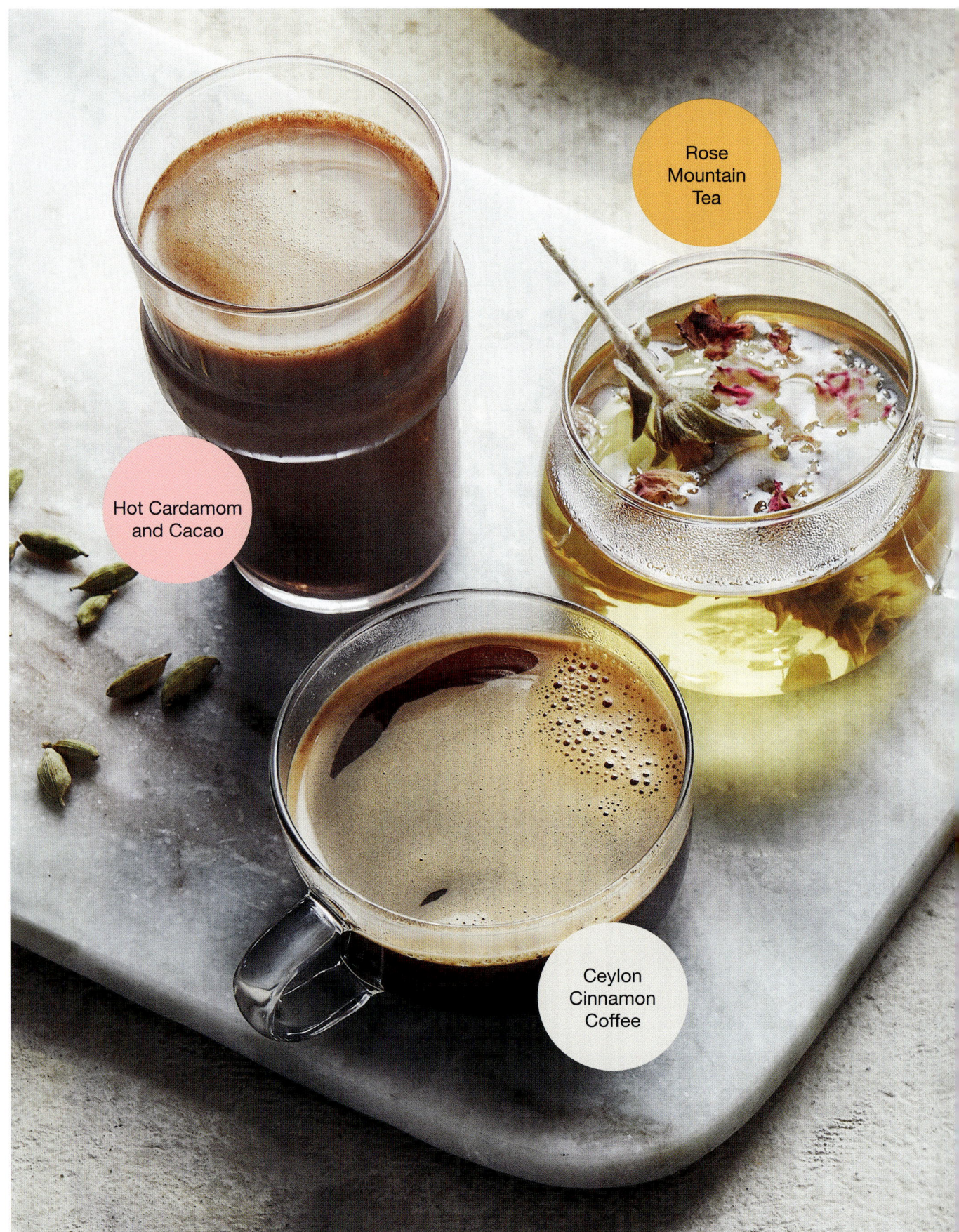

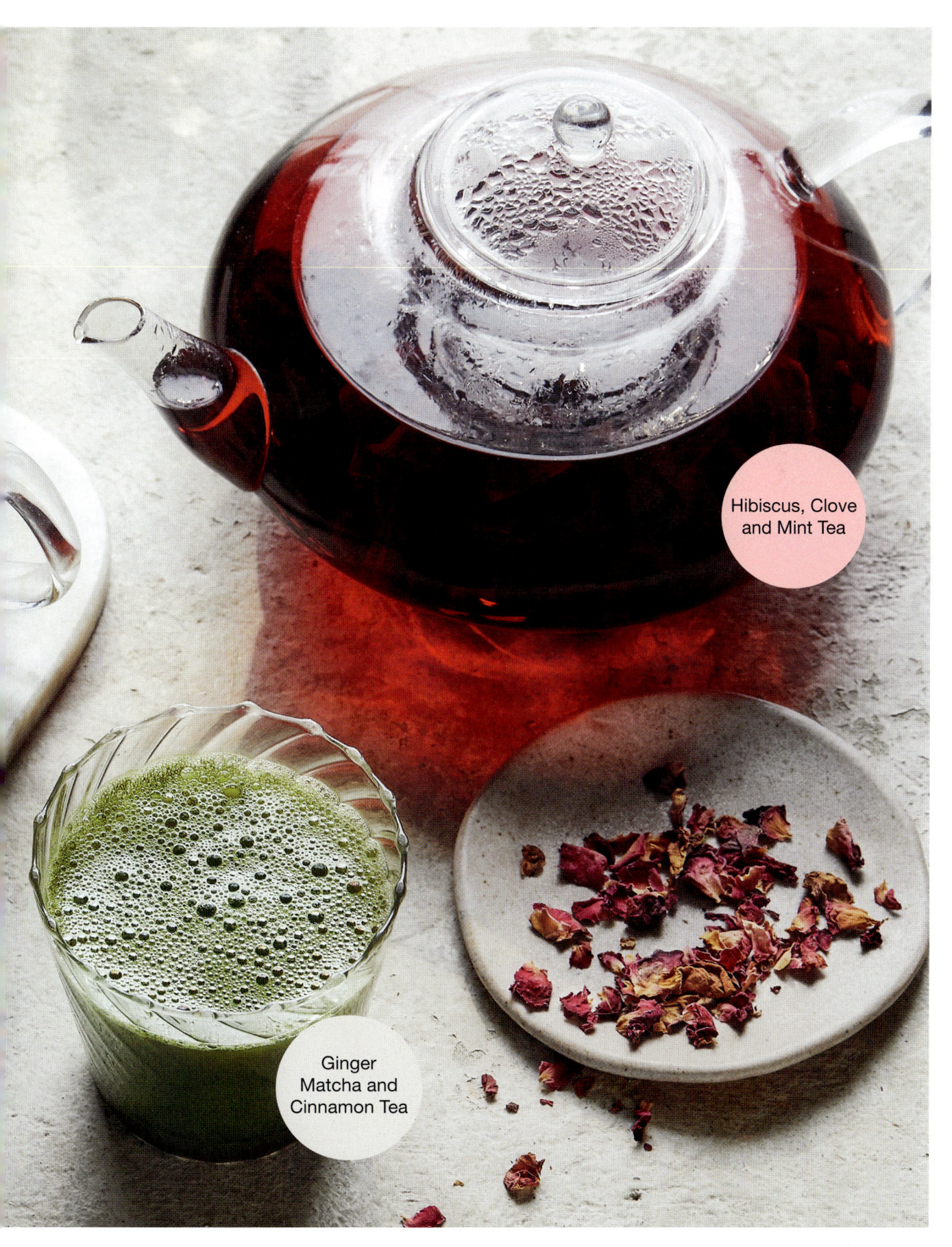

DRINKS TO LOWER INFLAMMATION

What we drink can have a significant effect on our inflammation levels. Alcohol, sugar-sweetened beverages and those with multiple additives are pro-inflammatory. But there are many delicious drinks to enjoy that are anti-inflammatory and help maintain balance. All are for 1 serving.

Hibiscus, Clove and Mint Tea

Also known as roselle or sour tea, hibiscus has been used for millennia as both a delicious beverage and an ancient medicinal therapy. It's packed with polyphenols and antioxidants that deliver a characteristic sharp, tangy taste.

Anthocyanins imbue it with a deep red colour and tannins, similar to those found in red wine, create a dry, slightly sour flavour. Reported benefits in the literature include reducing inflammation and lowering cholesterol with just 2–3 cups a day.

1–2 tsp dried hibiscus leaves
1–2 cloves
½ tsp raw or local honey (optional)
2–3 sprigs of mint

Steep the dried hibiscus leaves with the cloves in a cup of hot water (ideally you want it at 80°C or less, you can use water off the boil for around 10 minutes) for around 4 minutes. Remove the hibiscus leaves, but leave the cloves if you wish. Add ½ tsp of honey for sweetness, if you like, and some mint sprigs.

Ginger, Matcha and Cinnamon Tea

Super-concentrated in antioxidants and polyphenols like catechins, particularly epigallocatechin-3-gallate (EGCG), green tea has strong anti-inflammatory properties that have been shown in multiple studies to benefit heart and brain health.

Matcha is essentially the green tea leaves dried, pounded and blended into a fine powder that's easy to combine with water. If you enjoy the stronger taste, you'll get significantly more antioxidants than from loose green tea leaves, which have a lighter grassy flavour. Matcha has been found to reduce levels of inflammatory proteins such as TNF-a and IL-6, and it could even prevent non-alcoholic fatty liver disease (NAFLD) by reducing fat and inflammation in the liver. Look for ceremonial grade when purchasing.

Matcha is ideally brewed at around 70–80°C and requires whisking to combine with the water. Purists will probably shudder at this recipe, but the combination of sweet cinnamon and ginger mellows the bitter flavour in matcha and for first timers it could help you get used to the herbaceous taste.

1 tsp matcha powder
½ tsp ground ginger
½ tsp ground cinnamon
150ml hot water (off the boil, ideally around 80°C)
½ tsp raw honey (optional)

Combine the matcha, ginger and cinnamon in a large cup or bowl with half the water.

Whisk well and then add the remaining water with the honey if you want it sweeter.

Hot Cardamom and Cacao

Bitter, flavanol rich and delicious. Enjoying this drink every day could improve your heart and even make you smarter! But for some people the raw chocolate can be too bitter.

Like green tea, cacao powder also contains epicatechin, catechin and procyanidins, as well as alkaloids like theobromine which have significant anti-inflammatory properties. Its ability to modulate the production of inflammatory proteins and reduce inflammation has been shown in human and animal studies. In addition, because of the prebiotic fibres, cacao has been shown to help gut microbes become more 'tolerant' of inflammation.

I have a cacao drink in the afternoons as it's very low in caffeine and contains chemicals that boost blood flow to the brain. This recipe combines cardamom and cinnamon for a sweet antidote to the bitter compounds in the chocolate.

1 tbsp raw cacao powder
250ml hot water (off the boil, ideally around 80°C)
¼ tsp ground cardamom
½ tsp ground cinnamon
2 tsp collagen (optional)
1 tsp raw honey (optional)

Mix all the ingredients together in a large mug or small jug. Using a whisk or an electric frother is ideal as there's quite a lot of powder to combine into the liquid. You can also use a hot milk of your choice for a creamier, thicker drink.

Rose Mountain Tea

Also known as shepherd's tea, Olympus tea and Greek mountain tea, you can find mountain tea in speciality stores or online.

It's caffeine free and appears to be rich in phenolic acids, principally ferulic acid and chlorogenic acid and the flavone compound apigenin. These may contribute to its ability to lower levels of pro-inflammatory proteins like TNF-a and IL-6.

It has a flavour that resembles camomile, and I love combining the mountain tea, which looks like a sprig of dried wheat stem, with rose for hint of sweetness. Brew the water to 80°C to prevent burning the tea.

1 dried sprig of mountain tea
4–5 dried rose petals
200ml hot water (off the boil, ideally around 80°C)
Raw honey (optional)

Steep the mountain tea and rose petals in the hot water for 3–4 minutes, then remove the mountain tea sprig and rose petals and enjoy. Add some raw honey if you want a bit of sweetness.

Ceylon Cinnamon Coffee

Coffee contains over 100 compounds, including magnesium, vitamin B3, chlorogenic acid, cafestol and kahweol. A large number of studies have found that people who drink 2–3 cups of coffee a day have a lower risk of several cancers, neurological conditions like Parkinson's and Alzheimer's disease, and metabolic conditions including type 2 diabetes. These findings can be explained by the strong anti-inflammatory actions of these compounds.

I'm a purist and I enjoy a simple espresso or 'long black', a double espresso mixed with 100–150ml hot water. But there are some interesting ways in which to use other spices in coffee that would further enhance its benefits. My friends at Exhale Coffee, who source high-polyphenol coffee beans grown at altitude and medium roast them to preserve the health benefits and flavour, taught me this Moroccan recipe for cardamom coffee. Freshly grinding the spices releases a powerful flavour to match the intensity of the black coffee.

18g freshly ground coffee
250ml boiling water
Seeds from 1 cardamom pod, finely crushed
½ tsp freshly ground Ceylon cinnamon
1 tsp coconut sugar (optional)

Brew the coffee with the water and spices in a cafetière for 3–4 minutes. Pour and enjoy!

RESOURCES

My favourite store cupboard ingredients to keep in stock

These are the products that are worth investing in and you'll see featured throughout the recipes in this book.

FLAVOUR BOOSTERS:

Aged balsamic vinegar (not glaze, beware of sugars)
Aleppo pepper
Gochugaru (Korean) flakes
Smoked paprika – a real deep smoky flavour
Sweet paprika – very different flavour to smoked
Chilli oil – most use refined sunflower oil, I prefer cold-pressed rapeseed or olive oil where possible
Harissa – no sugar, using only olive oil
Sundried tomatoes – rich in antioxidants, I use the dried and oil based varieties to add umami and sweetness; look for ones stored in olive oil
Gochujang – try and source one with just one type of sugar, rather than multiple syrups and additives
Indian mild curry paste – no sugar or additives
Nutritional yeast – simple to get, very versatile to add saltiness and umami into your sauces and stews
White miso paste – a sweeter variety than the darker miso pastes; mix it into stews and dips
Thai green curry paste – no sugar or additives

PANTRY PROTEIN:

Canned anchovies, sardines – these make great toppers, source sustainably fished varieties
Cheese and yoghurt – yoghurt should have no more than three ingredients (milk, cultures and cream) and definitely not sugar (full-fat Greek is my favourite)
Dried mushrooms – when rehydrated and added to stock, rice or casseroles, they add a wealth of flavour
Lentil/chickpea/pea/brown rice/bean pastas – very easy to source and high in fibre and protein; you can easily get them online and in supermarket gluten free sections
Tahini – try and get it in glass jars and shake well before using so you don't get any clumps
Tofu – flavoured, smoked, firm, silken (see page 202)
Yuba/tofu knots – they are exceptionally high in protein and can be found online and in Asian speciality stores
Nut butter – peanut and almond
Pre-cooked Puy/beluga lentils – they keep in the cupboards for whenever you need a high-fibre protein boost
Shelled hemp seeds – I also have these to boost the protein of my salads and snacks
Dried, roasted fava beans/chickpeas/edamame – these usually come in little packs and are salted; great snack options and high in fibre too

ANTI-INFLAMMATORY PANTRY:

Extra virgin olive oil – on the bottle, look for a harvest date of less than 12 months, and more than 250mg polyphenols per kg
Cloves, Star Anise, Cinnamon sticks – add to hot water and throw into your curries
Cacao – look for single-origin, high-polyphenol varieties
Frozen berries – I always have a mix of these in the freezer for smoothies and snacks; blackcurrants and cranberry are highest in polyphenols
Frozen greens – spinach, peas and any leftover bagged salad I never got round to eating
Tomato purée / passata – these are concentrated anti-inflammatory compounds from tomatoes

Nutritional analysis of recipes

All values are given per portion unless otherwise specified.

BREAKFAST & BRUNCH

The Doctor's Daily Bread
Per 100g: Calories 296kcal, Protein 8.6g, Fat 18.4g, Carbs 20g, Fibre 8.3g, Sugars 4.2g

Overnight Protein Porridge with Cinnamon, Turmeric and Cacao
Calories 877kcal, Protein 36g, Fat 59.7g, Carbs 42.4g, Fibre 13.1g, Sugars 21.5g

Avocado Lentil Cakes with Smoked Salmon and Kimchi
Calories 524kcal, Protein 26.9g, Fat 35.8g, Carbs 19.5g, Fibre 8.1g, Sugars 2.9g

Crispy Chickpeas on Green Toast
Calories 683kcal, Protein 35.2g, Fat 30.1g, Carbs 58.4g, Fibre 19.1g, Sugars 5.1g

Feta, Red Pepper and Pomegranate
Calories 738kcal, Protein 24g, Fat 56.8g, Carbs 28.4g, Fibre 8.7g, Sugars 13.7g

Miso Beans on Toasted Rye
Calories 418kcal, Protein 20.8g, Fat 17.2g, Carbs 37.4g, Fibre 15.2g, Sugars 4.4

Pepper and Turmeric Tofu with Sauerkraut and Rye
Calories 381 kcal, Protein 18.4g, Fat 19g, Carbs 29.7g, Fibre 8.7g, Sugars 6.7g

Green Pesto Beans with Eggs and Hazelnuts
Calories 595kcal, Protein 29.1g, Fat 40.2g, Carbs 22.2g, Fibre 13.9g, Sugars 2.2g

Lentils, Eggs and Kimchi
Calories 500kcal, Protein 28.4g, Fat 28.4g, Carbs 28.6g, Fibre 8.2g, Sugars 4.3g

Smashed Chickpeas
Calories 254kcal, Protein 11.8g, Fat 11.9g, Carbs 20.4g, Fibre 8.7g, Sugars 1.7g

Paprika Pea Topper
Calories 298kcal, Protein 17.2g, Fat 9.6g, Carbs 27.7g, Fibre 15.8g, Sugars 3.5g

Eggs and Kraut
Calories 563kcal, Protein 22.6g, Fat 45.9g, Carbs 10.2g, Fibre 9.1g, Sugars 2.8g

One-pan Greens and Goats' Cheese with Pickled Red Onions
Calories 682kcal, Protein 36.9g, Fat 33.8g, Carbs 45.8g, Fibre 23.1g, Sugars 10.1g

High-protein Edamame and Pea Spread on Rye Toast
Calories 577kcal, Protein 33g, Fat 32.3g, Carbs 29.3g, Fibre 18.5g, Sugars 5.7g

Whipped Feta with Dill, Grapes, Chickpeas and Smoked Mackerel
Calories 689kcal, Protein 39.4g, Fat 43.9g, Carbs 29.4g, Fibre 9.4g, Sugars 10.6g

Overnight Pear and Pearl Barley Porridge with Star Anise
Calories 665kcal, Protein 24.1g, Fat 33g, Carbs 62.9g, Fibre 10.2g, Sugars 19.5g

Greens and Basil Tofu Scramble
Calories 441 kcal, Protein 23.4g, Fat 23.1g, Carbs 30.2g, Fibre 9.7g, Sugars 4.8g

Hot-smoked Salmon and Greens
Calories 456kcal, Protein 27g, Fat 23.8g, Carbs 19.5g, Fibre 8.1g, Sugars 5g

ONE-PAN DINNERS

3 Ways with Dairy: Go Sweet and Savoury 1 (cottage cheese)
Calories 252 kcal, 20.1 g fat, 8.1 g carbs, 7.9 g sugars, 1.2 g fibre, 9 g protein

3 Ways with Dairy: Go Sweet and Savoury 2 (Greek yoghurt)
Calories 510 kcal, 41.2 g fat, 18 g carbs, 14.5 g sugars, 5.2 grams fibre, 14.1 g protein

3 Ways with Dairy: Seed Crackers and Cheese
Calories 265 kcal, 21.6 g fat, 7 g carbs, 2.5 g sugars, 3 g fibre, 9.2 grams protein

3 Ways with Dairy: Berry and Dairy
Calories 226 kcal, 17.6 g fat, 5.7 g carbs, 4.1 g sugars, 3.6 g fibre, 9.5 g protein

Thai Green Curry Lentil and Hake Traybake
Calories 534kcal, Protein 49.6g, Fat 19.8g, Carbs 32.5g, Fibre 13.9g, Sugars 9.4g

Monkfish with Capers, Olives and Tomatoes
Calories 410kcal, Protein 35.8g, Fat 13.8g, Carbs 27.5g, Fibre 16.2g, Sugars 6.5g

Coconut Prawn Stew with Thai Green Paste
Calories 419kcal, Protein 27.3g, Fat 24.3g, Carbs 18.6g, Fibre 8.1g, Sugars 10.6g

Quick Kale Curry with Lentils
Calories 910 kcal, Protein 41.5g, Fat 49.7g, Carbs 67.2g, Fibre 14g, Sugars 6.8g

Smoky Masala Red Beans
Calories 358 kcal, Protein 21.2g, Fat 10.9g, Carbs 38.7g, Fibre 10g, Sugars 8.9g

Monkfish with Harissa Chickpeas and Spinach
Calories 321kcal, Protein 37.3g, Fat 5.8g, Carbs 23.9g, Fibre 12g, Sugars 4.1g

Haricot Bean and Feta Fish Stew
Calories 510kcal, Protein 33.6g, Fat 26.8g, Carbs 26.8g, Fibre 13.8g, Sugars 6.6g

Red Bean Stew with Chocolate and Spices
Calories 540 kcal, Protein 28.8g, Fat 19.7g, Carbs 54.2g, Fibre 15.7g, Sugars 13.6g

Harissa, Honey and Lentils with Monkfish
Calories 453kcal, Protein 41.7g, Fat 13.9g, Carbs 34.2g, Fibre 12.1g, Sugars 9.9g

Paprika, Peanut and Okra Stew with Cinnamon
Calories 754 kcal, Protein 40.5g, Fat 36.9g, Carbs 54.3g, Fibre 21.6g, Sugars 15.6g

Sundried Tomato and Red Pepper Beans with Hake
Calories 754kcal, Protein 50.2g, Fat 36.7g, Carbs 44.3g, Fibre 23g, Sugars 8.6g

Sticky Sweet Chilli Salmon with Roasted Cauliflower
Calories 445kcal, Protein 38.2g, Fat 19.5g, Carbs 25g, Fibre 8.3g, Sugars 12.7g

Lazy Coconut Fish Curry
Calories 750kcal, Protein 51.2g, Fat 43.3g, Carbs 32.7g, Fibre 12g, Sugars 5.9g

Rich and Silky Beans with Nachos
Calories 1066kcal, Protein 36.9g, Fat 47.7g, Carbs 109.2g, Fibre 26.4g, Sugars 21.3g

Spicy Gochujang Bake with Cod and Toasted Peanuts
Calories 622kcal, Protein 47.3g, Fat 22.6g, Carbs 51.2g, Fibre 12.5g, Sugars 18.4g

Sweet Spring Harissa Beans with Pecorino
Calories 468kcal, Protein 24.5g, Fat 21.1g, Carbs 36.4g, Fibre 17.3g, Sugars 14.3g

Smoky Paprika Lentils with Hake and Dill
Calories 429kcal, Protein 34.7g, Fat 16.3g, Carbs 31.1g, Fibre 10g, Sugars 5.1g

HIGH-PROTEIN DIVERSITY BOWLS

Salmon Tikka Bowls with a Quick Fennel and Cabbage Pickle
Calories 622kcal, Protein 46.9g, Fat 31.7g, Carbs 33.6g, Fibre 7.4g, Sugars 9.7g

Air-fried Cajun Chicken with Fennel Slaw and Watermelon
Calories 414kcal, Protein 26.3g, Fat 19.8g, Carbs 29g, Fibre 7.4g, Sugars 9.8g

Chipotle and Honey Air-fried Tofu Bowls with Black Beans and Pineapple
Calories 711 kcal, Protein 33.1g, Fat 32.3g, Carbs 66.1g, Fibre 11.5g, Sugars 19.5g

5 Spice Mince Bowls with Kimchi Mayo
Calories 1039 kcal, Protein 37.1g, Fat 75.6g, Carbs 46.3g, Fibre 12.7g, Sugars 7.1g

Pinto Bean Bowl with Spicy Prawns, Sweet Potato and Corn
Calories 642kcal, Protein 38.9g, Fat 26.8g, Carbs 58.2g, Fibre 6.5g, Sugars 7.9g

Spicy Gochujang Bowls with Green Apple Slaw and Brown Rice
Calories 707kcal, Protein 41.5g, Fat 36.2g, Carbs 47.7g, Fibre 12.1g, Sugars 16g

Paccheri with Red Mullet and Pistachio
Calories 759kcal, Protein 47.3g, Fat 33.2g, Carbs 63g, Fibre 9.8g, Sugars 7.7g

Plant-powered Lasagne with Mushroom and Tofu
Calories 771 kcal, Protein 43.7g, Fat 36.1g, Carbs 61.4g, Fibre 12.9g, Sugars 11.5g

Rupy's High-protein Rigatoni
Calories 1194kcal, Protein 56.7g, Fat 58.3g, Carbs 90.3g, Fibre 22.1g, Sugars 12.6g

Tomato, Caper and Fish Stew with Orecchiette
Calories 514kcal, Protein 38.6g,

Fat 8.7g, Carbs 64.8g, Fibre 11g, Sugars 10.7g

FRESH & LIGHT PLATES

Thai-style Pomelo Salad with Crispy Tofu
Calories 711 kcal, Protein 34g, Fat 39.9g, Carbs 50.8g, Fibre 6.4g Sugars 21.1g

Silken Soup with Crispy Masala Chickpeas and Soft Herbs
Calories 554kcal, Protein 30.2g, Fat 34.3g, Carbs 25.3g, Fibre 11.1g, Sugars 2.5g

Heritage Tomatoes, Strawberries and Feta
Calories 351kcal, Protein 9.1g, Fat 29.9g, Carbs 9.1 g, Fibre 4.5g, Sugars 8.3g

Salmon, Squash and Grilled Peach Salad with Tahini Herb Dressing
Calories 778kcal, Protein 26.6g, Fat 56.6g, Carbs 19.8g, Fibre 5.2g, Sugars 12.6g

Crispy Bean and Kraut Salad with Pumpkin Seeds
Calories 455kcal, Protein 18.9g, Fat 29.7g, Carbs 21.1g, Fibre 13.8g, Sugars 3.7g

Orange and Olive Freekeh with Grilled Trout
Calories 575kcal, Protein 42.5g, Fat 23.6g, Carbs 43.3g, Fibre 9.9g, Sugars 13.8g

Smoked Tofu, Avocado and Chicory Salad with Mustard Tahini Dressing
Calories 527 kcal, Protein 24.9g, Fat 40.2g, Carbs 12.3g, Fibre 8g, Sugars 2.1g

MEATLESS MIDWEEK

Miso Mushroom Soba Broth with Crispy Chilli Tofu
Calories 1068 kcal, Protein 49.8g, Fat 49.2g, Carbs 101.1g, Fibre 10.8g, Sugars 5.9g

Spicy Thyme Lentil Coconut Curry
Calories 588kcal, Protein 35.5g, Fat 32.4g, Carbs 31.4g, Fibre 14.6g, Sugars 5.2g

Sweet Chilli Cashew and Celery Stir-fry
Calories 548kcal, Protein 29g, Fat 27.9g, Carbs 39.8g, Fibre 10.7g, Sugars 15.5g

Lazy Ginger and Peanut Thai Curry
Calories 787kcal, Protein 50.3g, Fat 28.4g, Carbs 71g, Fibre 22.9g, Sugars 9.7g

Braised Shiitake and Broccoli with Crispy Chilli Yuba
Calories 558kcal, Protein 38.2g, Fat 27.6g, Carbs 36.6g, Fibre 5.3g, Sugars 8.9g

Almond and Cauliflower Curry with Crispy Tofu
Calories 1025 kcal, Protein 35g, Fat 74g, Carbs 47.9, Fibre 13.8g, Sugars 13.5g

Butter Bean and Miso Soup with Crispy Tempeh
Calories 555kcal, Protein 37.6g, Fat 29g, Carbs 25.7g, Fibre 20.4g, Sugars 3.5g

Harissa-toasted Quinoa Salad with Labneh
Calories 453kcal, Protein 16.6g, Fat 28g, Carbs 31g, Fibre 5g, Sugars 7.4g

Green Cashew Tofu Curry
Calories 1260 kcal, Protein 41.3g, Fat 90.5g, Carbs 65.6g, Fibre 9.1g, Sugars 11.3 g

Stir-fried Celery with Sweet and Spicy Yuba
Calories 584kcal, Protein 38.5g, Fat 34.7g, Carbs 27.6g, Fibre 3.7g, Sugars 12.3g

Herby Mushroom and Bean Gratin
Calories 754kcal, Protein 37.6g, Fat 43.8g, Carbs 44.3g, Fibre 16.1g, Sugars 8.7g

Spicy 'Meaty' Tacos with Avo Lime-soured Cream
Calories 835kcal, Protein 41.1g, Fat 51.6g, Carbs 40.9g, Fibre 21.2g, Sugars 16 g

Plant Protein Stir-fry with Greens
Calories 689kcal, Protein 69.6g, Fat 27.1g, Carbs 64.5g, Fibre 14.2g, Sugars 11.1g

Sumac and Legume Stew with Dried Mint and Garlic
Calories 437kcal, Protein 21.4g, Fat 17.9g, Carbs 39.2g, Fibre 16.6g, Sugars 6.6g

Za'atar and Tahini Beans with Crispy Tofu
Calories 689 kcal, Protein 32.5g, Fat 37.2g, Carbs 47.1g, Fibre 18g, Sugars 11.4g

MIDWEEK MEAT & FISH

Cinnamon and Cumin Curry with Crispy Chicken
Calories 593kcal, Protein 45.6g, Fat 26.3g, Carbs 36.8g, Fibre 13.3g, Sugars 8.5g

Grilled Chicken Thighs with Miso White Beans, Radicchio and Hazelnuts
Calories 653kcal, Protein 43.4g, Fat 37.7g, Carbs 26.1g, Fibre 17.9g, Sugars 4.4g

Sage and Garlic Chicken Broth
Calories 563kcal, Protein 48.2g, Fat 25g, Carbs 31.9g, Fibre 8.7g, Sugars 3.2g

Tahini and Gochujang Noodle Broth with Turkey
Calories 739kcal, Protein 43.7g, Fat 36.5g, Carbs 54.4g, Fibre 9.1g, Sugars 10.3g

Takeaway-style Chicken
Calories 649kcal, Protein 44.3g, Fat 30.6g, Carbs 45.4g, Fibre 7.5g, Sugars 11g

Cinnamon and Lentil Chicken Soup
Calories 538kcal, Protein 31.5g, Fat 23.7g, Carbs 43.6g, Fibre 11.6g, Sugars 7.2g

Fermented Garlic Honey with Smoky Ancho Chilli, Star Anise and Cinnamon
Per 15g: Calories 42kcal, Protein 1.1g, Fat 0g, Carbs 66.4g, Sugars 65.4g, Fibre 0.9g

Apple, Ginger and Anise Sauerkraut
Per 100g: Calories 35kcal, Protein 1.1g, Fat 0.2g, Carbs 5.9g, Fibre 2.6g, Sugars 5.6g

Smoky Beets
Per 100g: Calories 31kcal, Protein 1.3g, Fat 0.3g, Carbs 4.2g, Fibre 2.9g, Sugars 3.7g

Tarragon and Thyme Beans with Spicy Sea Bass
Calories 540kcal, Protein 36.5g, Fat 29.4g, Carbs 25g, Fibre 14.9g, Sugars 3.8g

Coconut, Prawn and Pineapple Curry
Calories 435kcal, Protein 25g, Fat 22.7g, Carbs 29.5g, Fibre 6.2g, Sugars 18.3g

Spinach and Masala Cod with Spicy Fennel Oil
Calories 509kcal, Protein 39.9g, Fat 25.8g, Carbs 23.2g, Fibre 12.3g, Sugars 2.8g

Grilled Mackerel with Roasted Vegetables and Chilli-pea Pesto
Calories 1096kcal, Protein 40.9g, Fat 80.9g, Carbs 38.5g, Fibre 13.7g, Sugars 12.4g

Easy Tomato Curry with Prawns and Peas
Calories 415kcal, Protein 32.6g, Fat 14.4g, Carbs 31.4g, Fibre 15g, Sugars 8.7g

Asparagus and Wild Garlic Green Orzo with Salmon
Calories 806kcal, Protein 58.4g, Fat 32.2g, Carbs 62.8g, Fibre 15.8g, Sugars 4.5g

Masala Sea Bass Nuggets with Spiced Vegetables
Calories 736kcal, Protein 42.6g, Fat 51.1g, Carbs 21.1g, Fibre 10.5g, Sugars 10g

Sri Lankan-style Coconut Lentils with Grilled Sardines
Calories 674kcal, Protein 45.2g, Fat 38.4g, Carbs 33.1g, Fibre 7.7g, Sugars 5g

Radish, Caraway and Chard with Baked Salmon
Calories 651kcal, Protein 50.2g, Fat 37.8g, Carbs 21.6g, Fibre 11.7g, Sugars 5.1g

Ginger, Miso and Tamarind Prawns with Beluga Lentils
Calories 499kcal, Protein 38.4g, Fat 18.4g, Carbs 39.9g, Fibre 10.3g, Sugars 15g

SNACKS, TOPPERS & DRINKS

Fennel and Oregano Chia and Pumpkin Seed Crackers
Per 20g: Calories 109kcal, Protein 4.6g, Fat 8.3g, Carbs 2.8g, Fibre 2.3g, Sugars 0.2g

Edamame and Pea Dip with Chilli Oil
Per 100g: Calories 295kcal, Protein 13.2g, Fat 22.9g, Carbs 5.5g, Fibre 7.1g, Sugars 1.7g

Frozen Yoghurt, Peanut and Berry Bark
Per 100g: Calories 244kcal, Protein 6.8g, Fat 17.5g, Carbs 13g, Fibre 3.3g, Sugars 11.4g

Curried Hemp Seeds
Per 1 tbsp (15g): Calories 88kcal, Protein 4.6g, Fat 7g, Carbs 1.3g, Fibre 0.7g, Sugars 0.2g

Crispy Chilli Edamame
Calories 278kcal, Protein 16.3g, Fat 18.8g, Carbs 7.1g, Fibre 7.8g, Sugars 3.3g

Protein content by food

FOOD GROUP	FOOD	PROTEIN PER 100G	SOURCE
Cheeses	Cottage cheese	9.4	CoFID
Cheeses	Feta	15.6	CoFID
Cheeses	Queso blanco	20.4	USDA
Cheeses	Halloumi	23.9	CoFID
Cheeses	Cheddar	25.4	CoFID
Cheeses	Paneer	26	CoFID
Cheeses	Parmesan	36.2	CoFID
Meat	Mince (cooked)	24.7	CoFID
Meat	Sirloin (cooked)	26.6	CoFID
Meat	Chicken breast (cooked)	28.4	CoFID
Meat	Fillet steak (cooked)	29.1	CoFID
Nut butter	Almond butter	21	USDA
Nut butter	Peanut butter	22.8	CoFID
Nuts	Macadamia	7.9	CoFID
Nuts	Pecans	9.2	CoFID
Nuts	Hazelnuts	14.1	CoFID
Nuts	Brazil nuts	14.3	CoFID
Nuts	Walnut	14.7	CoFID
Nuts	Cashews	17.7	CoFID
Nuts	Pistachio	17.9	CoFID
Nuts	Peanut	25.8	CoFID
Nuts	Almonds	21.2	CoFID
Plant products	Tofu (steamed)	8.1	CoFID
Plant products	Tahini	18.5	CoFID, USDA
Plant products	Tempeh	20.7	CoFID
Plant products	Yuba (Tofu knots)	44.6	Branded - Tofu Tasty
Plant products	Nutritional yeast	47	Branded Engevita
Plant products	Dehydrated soya chunks/mince	52	Ocado (various brands)
Plant products	Maca powder	10-11	Ocado (various brands)
Plant products	Miso paste	10-12	Ocado (various brands)
Plant products	Bean/lentil pastas	14-16	Ocado (various brands)
Plant products	Cacao powder	23-27	Ocado (various brands)
Pulses (cooked)	Beluga lentils	6	CoFID
Pulses (cooked)	Black beans	6.03	USDA
Pulses (cooked)	White beans (canned)	7.1	CoFID
Pulses (cooked)	Chickpeas	7.7	CoFID
Pulses (cooked)	Green lentils	7.8	CoFID
Pulses (cooked)	Butter beans	8.1	CoFID
Pulses (cooked)	Red Lentils	8.1	CoFID
Pulses (cooked)	Split pea	8.3	CoFID
Pulses (cooked)	Chickpeas (canned)	8.4	CoFID
Pulses (cooked)	Kidney beans	8.6	CoFID
Pulses (cooked)	Black-eyed peas	8.8	CoFID
Pulses (cooked)	Sprouted lentils	8.8	Branded
Pulses (cooked)	Pinto beans	8.9	CoFID
Pulses (cooked)	Puy lentils	11	Branded - Merchant Gourmet
Pulses (cooked)	Edamame	12.2	CoFID
Pulses (cooked)	Soya beans	14	CoFID
Seafood (cooked)	Haddock	21.8	CoFID
Seafood (cooked)	Cod	22.8	CoFID
Seafood (cooked)	Salmon	25.2	CoFID
Seafood (cooked)	Pollock	27.4	CoFID, USDA
Seeds	Chia seeds	16.5	USDA
Seeds	Sesame seeds	18.2	CoFID
Seeds	Flaxseeds	18.3	USDA
Seeds	Sunflower seeds	19.8	CoFID
Seeds	Pumpkin seeds	24.4	CoFID
Seeds	Hemp seeds	31.6	CoFID
Soya products	Silken tofu	4.8–6.9	USDA
Vegetables (cooked)	Watercress	1	USDA
Vegetables (cooked)	Mushrooms	1.4	CoFID
Vegetables (cooked)	Potatoes	1.5	CoFID
Vegetables (cooked)	Kale	2.7	CoFID
Vegetables (cooked)	Brussels sprouts	3.1	CoFID
Vegetables (cooked)	Spinach	3.2	CoFID
Vegetables (cooked)	Corn	3.6	CoFID
Vegetables (cooked)	Broccoli	4.1	CoFID
Whole grains (cooked)	Barley	2.7	CoFID
Whole grains (cooked)	Brown rice	3.6	CoFID
Whole grains (cooked)	Teff	3.87	USDA
Whole grains (cooked)	Quinoa	4.4	USDA
Whole grains (cooked)	Oats	4.6	CoFID

Prebiotic content by food

Fruit	FOOD	TOTAL PREBIOTICS G/100G	FOS G/100G	INULIN G/100G	TOTAL FRUCTANS G/100G
Vegetable	Dandelion greens	24.3		13.5	
Vegetable	Artichoke (Jerusalem)	21	0.84	18	12.2
Vegetable	Garlic	19.3	1.2	12.5	17.4
Vegetable	Leek	12.8	1.07	6.5	3
Pulses	Lentils	12	0.333		0.15
Vegetable	Onion	10.6	2.01		4.3
Pulses	Chickpeas	8.9	0.07		0.16
Pulses	Red kidney beans	8	0.51		0.54
Pulses	White beans	8			
Pulses	Black-eyed peas	5			
Vegetable	Asparagus	5	0.43	2.5	
Pulses	Butter beans		0.22		0.14
Fruit	Apples		0.07		
Fruit	Banana		0.5	0.5	
Fruit	Blueberry		0.5		
Fruit	Cherry		0.32		
Fruit	Grapefruit				0.23
Fruit	Nectarine		0.89		0.21
Fruit	Peach, white				0.4
Fruit	Pear		0.56		0.33
Fruit	Raspberries		0.51		
Grains	Barley		0.2	0.2	
Grains	Oat		0.92		0.32
Grains	Rye		0.6	0.7	1.05
Grains	Wheat grain		2.21	2.5	
Nuts & seeds	Almonds				
Nuts & seeds	Chia seeds				
Nuts & Seeds	Flaxseeds				
Vegetable	Artichoke (globe)		0.4	4.4	1.2
Vegetable	Beetroot		0.36		0.4
Vegetable	Broccoli		0.78		
Vegetable	Brussel sprouts		0.82		0.27
Vegetable	Cabbage		0.82		
Vegetable	Chicory root		0.39	42	
Vegetable	Courgette				0.29
Vegetable	Fennel bulb		0.61		
Vegetable	Kale		0.51		
Vegetable	Lettuce, red		0.37		
Vegetable	Mushrooms		0.28		
Vegetable	Parsnip		0.39		
Vegetable	Potato				
Vegetable	Seaweed				
Vegetable	Spring onions		3.32		
Vegetable	Spinach, baby				0.14

"Sources
Boyd et al. 2023
Siva et al. Frontiers in nutrition. 2019
Jovanovic-Malinovska et al. *International journal of food properties*. 2014
Lockyer et al. Nutrition Bulletin. 2019 "

Polyphenol

FOOD GROUP	FOOD/DRINK	TOTAL POLYPHENOLS MG/100G	SOURCE
Spices & herbs	Cloves	16047.5	Phenol-explorer
Spices & herbs	Ceylan cinnamon	9700	Phenol-explorer
Pulses (raw)	Adzuki bean	8970	Mastura et al. International Food Research Journal. 2018
Cacao products	Cocoa, powder	5624.23	Phenol-explorer
Pulses (raw)	Lentils	3697.3	Phenol-explorer
Spices & herbs	Capers	3600	Phenol-explorer
Spices & herbs	Oregano, dried (wild marjoram)	3117	Phenol-explorer
Spices & herbs	Sage, dried	2919.67	Phenol-explorer
Nuts & Seeds	Chestnut	2756.67	Phenol-explorer
Spices & herbs	Rosemary, dried	2518.67	Phenol-explorer
Fruits	Black Elderberry	1950	Phenol-explorer
Cacao products	Dark chocolate	1859.88	Phenol-explorer
Spices & herbs	Common thyme, dried	1815	Phenol-explorer
Spices & herbs	Star anise	1810	Phenol-explorer
Nuts & Seeds	Walnuts	1574.82	Phenol-explorer
Nuts & Seeds	Flaxseed meal	1528	Pérez-Jiménez et al. Eur J Clin Nutr. 2013
Nuts & Seeds	Pistachio	1420	Phenol-explorer
Nuts & Seeds	Sunflower seeds	1400	Zujko et al. International Journal of Food Properties. 2011
Pulses (raw)	Black bean	1390.75	Phenol-explorer
Vegetables	Red swiss chard leaves	1320	Phenol-explorer
Nuts & Seeds	Pecan	1284	Phenol-explorer
Fruits	Prune	1195	Phenol-explorer
Vegetables	Globe artichoke, heads	1142.4	Phenol-explorer
Fruits	Black raspberry	980	Phenol-explorer
Fruits	Fig, dried	960	Phenol-explorer
Vegetables	White swiss chard leaves	830	Phenol-explorer
Fruits	Blackcurrant	820.64	Phenol-explorer
Cereals	Buckwheat, whole grain flour	791.39	Phenol-explorer
Nuts & Seeds	Hazelnut	671.8	Phenol-explorer
Fruits	Lingonberry	652	Phenol-explorer
Fruits	Blackberry	569.43	Phenol-explorer
Fruits	Bilberry	525	Phenol-explorer
Fruits	Lowbush blueberry	471.55	Phenol-explorer
Vegetables	Red cabbage	451.03	Phenol-explorer
Fruits	Plum	409.79	Phenol-explorer
Nuts & Seeds	Peanut	406.29	Phenol-explorer
Fruits	Strawberry	289.2	Phenol-explorer
Nuts & Seeds	Almond	287.09	Phenol-explorer
Fruits	Peach	279.08	Phenol-explorer
Fruits	Orange	278.59	Phenol-explorer
Beverages	Coffee, filter	266.7	Phenol-explorer

FOOD GROUP	FOOD/DRINK	TOTAL POLYPHENOLS MG/100G	SOURCE
Vegetables	Spinach	248.14	Phenol-explorer
Nuts & Seeds	Brazil nut	244	Phenol-explorer
Nuts & Seeds	Cashew nut	232.9	Phenol-explorer
Vegetables	Red pepper (sweet)	229.04	Phenol-explorer
Fruits	Highbush blueberry	223.4	Phenol-explorer
Vegetables	Brussel sprouts	220.75	Phenol-explorer
Alcoholic beverages	Red wine	215.48	Phenol-explorer
Fruits	Apple	200.96	Phenol-explorer
Vegetables	Broccoli	198.55	Phenol-explorer
Vegetables	Pak choy	193.45	Phenol-explorer
Fruits	Tangerine	192	Phenol-explorer
Fruits	Black grape	184.97	Phenol-explorer
Vegetables	Green pepper (sweet)	181.52	Phenol-explorer
Fruits	Kiwi	179.71	Phenol-explorer
Vegetables	Kale	176.67	Phenol-explorer
Fruits	Sweet cherry	174.9	Phenol-explorer
Vegetables	Red beetroot	164.1	Phenol-explorer
Olives	Green olive	161.24	Phenol-explorer
Fruits	Red raspberry	154.65	Phenol-explorer
Vegetables	Avocado	152.12	Phenol-explorer
Plant products	Tempeh	148	Pérez-Jiménez et al. Eur J Clin Nutr. 2010
Nuts & Seeds	Pumpkin seeds	140	Zujko et al. International Journal of Food Properties. 2011
Pulses (raw)	White bean	137.75	Phenol-explorer
Vegetables	Rocket (Arugula)	136.4	Phenol-explorer
Vegetables	Red chicory	129.5	Phenol-explorer
Olives	Black olives	117.17	Phenol-explorer
Vegetables	Red lettuce	114	Phenol-explorer
Fruits	Pear	107.91	Phenol-explorer
Beverages	Black tea	104.48	Phenol-explorer
Vegetables	Red onion	102.83	Phenol-explorer
Cereals	Rice, whole grain	94.52	Phenol-explorer
Cereals	Oat, whole grain flour	82.21	Phenol-explorer
Cereals	Rye, whole grain flour	71.97	Phenol-explorer
Beverages	Green tea	61.86	Phenol-explorer
Oils	Extra-vrigin olive oil	55.14	Phenol-explorer

INDEX

alcohol 50
almond butter: miso and almond butter dressing 185
almonds 26
  almond and cauliflower curry with crispy tofu 201
animal protein 22–3
appetite control 36
apples: apple, ginger and star anise sauerkraut 239
  green apple slaw 154
asparagus and wild garlic green orzo with salmon 250
avocados: avocado lentil cakes with smoked salmon and kimchi 76
  smoked tofu, avocado and chicory salad 183
  spicy 'meaty' tacos with avo and lime-soured cream 214

bake, spicy gochujang 137
bark, frozen yoghurt, peanut and berry 266
beans 24, 26, 30, 53
  crispy bean and kraut salad 179
  green pesto beans with eggs and hazelnuts 86
  grilled chicken thighs with miso white beans, radicchio and hazelnuts 227
  herby mushroom and bean gratin 213
  miso beans on toasted rye 82
  rich and silky beans with nachos 134
  smoky masala red beans 114
  sundried tomato and red pepper beans with hake 129
  sweet spring harissa beans with pecorino 138
  tarragon and thyme beans with spicy sea bass 241
  3 ways with beans 156
  za'atar and tahini beans with crispy tofu 220

see also individual types of beans
beetroots, smoky 239
berries 53, 58, 102
  frozen yoghurt, peanut and berry bark 266
black beans: chipotle and honey air-fried tofu bowls with black beans and pineapple 149
bone health 17
bread: crispy chickpeas on green toast 78
  the doctor's daily bread 72
  greens and basil tofu scramble 98
  high-protein edamame and pea spread on rye toast 93
  miso beans on toasted rye 82
  pepper and turmeric tofu with kraut and rye 84
  toast toppers 87
broccoli: braised shiitake mushrooms and broccoli with crispy chilli yuba 198
butter bean and miso soup with crispy tempeh 204

cabbage: fennel and cabbage pickle 145
  slaws 154, 214
cacao 27
  hot cardamom and cacao 275
  overnight protein porridge with cinnamon, turmeric and cacao 75
Cajun chicken, air-fried 146
capers: monkfish with capers, olives and tomatoes 108
  tomato, caper and fish stew with orecchiette 167
cardamom: hot cardamom and cacao 275
cashews: green cashew tofu curry 208
  sweet chilli cashew and celery stir-fry 195

cauliflower: almond and cauliflower curry with crispy tofu 201
  sticky sweet chilli salmon with roasted cauliflower 130
celery: stir-fried celery with sweet and spicy yuba 210
  sweet chilli cashew and celery stir-fry 195
Ceylon cinnamon coffee 275
chard: radishes, caraway and chard with baked salmon 256
cheese 24, 26
  feta, red pepper and pomegranate 81
  haricot bean and feta fish stew 118
  heritage tomatoes, strawberries and feta 175
  lemon feta sauce 185
  one-pan greens and goats' cheese with pickled red onions 90
  seed crackers with cheese 102
  sweet spring harissa beans with pecorino 138
  whipped feta with dill, grapes, chickpeas and smoked mackerel 94
  see also labneh
chicken: air-fried Cajun chicken 146
  cinnamon and cumin curry with crispy chicken 224
  cinnamon and lentil chicken soup 234
  grilled chicken thighs with miso white beans, radicchio and hazelnuts 227
  sage and garlic chicken broth 228
  takeaway-style chicken 233
chickpeas: crispy chickpeas on green toast 78
  monkfish with harissa chickpeas and spinach 116

silken soup with crispy masala chickpeas and soft herbs 172
  smashed chickpea toast toppers 87
  whipped feta with dill, grapes, chickpeas and smoked mackerel 94
chicory: smoked tofu, avocado and chicory salad 183
chillies: chilli, lime and tahini dressing 185
  chilli-pea pesto 246
  crispy chilli tofu 190
  crispy chilli yuba 198
  fermented garlic honey with smoky ancho chilli, star anise and cinnamon 238
  sticky sweet chilli salmon with roasted cauliflower 130
  sweet chilli cashew and celery stir-fry 195
Chinese 5 spice mince bowls with kimchi mayo 150
chipotle and honey air-fried tofu bowls 149
chocolate: hot cardamom and cacao 275
  red bean stew with chocolate and spices 121
cinnamon: Ceylon cinnamon coffee 275
  cinnamon and cumin curry 224
  cinnamon and lentil chicken soup 234
  fermented garlic honey with smoky ancho chilli, star anise and cinnamon 238
  ginger, matcha and cinnamon tea 274
  overnight protein porridge with cinnamon, turmeric and cacao 75
  paprika, peanut and okra stew with cinnamon 125

coconut milk: coconut, prawn and pineapple curry 242
   coconut prawn stew with Thai green paste 111
   lazy coconut fish curry 132
   spicy thyme lentil coconut curry 192
   Sri Lankan-style coconut lentils with griddled sardines 255
coffee, Ceylon cinnamon 275
crackers, fennel, oregano, chia and pumpkin seed 262
crispy bean and kraut salad 179
crispy chickpeas on green toast 78
curry 126
   almond and cauliflower curry with crispy tofu 201
   cinnamon and cumin curry with crispy chicken 224
   coconut, prawn and pineapple curry 242
   curried hemp seeds 270
   easy tomato curry with prawns and peas 249
   green cashew tofu curry 208
   lazy coconut fish curry 132
   lazy ginger and peanut Thai curry 197
   masala sea bass nuggets with spiced vegetables 252
   quick kale curry with lentils 112
   salmon tikka bowls 145
   silken soup with crispy masala chickpeas 172
   smoky masala red beans 114
   spicy thyme lentil coconut curry 192
   spinach and masala cod with spicy fennel oil 244
   Thai green curry lentil and hake traybake 107

dairy 25, 102
dips 156, 264
the doctor's daily bread 72
dressings 176, 183–5
drinks to lower inflammation 274–5

edamame beans: crispy chilli edamame 270
   edamame and pea dip with chilli oil 264
   high-protein edamame and pea spread on rye toast 93
eggs 26
   eggs and kraut 89
   green pesto beans with eggs and hazelnuts 86
   lentils, eggs and kimchi 86
energy 16
exercise 67

fasting 68
fat, high-fat diets 50
fennel: fennel and cabbage pickle 145
   fennel slaw 146
fennel seeds: fennel oils 244, 264
   fennel, oregano, chia and pumpkin seed crackers 262
ferments 29, 52, 238–9
fibre 39–41, 51
fish 24, 62
   asparagus and wild garlic green orzo with salmon 250
   avocado lentil cakes with smoked salmon and kimchi 76
   grilled mackerel with roasted radish and chilli-pea pesto 246
   haricot bean and feta fish stew 118
   harissa, honey and lentils with monkfish 122
   hot-smoked salmon and greens 101
   lazy coconut fish curry 132
   masala sea bass nuggets with spiced vegetables 252
   monkfish with capers, olives and tomatoes 108
   monkfish with harissa chickpeas and spinach 116
   orange and olive freekeh with grilled trout 180
   paccheri with red mullet and pistachio 158
   radishes, caraway and chard with baked salmon 256
   salmon, squash and grilled peach salad 176
   salmon tikka bowls 145
   smoky paprika lentils with hake and dill 140
   spicy gochujang bake with cod and toasted peanuts 137
   spinach and masala cod 244
   Sri Lankan-style coconut lentils with griddled sardines 255
   sticky sweet chilli salmon with roasted cauliflower 130
   sundried tomato and red pepper beans with hake 129
   tarragon and thyme beans with spicy sea bass 241
   Thai green curry lentil and hake traybake 107
   tomato, caper and fish stew with orecchiette 167
   whipped feta with dill, grapes, chickpeas and smoked mackerel 94
freekeh, orange and olive 180
fruit 43

garam masala: masala sea bass nuggets with spiced vegetables 252
   silken soup with crispy masala chickpeas and soft herbs 172
   spinach and masala cod with spicy fennel oil 244
garlic: fermented garlic honey 238
   sage and garlic chicken broth 228
germination 29
ginger: apple, ginger and star anise sauerkraut 239
   ginger, matcha and cinnamon tea 274
   ginger, miso and tamarind prawns with beluga lentils 259
   lazy ginger and peanut Thai curry 197
gochujang: spicy gochujang bake 137
   spicy gochujang bowls 154
   tahini and gochujang noodle broth with turkey 230
grains 25
gratin, herby mushroom and bean 213

greens 53, 58
   greens and basil tofu scramble 98
   hot-smoked salmon and greens 101
   one-pan greens and goats' cheese 90
   plant protein stir-fry with greens 216
gut health 32–53
   benefits of a healthy gut 36–7
   leaky gut 48–51
   strategies to improve 53
   supporting 10, 11

haricot bean and feta fish stew 118
harissa: harissa, honey and lentils with monkfish 122
   harissa-toasted quinoa salad with labneh 207
   monkfish with harissa chickpeas and spinach 116
   sweet spring harissa beans with pecorino 138
hazelnuts: green pesto beans with eggs and hazelnuts 86
   grilled chicken thighs with miso white beans, radicchio and hazelnuts 227
heart health 37
hemp seeds 26
   curried hemp seeds 270
herbs 43, 61
   herby mushroom and bean gratin 213
   silken soup with crispy masala chickpeas and soft herbs 172
   tahini herb dressing 176
hibiscus, clove and mint tea 274
honey: chipotle and honey air-fried tofu bowls 149
   fermented garlic honey 238
   harissa, honey and lentils with monkfish 122
hormones 36

inflammation: drinks to lower 274–5
   inflammation-fighting foods 57–65
   lowering 10, 11, 54–69
   what it is 56

kale: quick kale curry 112
kimchi: avocado lentil cakes with smoked salmon and kimchi 76
  kimchi mayo 150
  lentils, eggs and kimchi 86

labneh: harissa-toasted quinoa salad with labneh 207
  labneh and za'atar sauce 185
lasagne, plant-powered 161–2
lazy coconut fish curry 132
lazy ginger and peanut Thai curry 197
legumes: sumac and legume stew 219
lemons: lemon feta sauce 185
  preserved lemon and tahini dressing 184
lentil cakes: avocado lentil cakes with smoked salmon and kimchi 76
lentils 24, 27
  cinnamon and lentil chicken soup 234
  ginger, miso and tamarind prawns with beluga lentils 259
  harissa, honey and lentils with monkfish 122
  lentils, eggs and kimchi 86
  quick kale curry with lentils 112
  smoky paprika lentils with hake and dill 140
  spicy thyme lentil coconut curry 192
  Sri Lankan-style coconut lentils with griddled sardines 255
  Thai green curry lentil and hake traybake 107
limes: chilli, lime and tahini dressing 185
  lime-soured cream 214
linseeds: the doctor's daily bread 72
longevity 17

matcha: ginger, matcha and cinnamon tea 274
mayonnaise 150, 152
menopause 17, 37
mental health 36
metabolic health 17

microbes 35, 38–45
miso paste 27
  butter bean and miso soup with crispy tempeh 204
  ginger, miso and tamarind prawns with beluga lentils 259
  grilled chicken thighs with miso white beans, radicchio and hazelnuts 227
  miso and almond butter dressing 185
  miso beans on toasted rye 82
  miso mushroom soba broth with crispy chilli tofu 190
muscle health 17
mushrooms 65
  braised shiitake mushrooms and broccoli with crispy chilli yuba 198
  herby mushroom and bean gratin 213
  miso mushroom soba broth with crispy chilli tofu 190
  plant-powered lasagne with mushroom and tofu 161–2
  spicy 'meaty' tacos 214

nachos, rich and silky beans with 134
noodles: miso mushroom soba broth with crispy chilli tofu 190
  tahini and gochujang noodle broth with turkey 230
nut butters, three ways with 126
nutrition, understanding 10–11
nuts 25, 26, 43, 53, 60

oats: overnight protein porridge 75
oils 62
  spicy fennel oil 244
okra: paprika, peanut and okra stew 125
olives: monkfish with capers, olives and tomatoes 108
  orange and olive freekeh with grilled trout 180
onions, pickled red 90
orange and olive freekeh with grilled trout 180
paprika: paprika pea topper 87
  paprika, peanut and okra stew 125

smoky paprika lentils with hake and dill 140
pasta 27
  asparagus and wild garlic green orzo with salmon 250
  plant-powered lasagne with mushroom and tofu 161–2
  paccheri with red mullet and pistachio 158
  Rupy's high-protein rigatoni 164
peaches: salmon, squash and grilled peach salad 176
peanut butter: frozen yoghurt, peanut and berry bark 266
  lazy ginger and peanut Thai curry 197
  soy and peanut dressing 184
paprika, peanut and okra stew 125
  spicy gochujang bake with cod and toasted peanuts 137
pearl barley: overnight pear and pearl barley porridge 96
peas: chilli-pea pesto 246
  easy tomato curry with prawns and peas 249
  edamame and pea dip 264
  high-protein edamame and pea spread on rye toast 93
  paprika pea topper 87
peppers: feta, red pepper and pomegranate 81
  sundried tomato and red pepper beans with hake 129
pesto: chilli-pea pesto 246
  green pesto beans 86
pickles: fennel and cabbage pickle 145
  pickled red onions 90
pineapple: chipotle and honey air-fried tofu bowls with black beans and pineapple 149
  coconut, prawn and pineapple curry 242
pinto bean bowl with spicy prawns, sweet potato and corn 152
pistachios: the doctor's daily bread 72
plant-based diets 44–5
plant-based protein 8, 22–3, 28–9
polyphenols 42–5

pomegranate, feta, red pepper and 81
porridge: overnight pear and pearl barley porridge 96
  overnight protein porridge 75
prawns: coconut, prawn and pineapple curry 242
  coconut prawn stew with Thai green paste 111
  easy tomato curry with prawns and peas 249
  ginger, miso and tamarind prawns 259
  pinto bean bowl with spicy prawns, sweet potato and corn 152
prebiotic fibre 39–41
probiotics 52
protein 12–31
  benefits of eating enough 16–17
  daily requirements 18–20
  importance of 6, 15
  increasing 30
  plant-based 8, 22–3, 28–9
  portion sizes 23–7
  supplements 31
  what it is used for 14
  when to eat 21
pumpkin seeds: crispy bean and kraut salad with pumpkin seeds 179
  fennel, oregano, chia and pumpkin seed crackers 262

quinoa: harissa-toasted quinoa salad with labneh 207
radicchio: grilled chicken thighs with miso white beans, radicchio and hazelnuts 227
radishes, caraway and chard with baked salmon 256
red kidney beans: red bean stew with chocolate and spices 121
  smoky masala red beans 114
rose mountain tea 275
Rupy's high-protein rigatoni 164

salads: crispy bean and kraut salad 179
  fennel slaw 146
  green apple slaw 154
  harissa-toasted quinoa salad with labneh 207

salmon, squash and grilled peach salad 176
slaw 214
smoked tofu, avocado and chicory salad 183
Thai-style pomelo salad with crispy tofu 170
sauces 126, 184–5
sauerkraut 238–9
  crispy bean and kraut salad 179
  eggs and kraut 89
  pepper and turmeric tofu with sauerkraut and rye 84
seeds 25, 26, 43, 53, 60
  seed crackers with cheese 102
  three ways with seed butters 126
skin health 37
slaws 146, 154, 214
sleep 16, 51
smashed chickpea toast toppers 87
smoky beetroots 239
smoky masala red beans 114
smoky paprika lentils with hake and dill 140
soups and broths: butter bean and miso soup with crispy tempeh 204
  cinnamon and lentil chicken soup 234
  miso mushroom soba broth 19
  sage and garlic chicken broth 228
  silken soup with crispy masala chickpeas and soft herbs 172
  tahini and gochujang noodle broth 230
soy and peanut dressing 184
soya 27, 30
spices 43, 61
spicy fennel oil 244
spicy gochujang bake with cod and toasted peanuts 137
spicy gochujang bowls 154
spicy mayonnaise 152
spicy 'meaty' tacos 214

spicy thyme lentil coconut curry 192
spinach: monkfish with harissa chickpeas and spinach 116
  spinach and masala cod with spicy fennel oil 244
sprouting 29
squash: salmon, squash and grilled peach salad with tahini herb dressing 176
Sri Lankan-style coconut lentils with griddled sardines 255
stews 156
  coconut prawn stew with Thai green paste 111
  haricot bean and feta fish stew 118
  paprika, peanut and okra stew 125
  red bean stew with chocolate and spices 121
  sumac and legume stew 219
  tomato, caper and fish stew with orecchiette 167
sticky sweet chilli salmon with roasted cauliflower 130
stir-fries 126
  plant protein stir-fry with greens 216
  stir-fried celery with sweet and spicy yuba 210
  sweet chilli cashew and celery stir-fry 195
strawberries: heritage tomatoes, strawberries and feta 175
stress 51, 66
sugar 16, 50
supplements, protein 31
sweet chilli cashew and celery stir-fry 195
sweet potatoes: pinto bean bowl with spicy prawns, sweet potato and corn 152
sweet spring harissa beans with pecorino 138
sweetcorn: pinto bean bowl with spicy prawns, sweet potato and corn 152

tacos, spicy 'meaty' 214
tahini 27
  chilli, lime and tahini dressing 185
  mustard tahini dressing 183

preserved lemon and tahini dressing 184
  tahini and gochujang noodle broth with turkey 230
  tahini herb dressing 176
  za'atar and tahini beans with crispy tofu 220
takeaway-style chicken 233
tea: ginger, matcha and cinnamon tea 274
  hibiscus, clove and mint tea 274
  rose mountain tea 275
tempeh 26, 30, 202
  butter bean and miso soup with crispy tempeh 204
  crispy tempeh 192
  plant protein stir-fry with greens 216
  Rupy's high-protein rigatoni 164
  spicy 'meaty' tacos 214
  sweet chilli cashew and celery stir-fry 195
Thai curries: lazy ginger and peanut Thai curry 197
  Thai green curry lentil and hake traybake 107
Thai-style pomelo salad with crispy tofu 170
toast toppers 87
tofu 26, 27, 30, 202–3
  almond and cauliflower curry with crispy tofu 201
  chipotle and honey air-fried tofu bowls 149
  crispy chilli tofu 190
  crispy chilli yuba 198
  5 spice mince bowls with kimchi mayo 150
  green cashew tofu curry 208
  greens and basil tofu scramble 98
  pepper and turmeric tofu with sauerkraut and rye 84
  protein lasagne with mushroom and tofu 161–2
  silken soup with crispy masala chickpeas and soft herbs 172
  smoked tofu, avocado and chicory salad 183
  stir-fried celery with sweet and spicy yuba 210

Thai-style pomelo salad with crispy tofu 170
za'atar and tahini beans with crispy tofu 220
tomatoes: easy tomato curry with prawns and peas 249
  heritage tomatoes, strawberries and feta 175
  monkfish with capers, olives and tomatoes 108
  sundried tomato and red pepper beans with hake 129
  tomato, caper and fish stew with orecchiette 167
toppers 30, 156
traybake, Thai green curry lentil and hake 107
turkey: spicy gochujang bowls 154
  tahini and gochujang noodle broth 230

ultra-processed food 50

yoghurt 25, 102
  frozen yoghurt, peanut and berry bark 266
yuba 27
  crispy chilli yuba 198
  stir-fried celery with sweet and spicy yuba 210

References

INTRODUCTION
Meat replacements
https://pubmed.ncbi.nlm.nih.gov/36304815/

HEALTHY HIGH PROTEIN
Liver protein functions
doi: 10.1016/j.cub.2017.09.019
DOI: 10.1017/S0007114519003064

Daily protein turnover
doi: 10.1172/JCI118937
doi: 10.2215/CJN.04790516
DOI: 10.1024/0300-9831/A000064
doi: 10.1590/S0100-879X2012007500096

Daily protein intake recommendations
DOI:10.1016/j.jamda.2013.05.021
https://www.ncbi.nlm.nih.gov/pmc/articles/PMC5872778/
DOI: 10.1139/apnm-2015-0550
DOI: 10.1039/c5fo01530h
DOI: 10.1159/000499374

Timing, distribution of protein, metabolic benefits
DOI: 10.3945/ajcn.114.084053

Safety of higher protein consumption
DOI: 10.1093/jn/nxy197

Older adults and Protein
https://www.ncbi.nlm.nih.gov/pmc/articles/PMC7567142/
https://www.ncbi.nlm.nih.gov/pmc/articles/PMC4924200/

Protein adequacy
https://www.sciencedirect.com/science/article/pii/S0271531716000026?
https://www.mdpi.com/2072-6643/11/11/2661

Best plant-based proteins
https://cdnsciencepub.com/doi/full/10.1139/apnm-2021-0806

All plants contain protein
DOI: 10.1093/nutrit/nuy073

Benefits of protein at each meal
DOI: 10.3945/ajcn.114.084053

Plant-based protein and all-cause mortality
https://pubmed.ncbi.nlm.nih.gov/32699048/

Sleep quality and protein
DOI: 10.1093/nutrit/nuac061
https://doi.org/10.1038/s41430-024-01414-y

Distribution of protein
https://academic.oup.com/nutritionreviews/article/77/4/197/5307079

Protein intake and calorie intake reduction
https://www.ncbi.nlm.nih.gov/pmc/articles/PMC8399074/

Protein and appetite
https://www.ncbi.nlm.nih.gov/pmc/articles/PMC5872778/

Protein leverage hypothesis
https://www.nature.com/articles/s41430-023-01276-w#
https://ajcn.nutrition.org/article/S0002-9165(23)05376-5/fulltext

Markers of cognition in older adults
https://www.sciencedirect.com/science/article/pii/S0002916522001241

Protein intake reduces appetite
https://pubmed.ncbi.nlm.nih.gov/14522731/
https://pubmed.ncbi.nlm.nih.gov/33747991/

Protein at breakfast
https://pubmed.ncbi.nlm.nih.gov/36615743/

Sarcopenia
https://www.ncbi.nlm.nih.gov/pmc/articles/PMC4066461
https://doi.org/10.1359/JBMR.040204

Menopause and protein
https://pubmed.ncbi.nlm.nih.gov/24522467/
https://obgyn.onlinelibrary.wiley.com/doi/10.1111/1471-0528.17290?af=R

https://www.ncbi.nlm.nih.gov/pmc/articles/PMC7098934/
https://www.ncbi.nlm.nih.gov/pmc/articles/PMC8308420/

Muscle protein synthesis and extra protein
https://examine.com/research-feed/study/1al6rd/

Reduced all-cause mortality with plant-based protein
https://www.ncbi.nlm.nih.gov/pmc/articles/PMC7374797/

Soya supplements
https://www.sciencedirect.com/science/article/pii/S0890623820302926#

Carefully planned plant-based protein intake
https://pubmed.ncbi.nlm.nih.gov/37603200/
https://www.ncbi.nlm.nih.gov/pmc/articles/PMC10655824/#

Minimally processed soya
https://pubmed.ncbi.nlm.nih.gov/35325028/

Protein digestibility
https://www.ncbi.nlm.nih.gov/pmc/articles/PMC6723444/

Food combinations
https://www.sciencedirect.com/science/article/pii/S000291652323823X

Fermenting to increase protein
https://onlinelibrary.wiley.com/doi/10.1002/fsn3.846

BETTER GUT HEALTH
Microbe antimicrobial effects
https://www.ncbi.nlm.nih.gov/pmc/articles/PMC7126101/
https://www.ncbi.nlm.nih.gov/pmc/articles/PMC6412307/
https://www.frontiersin.org/journals/microbiology/articles/10.3389/fmicb.2019.02977/full

Microbes and depression
https://www.mdpi.com/2072-6643/16/7/1054

Microbes and health
https://www.bmj.com/content/361/bmj.k2179

Mushrooms as prebiotics
https://www.sciencedirect.com/science/article/abs/pii/S0924224409002295
https://www.ncbi.nlm.nih.gov/pmc/articles/PMC5618583/
https://www.ncbi.nlm.nih.gov/pmc/articles/PMC10608147

Gut microbes and oestrogen
https://pubmed.ncbi.nlm.nih.gov/28778332/

Gut microbes and appetite control
https://www.sciencedirect.com/science/article/pii/S0022316622107261
https://microbiomejournal.biomedcentral.com/articles/10.1186/s40168-021-01093-y

Gut microbes and skin health
https://pubmed.ncbi.nlm.nih.gov/37513540/
https://www.tandfonline.com/doi/full/10.1080/19490976.2022.2096995
https://www.mdpi.com/2227-9059/10/5/1037

Gut metabolites and health review
https://gut.bmj.com/content/71/5/1020
https://www.frontiersin.org/journals/microbiology/articles/10.3389/fmicb.2022.999001/full

Gut microbes and menopause
https://journals.asm.org/doi/10.1128/msystems.00273-22
https://www.mdpi.com/2077-0383/10/13/2916

Microbes and energy levels
https://www.ncbi.nlm.nih.gov/pmc/articles/PMC8839554/

Prebiotics and gut health
Boyd, C., Gieng, J., 'Determination of the prebiotic content of foods in the 2015–2016 Food and Nutrient Database for Dietary Studies (FNDDS)'.

Polyphenols in human health
https://www.ncbi.nlm.nih.gov/pmc/articles/PMC2835915/

Diet rapidly changes the gut microbiome
https://www.nature.com/articles/nature12820
https://www.mdpi.com/2072-6643/11/12/2862

Bile formation and secretion
https://www.ncbi.nlm.nih.gov/pmc/articles/PMC4091928/

Leaky gut and intestinal barrier
https://www.ncbi.nlm.nih.gov/pmc/articles/PMC6790068/
https://www.ncbi.nlm.nih.gov/pmc/articles/PMC8427160/

Sugar and intestinal permeability
https://pubmed.ncbi.nlm.nih.gov/29519916/

Stress and leaky gut
https://pubmed.ncbi.nlm.nih.gov/24153250/

Circadian clock and gut leakiness
https://www.ncbi.nlm.nih.gov/pmc/articles/PMC3688973/

Fermentation benefits
https://www.cell.com/cell/fulltext/S0092-8674(21)00754-6

Ancient ferments
https://www.ncbi.nlm.nih.gov/pmc/articles/PMC9227559/

LOWERING INFLAMMATION
Dietary inflammation index
https://pubmed.ncbi.nlm.nih.gov/23941862/
https://www.frontiersin.org/articles/10.3389/fnut.2021.647122/full
https://pubmed.ncbi.nlm.nih.gov/29439509/

Berries and inflammation
https://www.frontiersin.org/journals/pharmacology/articles/10.3389/fphar.2018.00078/full

Berries as senolytics
https://pubmed.ncbi.nlm.nih.gov/30279143/
https://www.ncbi.nlm.nih.gov/pmc/articles/PMC8756168/

Greens and dementia
https://www.neurology.org/doi/10.1212/WNL.0000000000207176

African greens
https://www.researchgate.net/publication/357300469_Anti-inflammatory_and_Anti-cancer_properties_of_selected_green_Leafy_vegetables_-_review

Nuts
https://www.ncbi.nlm.nih.gov/pmc/articles/PMC4350958/

Rosemary as nutraceutical
https://pubmed.ncbi.nlm.nih.gov/37809749/
https://onlinelibrary.wiley.com/doi/epdf/10.1002/ptr.6648?

Fish and resolvins
https://pubmed.ncbi.nlm.nih.gov/29757195/
https://pubmed.ncbi.nlm.nih.gov/35268778/

Olive oil
https://jamanetwork.com/journals/jamanetworkopen/fullarticle/2818362

Mushrooms
https://www.ncbi.nlm.nih.gov/pmc/articles/PMC5618583/
https://www.ncbi.nlm.nih.gov/pmc/articles/PMC10183216/

Coffee
https://www.bmj.com/content/359/bmj.j5024

Hibiscus
https://pubmed.ncbi.nlm.nih.gov/33507846/

Green tea
https://www.ncbi.nlm.nih.gov/pmc/articles/PMC7796401/
https://pubmed.ncbi.nlm.nih.gov/34204055/

Cacao
https://pubmed.ncbi.nlm.nih.gov/28649251/

Mountain tea
https://pubmed.ncbi.nlm.nih.gov/22274814/
https://www.mdpi.com/1420-3049/25/16/3763

Stress
https://www.ncbi.nlm.nih.gov/pmc/articles/PMC3860380/
https://pubmed.ncbi.nlm.nih.gov/19488073/
https://www.ncbi.nlm.nih.gov/pmc/articles/PMC3781604/

Exercise
https://pubmed.ncbi.nlm.nih.gov/18923185/

Fasting and autophagy
https://www.ncbi.nlm.nih.gov/pmc/articles/PMC6347410/
https://www.nature.com/articles/nm.3804

Acknowledgements

Having the chance to write books is a privilege I deeply appreciate. From the age of 11, I knew I wanted to write and had a natural talent for it, though I didn't quite imagine myself as a traditional writer.

As an adult, allowing myself the freedom to pursue my passions and express them through various creative outlets led me to write recipes, produce cooking shows, and ultimately, become an author.

While perseverance and self-permission to explore this new career have been essential, my deepest gratitude goes to my family and loved ones, who have supported me throughout the years. Without their encouragement, I probably wouldn't be here writing the acknowledgements for my fifth book.

The greatest thanks to my parents whose sacrifices I now have a greater understanding of and appreciation for, since gaining the new perspective of a father. My wife Rochelle, baby sister Jasmin and my in-laws, Carla and Franco, for proofreading the text for clarity. I appreciate you all.

My Doctor's Kitchen team are phenomenal and I'm so grateful for you all. Special thanks to Karen for being the organisational rock you always are, helping maintain my sanity and making sure everything runs as smooth as possible for me. Órfhlaith for testing and providing feedback on some of these recipes; the energy and enthusiasm you bring to our mission is amazing and deeply appreciated. Hugo for never failing to find a solution for anything I throw at you, whether it's building lunch tables, generating QR codes or squashing technical bugs, your ability to remain calm, provide reassurance and fix things is incredible. Sakina for being our research whizz, helping with the nutritional values for this book and bringing the excitement and love for all things food, nutrition and medicine to the team. If we continue to be committed, curious and energetic, nothing can stop Doctor's Kitchen from helping millions of lives.

Thanks to my literary agent Carly Cook and manager Bev James for being an incredible support network during this entire process and for the many years we've worked together. Your enthusiasm and encouragement are so appreciated.

Thanks to the wonderful team at Ebury led by Laura Higginson and Stephanie Milner, supported by editor Vicky Orchard and assistant editor Samuel Heaton, designer Claire Rochford and art director Loulou Clark for trusting me with the freedom to choose a topic and title that I think is misunderstood and underserved. I hope we can bring clarity to this complicated subject and get people eating healthily. Thanks to the food shoot team led by Andrew Burton and Pippa Leon, with Max Robinson for bringing these recipes to life and making them shine beautifully across the pages, it was a pleasure to work with all of you.

Special shout out to Dr Ayan Panja for proofreading my original script and brainstorming some title ideas with me, along with Dr Tara Swart, in the very early part of this process. I really appreciate your feedback and ideas, you're both amazing people and I value your love and guidance.

Special thanks to my food testers Nicola Graimes and Eden Owen-Jones for providing much valued feedback and tweaks to the recipes to make sure they work perfectly and taste delicious.

And of course to my Doctor's Kitchen community. Bless you. Whether this is your first interaction with my writing or you're a diehard fan who subscribes to our weekly newsletters, watches the YouTube channel, listens to my podcasts, uses our app and avidly cooks Doctor's Kitchen recipes every week. I have so much appreciation for you all, and I hope to continue to play a small part in your health journey each week.

And finally, to myself. Keep going Rupy. Believe in yourself. You got this.

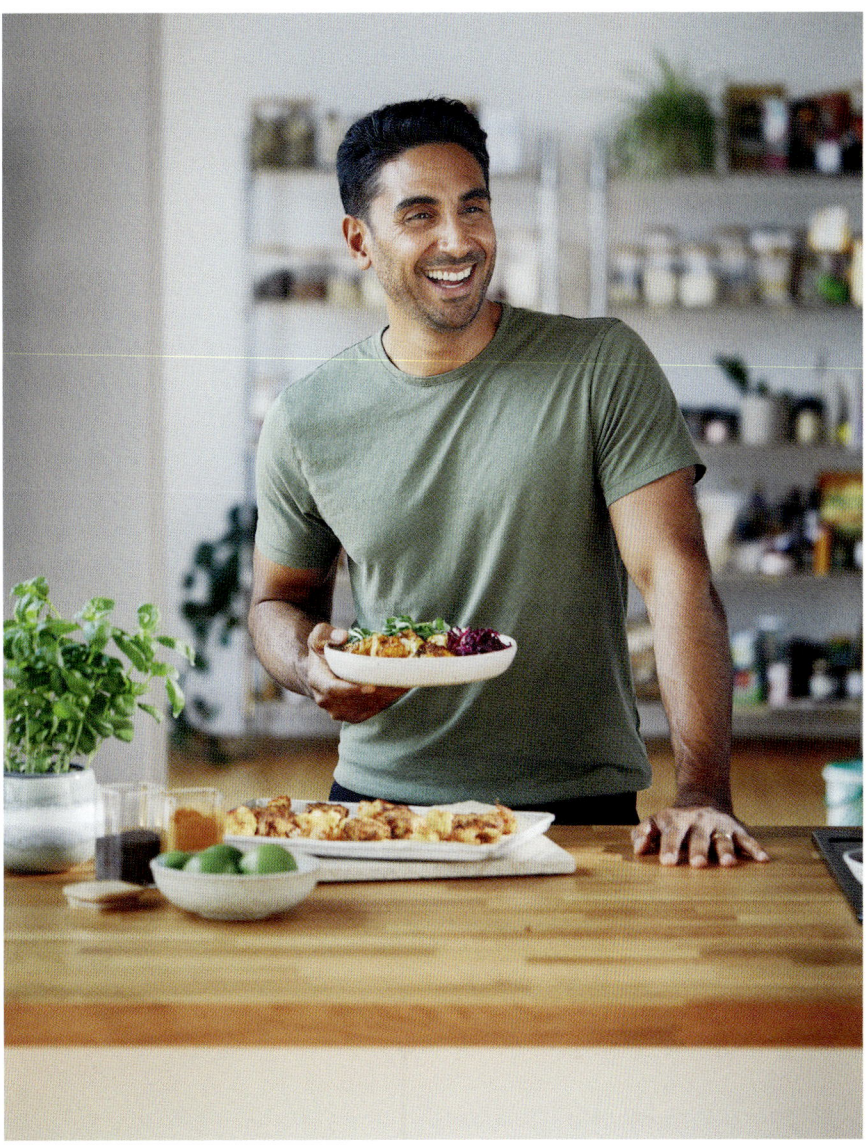

Dr Rupy is a London-based doctor, specialising in General Practice and Emergency Medicine, who is on a mission to reverse the tidal wave of preventable lifestyle disease one plate of delicious food at a time. He has a Masters in Nutritional Medicine and is the founder of Europe's first Culinary Medicine programme for medical schools, as well as hosting one of Europe's top health and wellness podcasts. He is a Sunday Times bestselling author and regularly appears on national television.

Ebury Press

UK | USA | Canada | Ireland | Australia
India | New Zealand | South Africa

Ebury Press is part of the Penguin Random House group of companies whose addresses can be found at global.penguinrandomhouse.com

Penguin Random House UK
One Embassy Gardens, 8 Viaduct Gardens, London SW11 7BW

penguin.co.uk
global.penguinrandomhouse.com

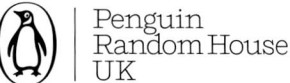

First published by Ebury Press in 2025

5

Copyright © Rupy Aujla 2025
Photography © Andrew Burton 2025

The moral right of the author has been asserted.

No part of this book may be used or reproduced in any manner for the purpose of training artificial intelligence technologies or systems. In accordance with Article 4(3) of the DSM Directive 2019/790, Penguin Random House expressly reserves this work from the text and data mining exception.

Publishing Director: Stephanie Milner
Project Editor: Vicky Orchard
Design: Claire Rochford
Photography: Andrew Burton
Food Stylist: Pippa Leon
Prop Stylist: Max Robinson

Colour origination by Altaimage Ltd
Printed and bound in Germany by Mohn Media

The authorised representative in the EEA is Penguin Random House Ireland, Morrison Chambers, 32 Nassau Street, Dublin D02 YH68.

A CIP catalogue record for this book is available from the British Library

ISBN 9781529148848

Penguin Random House is committed to a sustainable future for our business, our readers and our planet. This book is made from Forest Stewardship Council® certified paper.